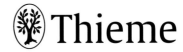

Clinical Endodontics

A Textbook

3rd edition

Leif Tronstad, LDS, DMD, MS, PhD
Professor Emeritus
University of Oslo
Faculty of Dentistry
Oslo, Norway

572 illustrations

Thieme
Stuttgart · New York

Library of Congress Cataloging-in-Publication Data

Tronstad, Leif.
Clinical endodontics : a textbook / Leif Tronstad.—3rd rev. ed.
    p. ; cm.
Includes bibliographical references and index.
ISBN 978-3-13-768103-8 (alk. paper)
1. Endodontics-Textbooks. I. Title.
[DNLM: 1. Dental Pulp Diseases–therapy.
2. Endodontics–methods. WU 230 T854c 2008]
RK351.T76 2008
617.6'342–dc22

Important note: Medicine is an ever-changing science undergoing continual development. Research and clinical experience are continually expanding our knowledge, in particular our knowledge of proper treatment and drug therapy. Insofar as this book mentions any dosage or application, readers may rest assured that the authors, editors, and publishers have made every effort to ensure that such references are in accordance with **the state of knowledge at the time of production of the book.**

Nevertheless, this does not involve, imply, or express any guarantee or responsibility on the part of the publishers in respect to any dosage instructions and forms of applications stated in the book. **Every user is requested to examine carefully** the manufacturers' leaflets accompanying each drug and to check, if necessary in consultation with a physician or specialist, whether the dosage schedules mentioned therein or the contraindications stated by the manufacturers differ from the statements made in the present book. Such examination is particularly important with drugs that are either rarely used or have been newly released on the market. Every dosage schedule or every form of application used is entirely at the user's own risk and responsibility. The authors and publishers request every user to report to the publishers any discrepancies or inaccuracies noticed. If errors in this work are found after publication, errata will be posted at www.thieme.com on the product description page.

Some of the product names, patents, and registered designs referred to in this book are in fact registered trademarks or proprietary names even though specific reference to this fact is not always made in the text. Therefore, the appearance of a name without designation as proprietary is not to be construed as a representation by the publisher that it is in the public domain.

© 2009 Georg Thieme Verlag,
Rüdigerstrasse 14, 70469 Stuttgart, Germany
http://www.thieme.de
Thieme New York, 333 Seventh Avenue,
New York, NY 10001, USA
http://www.thieme.com

Cover design: Thieme Publishing Group
Typesetting by Sommer Druck, Feuchtwangen
Printed in Germany by Graphisches Centrum Cuno GmbH,
    Calbe (Saale)

ISBN 978-3-13-768103-8   1 2 3 4 5 6

To
Anne-Grethe
and to Nora, Greger, Ulrik, Andrea, Kristin,
and Karl-Henrik

Preface to the Third Edition

The scope of the third edition of *Clinical Endodontics* is as before to be a simple, yet comprehensive textbook in endodontics that serves as an introductory text for dental students and as a suitable refresher source for general practitioners, postdoctoral students, and endodontists. With this concept in mind, *Clinical Endodontics* summarizes the biology of the endodontium and the apical periodontium and deals with the etiology and pathogenesis of endodontic diseases. Examination methods, diagnoses, treatment principles, and prognosis of endodontic treatment are discussed, and main endodontic techniques are described. The format of the previous editions has been kept, and new relevant information has been added to the text. The lists of references following each chapter have been updated. I again extend my thanks to friends and colleagues who have contributed illustrational material to the book.

Oslo, Summer 2008   *Leif Tronstad*

Table of Contents

1

The Endodontium

Structure

The endodontium comprises the dentin and pulp of the tooth. Both tissues develop from the dental papilla, and although the dentin mineralizes and the pulp remains a soft tissue, they maintain an intimate structural and functional relationship throughout the life of the tooth.

All the cells of the endodontium are located in the pulp and only cellular extensions, odontoblast processes, and nerve endings are found in the dentin. Thus, tissue reactions in the dentin are dependent to a great extent on the activity of cells in the pulp. Conversely, pulpal reactions may be significantly modified by tissue changes in the dentin.

The Dentin
Composition and Morphology

The dentin is composed of approximately 70% inorganic material in the form of hydroxyapatite crystals. The organic matrix, about 15–20%, consists of collagen. Noncollagenous proteins constitute 1–2% of the tissue, whereas the remaining 10–12% is water.

The dentin of the fully formed tooth is called *primary dentin*. It constitutes the bulk of the tooth and is especially characterized by the presence of *dentinal tubules* (**Fig. 1.1**). The tubules generally extend from the area of the dentin–enamel and

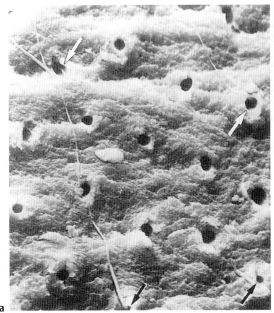
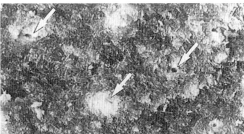
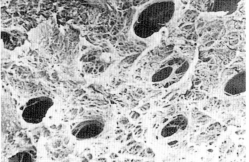

Fig. 1.1 Scanning electron micrographs of fractured coronal dentin from an impacted canine in a 13-year-old.
a Dentin from the middle area of the crown with crosscut dentinal tubules (diameter: 2 μm). Fibers are seen leaving some of the tubules (× 1700).

b Dentin near the enamel–dentin junction (mantle dentin) with crosscut dentinal tubules (arrows). Note small diameter (0.5 μm) of the tubules (× 1700).
c Predentinal surface with intertubular fibrous matrix (× 2600).

the dentin–cementum junctions to the pulp. The tubules are surrounded by *peritubular dentin*, which is a dense, highly mineralized tissue with a noncollagenous matrix. Between the tubules we find the *intertubular dentin*, which consists of mineralized collagen. Unmineralized *predentin* lines the pulpal aspect of the dentin.

Unmineralized matrix may also be seen inside the mineralized primary dentin. Well known is *interglobular dentin*, which occurs when mineralizing globules fail to coalesce. From a clinical point of view, it is more important that the buccal and lingual portions of the incisal dentin not always unite, but leave an unmineralized central streak or a soft tissue-containing space, sometimes extending all the way to the incisal dentin–enamel junction (**Fig. 1.2**). Clearly, in such teeth, an apparent uncomplicated crown fracture will cause exposure of the pulp.

Dentinogenesis continues, but at a slower rate, even after the teeth are fully formed. This dentin is called *physiologic secondary dentin* and it differs from the primary dentin in that its structure and composition may vary within the tooth and from

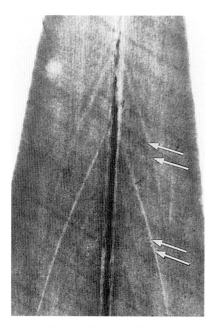

Fig. 1.2 Microradiograph of an incisor from an 11-year-old. Accentuated incremental lines of buccal and lingual dentin (arrows) meet at the radiopaque central streak, but do not join because of a slit in the dentin at this location.

one tooth to the next. As will be discussed later (see p. 26), increased secondary dentin formation in localized areas of the tooth may occur in response to external irritation. The structure of this tissue will depend on the severity of the irritation and the degree of tissue injury in the pulp and appears to be completely unpredictable (**Fig. 1.3**). As a rule, the secondary dentin formed in response to external irritants is more irregular than the physiologic secondary dentin.

Dentinal Tubules

It is well established that the dentinal tubules may serve as portals of entry for external irritants into the pulp. Thus, from a clinical point of view, the tubules are the most important and interesting component of the dentin.

In the crown of the tooth, the dentinal tubules generally extend from the area of the dentin–enamel junction to the pulp. In the root, the most peripheral dentin is atubular and the tubules thus begin in an area slightly pulpal to the dentin–cementum junction and extend to the pulp. The diameter of the tubules varies from $0.5\,\mu m$ in the peripheral dentin to $3–4\,\mu m$ near the pulp. In the bulk of the dentin they have a diameter of about $2\,\mu m$. Due to the much larger peripheral than pulpal surface of the dentin, the number of tubules per square millimeter area increases dramatically in a pulpal direction. Thus, at the dentin–enamel junction, the number of tubules is about 8000 per mm^2, halfway between the dentin–enamel junction and the pulp it is $20\,000–30\,000$ per mm^2, and near the pulp the number may be as high as $50\,000–60\,000$ per mm^2. Similarly, the total volume of the dentinal tubules increases in a pulpal direction and may constitute up to 80% of the total volume of the coronal dentin near the pulp.

The dentinal tubules contain tissue fluids (dentin liquor) which is fluid from the pulp tissue filling out the hollows of the dentin. Odontoblastic processes are present in most tubules and they are especially well visualized close to the pulp. Unmyelinated nerve endings may be present as well, usually in intimate contact with the odontoblastic processes (**Fig. 1.4**). In addition, unmineralized and mineralized collagen fibers are seen in many tubules at all levels of the dentin (**Fig. 1.5**).

Mineralized deposits of various structure and appearance occur in the dentinal tubules under various clinical conditions. Sometimes these deposits have the appearance of peritubular dentin,

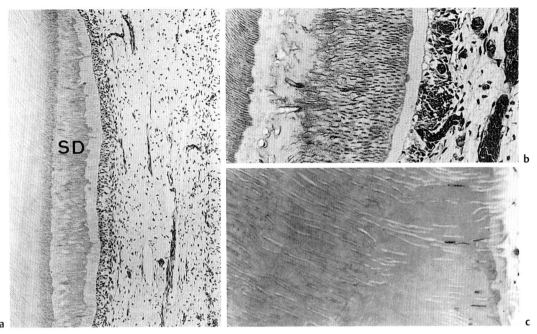

Fig. 1.3 Localized secondary dentin formation as a result of external irritation (hematoxylin-eosin).
a Secondary dentin (SD) with regular tubular structure indicating mild stimulation of odontoblasts.
b Secondary dentin with an atubular, cell-containing zone at the dentin–secondary dentin interface due to severe disturbance of odontoblast function. The cells have recovered and have continued to lay down tubular dentin.
c Secondary dentin with few tubules due to death of most odontoblastic cells.

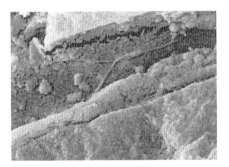

Fig. 1.4 Scanning electron micrograph of a tubule from circumpulpal dentin in a 21-year-old. In addition to the odontoblastic process, a slim fiber which divides into two branches and which is interpreted as a nerve fiber is present (×9000).

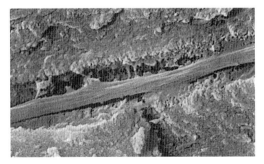

Fig. 1.5 Scanning electron micrograph of a tubule from the coronal dentin of a 42-year-old. A fiber consisting of fibrils with the cross-banding typical of collagen visible on their surface is present in the tubule (×10000).

and have generally been regarded as resulting from a continuous formation of the peritubular dentin (**Fig. 1.6**). This is probably a misconception since peritubular dentin is a developmental and not an acquired structure and since it forms in full thickness concomitantly with the intertubular dentin. Toward the lumen of the tubule, the peritubular dentin appears to be lined by an organic sheath which has been termed the *lamina limitans* (**Fig. 1.6**). A proper term for tubular deposits inside the lamina limitans would therefore be *intratubular dentin*.

Age Changes

Both macroscopic and microscopic changes occur in the dentin with increasing age, and both types of changes are of considerable clinical importance.

The macroscopic age changes are characterized by the lifelong formation of physiologic secondary dentin which continually modifies the size and to some extent the shape of the pulp chamber and the root canal. At first these changes are beneficial in that they give the root canal a size and form that enhances the possibilities for successful en-

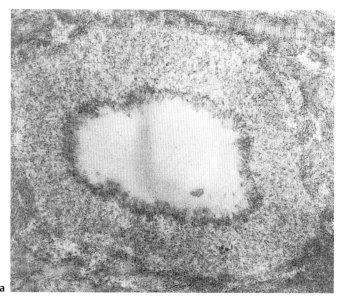

a

Fig. 1.6
a **Electron micrograph of a cross-cut tubule from partly demineralized root dentin.** An electron-dense line (lamina limitans) is recognized between the peritubular dentin matrix and the material beginning to occlude the tubule (× 20 000).
b Crosscut tubule from undemineralized dentin occluded with material (intratubular dentin) with electron density different from that of peritubular dentin (PD) (× 19 000).

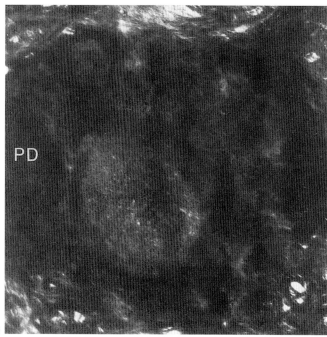

PD

b

dodontic treatment. However, in old age, the root canals may be obliterated to such an extent that necessary endodontic treatment becomes extremely difficult. Physiologic secondary dentin formation also occurs on the walls of lateral and accessory root canals, often causing a complete occlusion of these narrow spaces. This is the reason why accessory canals, for instance, in the furcation area of molar teeth which may be readily demonstrable in young teeth are evident only in rare instances during endodontic treatment of adult patients.

The microscopic age changes of the dentin are characterized by the fact that an increasing number of dentinal tubules become obliterated by mineralized tissue. The occluding material is homogenous and consists of a noncollagenous matrix and small hydroxyapatite crystals. Its appearance is similar to that of peritubular dentin, but as a rule it can be distinguished from this tissue by a difference in density or by the presence of the *lamina limitans* (**Fig.1.6**). From a clinical point of view, it is important to know that the formation of the age-related intratubular dentin starts at the apex of the tooth and continues in a coronal direction with increasing age. In the coronal dentin, the intratubular mineralization will not lead to a complete obliteration of the tubules until the patient is in his 70s. The process is so closely related to age that the coronal extent of the tubular occlusion is used in forensic dentistry for age determination purposes.

Thus, the microscopic dentinal changes that occur as a result of aging render the root of the tooth homogenous with few patent dentinal tubules. Conceivably, this may facilitate endodontic treatment of nonvital teeth where dentinal tubule infection is a definite problem. The tubules of the coronal dentin, on the other hand, will not be significantly affected by the aging process until the patient is old.

The Dental Pulp

Morphology
The dental pulp consists of a richly vascularized and highly innervated connective tissue (**Fig.1.7**). It is surrounded by dentin and has a form that mimics the outer contour of the various teeth (**Fig.1.8**). The pulp tissue is in communication with the periodontium and the rest of the body through the apical foramen and accessory canals near the apex of the root (**Fig.1.9**). Accessory canals are also found laterally in the root and in the furcation area of molar teeth. However, from a practical–clinical point of view, the pulp is an end organ without collateral circulation.

Cells, Fibers, and Ground Substance
The most characteristic element of the dental pulp is the dentin-forming cell, the *odontoblast*. The odontoblasts are tightly packed, regularly aligned, polarized cells located at the periphery of the pulp with cytoplasmic processes extending into the tubules of the predentin and dentin. This continuous sheet of odontoblasts at the pulp periphery has been termed the *odontoblastic layer* (**Fig.1.10**). Ultrastructurally the odontoblasts are shown to be similar to other connective tissue cells and their identity is mainly determined by their location. The odontoblasts are static postmitotic cells, apparently incapable of further cell division. Also, the rate of repopulation of the

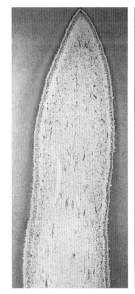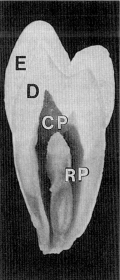

Fig. 1.7   Fig. 1.8

Fig. 1.7 Coronal pulp in the incisor tooth of a monkey. The odontoblast layer bordering the lightly stained predentin as well as cell-free and cell-rich subodontoblastic zones can be recognized (hematoxylin-eosin).

Fig. 1.8 Overview of the tooth with enamel (E), dentin (D), coronal pulp (CP), and root pulp (RP). Note that the pulpal cavity has a shape which mimics the outer contour of the tooth.

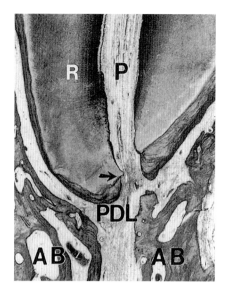

Fig. 1.9 Apical part of the root of a human incisor (R) with pulp (P), periodontal ligament (PDL), and alveolar bone (AB). Note that the apical foramen (arrow) is located laterally to the anatomical apex of the tooth (hematoxylin-eosin).

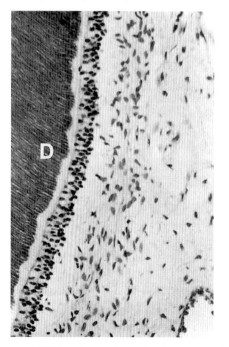

Fig. 1.10 Dentin–pulp interface in a monkey incisor. Adjacent to the dentin (D), the unmineralized (and unstained) predentin, the odontoblast layer, the cell-free zone, and the cell-rich zone can be seen (hematoxylin-eosin).

odontoblast layer is extremely slow under physiological conditions. Probably most and possibly all odontoblasts seen in teeth in older individuals are the original cells. The cell bodies of the odontoblasts are united in certain areas by cell-to-cell junctions. This may allow the odontoblasts to function as a syncytium, a continuous layer of cells.

Another trait of pulp identity is the subodontoblastic region. In the coronal pulp this region is characterized by a cell-free zone and a cell-rich zone beneath the odontoblastic layer (**Figs.1.7, 1.10**). The cells of the subodontoblastic region differ from the odontoblasts in that they have a bipolar, sometimes multipolar arrangement. Structurally, the cells resemble fibroblasts of the central pulp, and like the odontoblasts, they are identified by their location. It has been speculated that the subodontoblastic cells have specific functions, for instance, that they are "preodontoblasts" capable of proliferation and differentiation into new odontoblasts. This theory and others have not been substantiated. However, it is known that they are involved in the elaboration of collagen and ground substance like the cells of the rest of the pulp.

In the bulk of the pulp tissue, three main types of cells are seen: inactive mesenchymal cells, fibroblasts, and fibrocytes. The mesenchymal cells are thought to be multipotential in that when they are stimulated and undergo cell division, their daughter cells may develop into any of the mature connective tissue cells, including odontoblasts. The fibroblasts are the most numerous cells in the pulp and are responsible for ground substance and collagen production, collagen degradation, and turnover. The fibrocytes possibly play a role in the maintenance of collagen fibers.

As will be discussed in some detail later, the pulp has cells that under certain circumstances can develop into hard tissue–producing cells. Thus, after pulp capping, the dentin bridge is formed by new odontoblasts (see **Fig. 5.11**). Cementum- and bone-like tissues as well as more structureless hard tissues may form in the pulp as well. However, it is not quite clear at present which of the cells in the pulp are capable of differentiation into hard tissue-producing cells.

Other stable cellular elements in the pulp either belong to the vascular or the neural system. In addition, inflammatory cells such as lymphocytes, plasma cells, and macrophages are occasionally seen. Mast cells appear to be a rare occurrence in the healthy pulp.

The ground substance of the pulp has a mucoid consistency. It serves as a matrix in which cells, fibers, and blood vessels are embedded. It is organized as a heterogenous colloid with soluble and insoluble components. The main molecular components are proteoglycans which consist of a glycosaminoglycan linked to a protein molecule. Their major functions have been recognized to be the protection of the cellular elements and capillaries of the pulp, their interaction with collagen to form aggregates possibly involved in dentin matrix formation, as well as control or inhibition of mineralization.

The pulp has two main types of fibers, collagen fibers and elastic fibers, the latter always being confined to the walls of larger blood vessels. Thus, the fibers of the intercellular matrix of the pulp are collagenous in nature. The fibers of the young pulp are small and far from numerous. They are distributed diffusely within the tissue and are often covered by a glycosaminoglycan sheath. In the mature pulp, larger fiber bundles can be seen as well, especially along blood vessels in the root pulp. These fibers are usually devoid of a glycosaminoglycan sheath.

Vascular Supply

Blood vessels the size of arterioles branch off the dental artery and enter the pulp through the apical foramen and possibly through accessory canals (**Fig. 1.11**). Inside the pulp the main arterioles are seen in a central location extending to the coronal pulp. They give off branches that spread in the tissue, diminish in size, and finally become capillaries. An extensive capillary network is formed in the subodontoblast and odontoblast areas of the pulp. The capillaries provide the odontoblasts and other cells of the pulp with an adequate supply of nutrients. The blood then passes from the capillaries to postcapillary venules and to gradually larger venules toward the central region of the pulp where they are seen alongside the arterioles. Two to three venules leave the pulp through the apical foramen and possibly through accessory canals. Outside the tooth the pulp venules join with vessels that drain the periodontal ligament and alveolar bone.

Multiple arteriovenous anastomoses exist in the pulp. These direct connections between arterioles and venules make it possible for the circu-

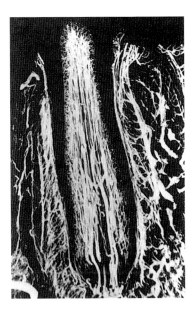

Fig. 1.11 Microangiograph showing vasculature in the pulp of a dog incisor. The main vessels are located centrally in the pulp and an extensive capillary network is seen, especially in the subodontoblast and odontoblast regions.

lating blood to bypass the capillary plexus. They play an important role in the regulation of pulpal blood flow.

The vascular pattern described above is basically found in all single-rooted teeth and in each root of multirooted teeth. Thus, in multirooted teeth, an alternate blood supply is generally available, resulting in extensive anastomoses in the coronal pulp. However, the main venous drainage sometimes occurs through one root in these teeth. Blood vessels which communicate with the pulp through accessory or lateral canals do not contribute significantly as a source of collateral circulation, except possibly in the apical 1–2 mm of the root canal.

The existence of lymphatic vessels in the pulp is a matter of dispute due to limitations in available investigative techniques. Recent ultrastructural studies suggest that lymphatic capillaries arise in the peripheral areas of the pulp and join other lymph vessels to form collecting channels that leave the pulp through the apical foramen. Moreover, there is evidence of anastomoses between lymphatics from the pulp, the periodontal ligament, and the alveolar bone in the periapical area.

Innervation

The innervation of the pulp comprises afferent nerves which conduct sensory impulses (A-fibers) and autonomic nerves (C-fibers) that are mainly involved in neurogenic modulation of the blood flow but also in transmission of pain (see p.66). The A-fibers are of the trigeminal system. They are myelinated, surrounded by Schwann cells, and enter the pulp in bundles with the blood vessels through the apical foramen. The C-fibers constitute the majority of the pulpal nerves. They are unmyelinated and enclosed singly or in groups by Schwann cells, and enter the pulp with the sensory fibers. Some branching of the nerves occurs in the root pulp and the branching becomes extensive in the coronal pulp. Beneath the cell-rich zone is the plexus of Raschkow, which consists of a large number of both myelinated and unmyelinated nerve axons. From this plexus some sensory nerves without their myelin sheath but still inside their Schwann cells approach the odontoblastic layer. Near the odontoblasts, terminal axons leave their Schwann cells and pass between the odontoblasts to the predentin, and in some instances enter the dentinal tubules, where they end in close proximity of the odontoblastic process (**Fig.1.5**). Nerve endings may also be trapped in the miner-alized dentin between the tubules. However, most of the sensory nerves end in the odontoblastic layer or they pass between the odontoblasts and return to the area of Raschkow's plexus.

The physiological need for the vast number of nerves in the periphery of the coronal pulp is not immediately understood. In all likelihood they have proprioceptive functions. Thus, it has been shown that patients readily bite three times as hard on pulpless teeth as on teeth with intact pulps.

Age Changes

As discussed above, continued formation of physiologic secondary dentin over the years will lead to a reduction in the size of the pulp chamber and the root canal. Certain changes which occur in the pulp tissue can be related to the aging process as well. A striking observation is a reduced or missing odontoblastic layer in teeth from older individuals (**Fig.1.12**). Fibrosis of the pulp is commonly seen and a reduced number of cells is present between the fiber bundles. Arteriosclerotic changes may occur in the pulp vessels, and capillaries and precapillaries commonly calcify. Nerve endings regularly calcify as well. Intrapulpal mineralizations increase with age and especially diffuse calcifica-

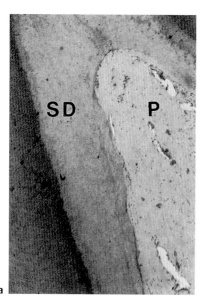
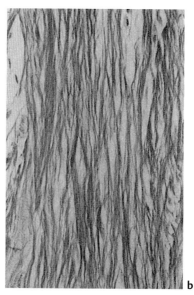

Fig. 1.12
a Coronal pulp (P) from the incisor of a 71-year-old. Large amounts of secondary dentin (SD) have formed. Almost no odontoblasts are present and the pulp is generally poor in cells (hematoxylin-eosin).

b Root pulp poor in cells and rich in fibers (van Gieson stain).

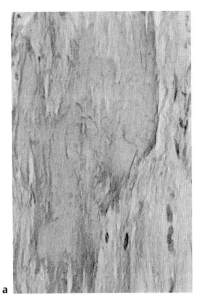

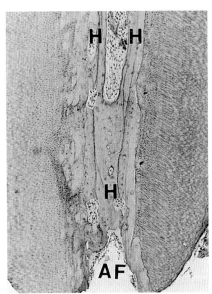

a

b

Fig. 1.13
a **Diffuse calcifications in root pulp** (van Gieson stain).

b Cellular (cementum-like) hard tissue (H) in the root canal near the apical foramen (AF) (hematoxylin-eosin).

tions along the vessels of the root pulp are considered to be an age-related phenomenon (**Fig. 1.13**).

Age reduces the functional capacities of a tissue. It is conceivable, therefore, that the age of a patient may affect unfavorably the outcome of certain endodontic procedures like pulp capping and pulpotomy.

Reaction Patterns

Pulpitis
Like other connective tissues in the body, the pulp reacts to irritants with inflammation (**Fig. 1.14**). However, the pulp has certain characteristics that make it unique and that may alter this tissue response—sometimes dramatically. Tumor (swelling) is one of the cardinal signs of inflammation. When the pulp becomes inflamed, anatomical limitations, that is, the hard root-canal walls, will preclude an increase in tissue volume. In addition, the pulp almost completely lacks a collateral circulation. These two factors place the pulp at a considerable disadvantage in dealing with edema, necrotic tissue, and foreign material. On the other hand, the pulp is the only connective tissue that has the ability, at least to a certain extent, to protect itself from external irritants by the formation of intratubular and secondary dentin.

In the classic view of pulpal inflammation, immense importance was given to the influence of the anatomical environment on the pulp. It was assumed that with a local inflammation in the pulp there would be an increased blood flow to the inflamed area. The vasodilation and increased capillary pressure and permeability induced by the inflammation would result in an increased filtration from the capillaries into the tissue, which in turn would cause steadily increasing tissue pressure (**Fig. 1.15**). Gradually, as the pressure outside the vessels rose, the thin-walled vessels were compressed. This would lead to a decrease in blood flow as well as an increase in venous pressure, which in turn would result in increased capillary pressure and a further increase in the filtration from the capillaries to the tissue. Thus, a vicious circle seemed to develop, resulting in a steady increase in tissue pressure. Consequently,

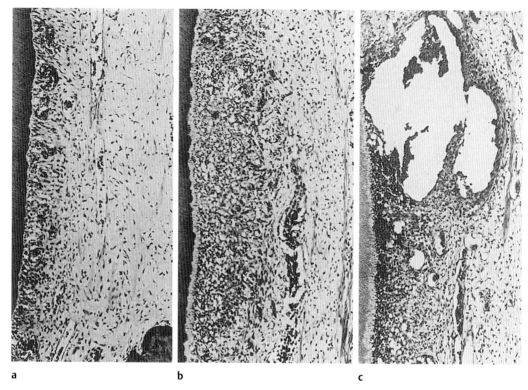

a   b   c

Fig. 1.14 Local inflammatory responses to external irritation in the pulp of monkey teeth (hematoxylin-eosin).
a Mild inflammation with filled capillaries in the odontoblast layer and few inflammatory cells.

b Moderate inflammation with accumulation of inflammatory cells in the affected area of the pulp.
c Severe inflammation with abscess formation.

since the pulp lacks the possibility of expansion, the final result of the increase in tissue pressure was then thought to be a choking or strangulation of the pulpal vessels at the apical foramen, leading to a stagnation of the blood circulation with resultant ischemia and necrosis.

However, modern research has not supported the strangulation theory. For example, in experiments where the tissue pressure of the pulp is measured, it has been found that a pressure increase in one area of the pulp does not cause a pressure increase in the rest of the pulp. It has also been shown that when local inflammation is induced in the pulp, the tissue pressure increases only in the inflamed area and not in the entire pulp cavity. Experiments with in vivo microscopy have confirmed that an injury in the coronal pulp results in local circulatory disturbances and, if the injury is severe enough, to complete stasis in the

vessels in and near the injured area. The circulation in the root pulp, by contrast, is unaffected in these experiments. Experimental studies on the healing of pulpal inflammation have confirmed these findings (**Fig. 1.16**), and presently there is convincing evidence that even severe inflammatory changes in a limited area of the pulp do not result in a circulatory stoppage in the entire pulp.

Based on these and other studies, a modern theory on the hemodynamics of pulpitis has developed. The pulp normally has a relatively high blood flow which is not significantly influenced by vasodilator substances. Thus, only minor increases in blood flow occur during pulp inflammation, and only locally in the inflamed area (**Fig. 1.17**). The increase in capillary permeability, therefore, appears to be considerably more important than the increase in blood flow for the inflammatory response in the pulp. Two possibil-

VASCULAR REACTIONS IN THE INFLAMED PULP

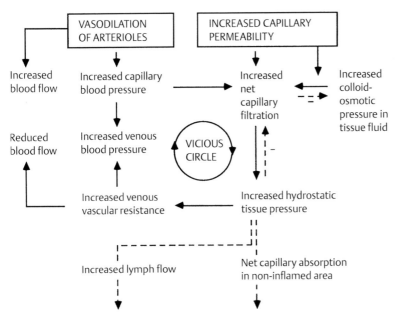

Fig. 1.15 Diagram illustrating the so-called vicious circle of local pulpal inflammation. Broken lines suggest mechanisms which may break the circle.

ities exist for the transport of edematous fluids away from an inflamed area in the pulp: 1) lymphatics, and 2) blood vessels in the adjacent uninflamed tissue. Increased drainage into lymphatic vessels from inflamed areas is known to occur in other tissues. In the pulp the lymphatic flow would be further aided by a positive pressure gradient between the inflamed area and the adjacent uninflamed tissue. Because of the positive pressure gradient, transport of fluids will also occur through the tissue itself to adjacent uninflamed tissue which has normal structural characteristics and where no changes in capillary pressure or permeability have occurred. Here there will be a net absorption of fluids from the tissue into the vessels, thus preventing an increase in tissue pressure in the uninflamed areas of the pulp. A generalized edema of the pulp during inflammation, therefore, is prevented by a localized increase in the tissue pressure in the inflamed area, by an increased lymphatic flow, and by a net absorption into the capillaries of the uninflamed tissue adjacent to the inflamed area of the pulp.

Thus, the modern view of the reaction pattern of the pulp is as follows: The pulp reacts to irri-

tants with local inflammation in an area of the tissue that is subjected to the irritants. The inflammation may remain as a local inflammation for a long time, sometimes for years, if the irritants are mild. If the irritants are removed, for example, if a carious lesion is excavated and a restoration placed in the tooth, the local inflammation may heal (**Figs. 1.18**, **1.40**, **1.41**). The resistance of the pulp to irritants and its ability for repair are considerable. Still, if the irritants are long-lasting and strong enough, the inflammation will spread in the pulp. In most instances the process progresses rather slowly from the periphery where the irritants reach the pulp, toward the central pulp, the root pulp, and the periapical tissues.

Successive necrosis of the tissue in the direction of the apical foramen then takes place (**Fig. 1.18**).

Pathogenesis of Pulpitis

Inflammation in the pulp develops in the same manner as in other tissues. The cellular phase is dominated at first by neutrophilic leukocytes; lymphocytes, macrophages, and plasma cells appear later. The last cell types, however, dominate

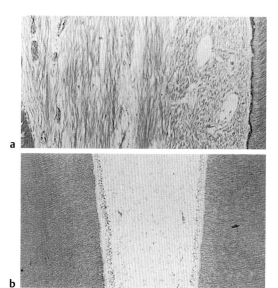

Fig. 1.16 Monkey incisor where severe inflammation was induced experimentally in the coronal pulp (van Gieson stain). After 90 days, repair occurred with the formation of fibrous tissue in the coronal pulp.
a No odontoblasts are seen and the root canal walls are covered by a cementum-like tissue.
b The root pulp appears to be unaffected by the extensive tissue reactions further coronally. The odontoblast layer is intact and the tissue remains rich in cells and poor in fibers.

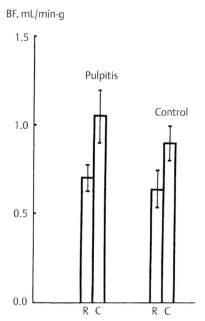

Fig. 1.17 Diagram showing blood flow in mL/min × g in the coronal pulp (C) and root pulp (R) of healthy (control) and inflamed dogs' teeth. Experimentally induced pulpitis in the coronal pulp gave only a slight increase in blood flow in the inflamed area, whereas in the root pulp no difference in blood flow was registered between inflamed and healthy teeth.

the histological picture during sustained pulp inflammation, giving it the character of a chronic inflammation.

Thus, following the vascular phase of the inflammatory reaction, which in the pulp is characterized by a rather slight increase in blood flow, dilation and increased permeability of the capillaries, and accumulation of fluids in the tissue, the neutrophilic leukocytes are attracted to the area by chemotaxis (**Fig. 1.19**). They pass through intercellular gaps in the vessel walls and accumulate in the tissue, where they function as phagocytes. If at this time the irritants can be removed, there is a considerable potential for repair. If not, probably more neutrophilic leukocytes will arrive on the scene. These cells have a life span of only a few hours and will soon start to break down, releasing toxic cellular components and proteolytic enzymes which may destroy cells, fibers, and ground substance in the inflamed area of the pulp. If the tissue destruction is severe enough, it may be rec-

ognized clinically as a drop of pus when the pulp chamber is opened (**Fig. 1.20**). If the leukocytic breakdown occurs slowly, encapsuled abscesses can form and may be seen microscopically. This encapsulation of the destroyed tissue may for a time delay further tissue destruction. Sometimes even calcification of the abscess membrane is seen (**Fig. 1.21**). It is not known whether or not pulpal repair may occur at this stage of the inflammatory process.

Gradually, the scene is no longer dominated by neutrophilic leukocytes, but by lymphocytes that have come to the inflamed area, left the capillaries, and aggregated in the tissue. The inflammation is now no longer *acute*, but *chronic*, and in addition to the lymphocytes, macrophages and plasma cells will typically be seen in the inflamed area (**Fig. 1.22**). Both B lymphocytes and T lymphocytes have been recognized in the pulp, representing the humoral- and cell-mediated systems of immunity. Invasion of the pulp tissue by anti-

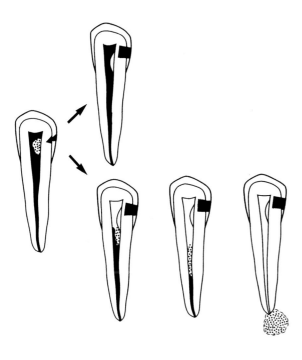

Fig. 1.18 Diagram illustrating the possible outcome of reparative treatment of a carious lesion with corresponding local inflammation in subjacent pulp (left). When the irritants are removed and the cavity is restored, the local inflammation will usually heal (top). However, if enough bacteria have reached the pulp, the inflammation will spread in spite of the placement of a restoration, slowly leading to complete pulpal necrosis and the development of an apical periodontitis.

genic products may be inhibited by the complexing of these products with antibodies and the formation of antigen–antibody complexes which in turn are phagocytized and digested, especially by macrophages. However, lymphocytes may also have a destructive effect on the pulp tissue, either through direct cytotoxic activity or through biologically active and destructive cytokines. Macrophages can lead to tissue destruction as well through the production of cytokines, collagenase, and other products. Thus, the immune response may inflict further damage to an already injured pulp. This again may result in an increased chemotactic activity and attraction of neutrophilic leukocytes. An acute inflammatory reaction may then be superimposed on the chronic inflammation. This is a rather common occurrence in inflamed pulps, although in many instances an acute episode will be caused by new external irritants reaching the pulp tissue.

Pulpal inflammation is, therefore, a dynamic process. Various stages of the inflammatory process can often be observed in different areas of the same pulp. A typical observation would be necrosis of the tissue in the area where the inflammation started. The tissue subjacent to this area may be inflamed, dominated by the cells typical of a chronic inflammation. Also, in this area one

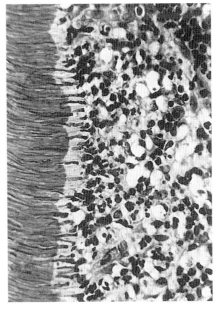

Fig. 1.19 Neutrophilic leukocytes in pulp tissue responding to external irritants reaching the pulp through exposed dentinal tubules (hematoxylin-eosin).

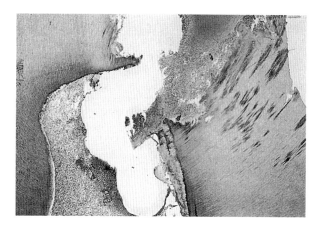

Fig. 1.20 A drop of pus from a pulpal abscess is seen in a carious cavity (hematoxylin-eosin).

or more encapsulated microabscesses may be seen. Apical to the inflamed area, noninflamed pulp tissue will be present (**Fig.1.23**). Without treatment, the inflammation (and later the necrosis) will gradually spread in an apical direction until the entire pulp becomes necrotic. A total pulpitis in the sense that the entire pulp is infiltrated by inflammatory cells does not seem to occur.

A rare variation in the development of pulp inflammation is the formation of a *pulp polyp*. Under particularly favorable circumstances, the successive breakdown of the pulp can stop temporarily when a carious attack or a traumatic injury has resulted in an opening of the pulp cavity. Instead of becoming necrotic, the pulp tissue may start to proliferate. A *proliferating pulpitis* or a pulp polyp then develops (**Fig.1.24**). On the sur-

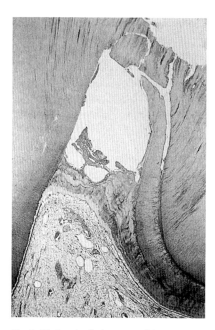

Fig. 1.21 A pulpal abscess subjacent to a carious lesion is "walled off" by calcified tissue (hematoxylin-eosin).

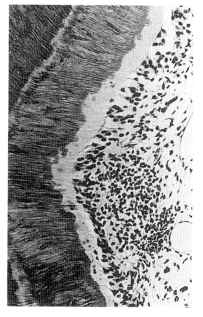

Fig. 1.22 Accumulation of inflammatory cells typical of chronic inflammation is seen in the pulp of a monkey tooth subjacent to secondary dentin (hematoxylin-eosin).

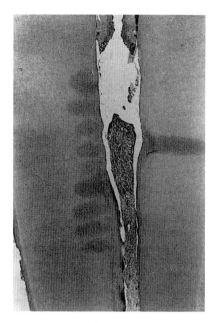

Fig. 1.23 Section from a tooth where pulp has been exposed to the oral cavity for some time. The tissue in the pulp chamber and coronal half of the root canal is necrotic. Subjacent to the necrotic tissue, the pulp is severely inflamed. In the apical area of the root canal the pulp tissue is still uninflamed (hematoxylin-eosin).

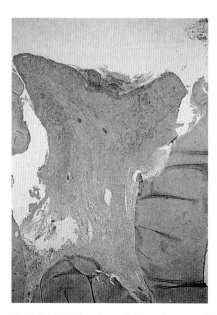

Fig. 1.24 Proliferation of tissue from molar root pulp, leading to the formation of a pulp polyp (hematoxylin-eosin).

face the pulp polyp normally has a necrotic layer, but in some instances it becomes epithelialized. However, the epithelial lining does not give the protection seen in the gingiva. It is infiltrated with inflammatory cells, is ulcerated, and bleeds easily when touched. Occasionally a pulp polyp may reach the gingiva, and a tissue bridge between the gingiva and the pulp is established. A pulp polyp may last for a relatively long time, but the end result will always be total tissue breakdown as described above.

Etiology of Pulpitis

Inflammation of the pulp can be caused by many etiological factors. For clinical–practical reasons the following division can be made:
1. Infectious pulpitis, due to caries or exposure of the dentin or pulp to the oral cavity;
2. Traumatic pulpitis, due to traumatic injuries of the teeth; and
3. Iatrogenic pulpitis, due to improper and sometimes proper dental treatment.

Dental Caries

When a carious lesion has reached the dentin, the dentinal tubules are portals of entry for bacteria, bacterial products, tissue breakdown products, and irritants from the saliva and the oral cavity. Even in teeth with enamel caries without macroscopic loss of tissue, a few inflammatory cells may be seen in the pulp underneath the lesion, and under dentin caries, inflammatory foci, sometimes with abscesses, may be seen (**Fig. 1.25**).

It has been assumed that although there are microorganisms in the dentinal tubules of a carious lesion, the pulp will not be infected as long as it is vital. Rather, it is bacterial products that initially cause the inflammation, either through a direct cytotoxic effect or indirectly by their antigenic properties. The classic opinion is that not until the pulp injury is so severe that a localized area of necrosis has developed will it be possible for bacteria to enter the pulp cavity. Bacteria will then establish colonies in the necrotic tissue and the pulp will become infected. However, from recent studies it appears that invasiveness is an important aspect of the virulence of many endodontopathic bacteria. Thus, during the spread of inflammation in the pulp, bacteria may be present both in the part of the pulp that has become necrotic and in the superficial layer of the subjacent vital tissue. The front of infection, in other words,

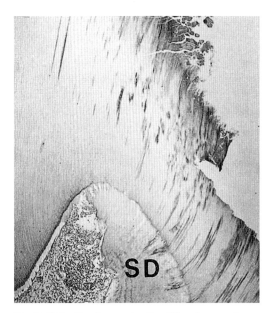

Fig. 1.25 Section from a tooth with a deep carious lesion. Large amounts of secondary dentin (SD) have formed. The pulp is severely inflamed (hematoxylin-eosin).

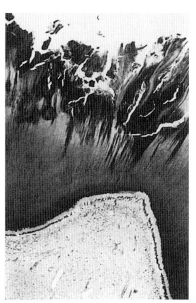

Fig. 1.26 Section from a tooth with a deep carious lesion. Secondary dentin formation is not evident and the pulp is not inflamed (hematoxylin-eosin).

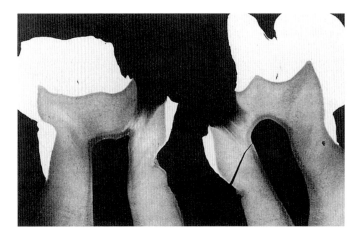

Fig. 1.27 Microradiograph of a tooth with a deep carious lesion. A hypermineralized (sclerotic) zone has formed in the primary dentin between the carious lesion and the pulp.

will be at the transition zone between the necrotic and vital (inflamed) pulp tissue.

While marked inflammatory reactions can be observed in the pulp of teeth with only superficial carious lesions, it is also possible to find teeth with much more severe carious attacks without pulpal inflammation (**Fig. 1.26**). One reason for this seemingly illogical occurrence is that products from the carious lesion may stimulate the pulp to produce intratubular dentin, resulting in a sclerosis of the tubules. A zone of sclerosis is formed in the dentin between the peripheral area of destruction and the pulp (**Fig. 1.27**). The intratubular deposits in the zone of sclerosis consist of small hydroxyapatite crystals that may obliterate the tubules completely. The deposits are identical with those seen in age-changed dentin (**Fig. 1.6**). Peripherally to the sclerotic zone, additional intratubular mineralized deposits may be found. These deposits vary considerably in quality and appearance. Usually they consist of large, irregularly arranged, needle-shaped hydroxyapatite crystals, or large, rhomboid-shaped whitlockite crystals (**Fig. 1.28**). These irregular deposits are in all likelihood not formed by pulpal cells, but result from a passive reprecipitation of minerals that were dissolved in the more peripheral parts of the carious dentin.

The sclerotic zone of the dentin may become an effective barrier which prevents the passage of irritants from the carious lesion to the pulp. The barrier may even be so effective that repair of pulpal inflammation that had developed prior to the formation of the barrier may occur. A permanent repair without treatment is still unthinkable, since an untreated carious process will proceed and gradually break through the sclerotic zone of the dentin so that irritants can reach the pulp once again. Moreover, in most instances the sclerotic zone of the dentin is less than perfect. It may reduce, but usually will not entirely stop, the irritants from the carious lesion reaching the pulp. Also, it should be remembered that the carious process spreads not only in a pulpal direction in the dentin, but in a lateral direction as well, especially in the area near the enamel–dentin junction. This results in irritants reaching the pulp through newly exposed dentinal tubules where intratubular sclerosis has not yet formed. Therefore, *from a clinical point of view it must be assumed that the pulp is inflamed to some extent in all teeth with active carious lesions.*

It is important to note that the sclerotic zone is formed in the primary dentin (**Fig. 1.27**). The secondary dentin, which as a rule also forms in the pulp under a carious lesion, will not, however, constitute an effective barrier against the external irritants (**Fig. 1.25**). On the contrary, when the carious process has broken through to the secondary dentin, the pulp will unquestionably be inflamed. Gradually, the carious process will also break through to the pulp and cause a pulp exposure (**Fig. 1.29**). At that time the inflammation is usually irreversible with today's treatment methods.

As is evident from the above, the pulp reaction in carious teeth may vary considerably, and it is virtually impossible with clinical means to have

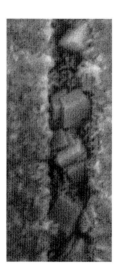

Fig. 1.28 Scanning electron micrograph of a dentinal tubule with whitlockite crystals as seen in carious dentin (×17 500).

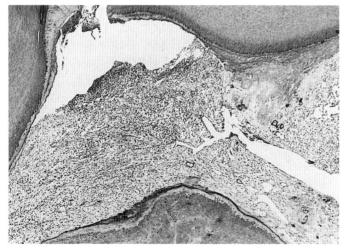

Fig. 1.29 Section from a tooth with pulp exposure due to caries. The pulp tissue subjacent to the exposure is severely inflamed (hematoxylin-eosin).

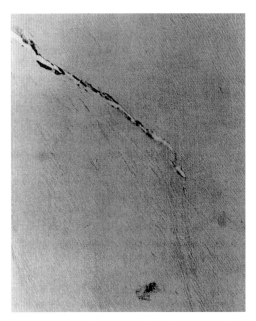

Fig. 1.30 Section from a tooth with an enamel–dentin crack filled with bacterial plaque. The crack runs at an angle to the dentinal tubules, and many tubules which are opened up by the crack contain bacteria as well (Brown–Brenn stain).

an opinion of its severity until the tooth gives a negative sensitivity response which suggests pulp necrosis. The therapeutic implications of this unclear diagnostic situation are discussed in Chapter 5.

Dentin Exposed to Oral Cavity

Other etiological factors leading to an infectious pulpitis are conditions that contribute to the exposure of the dentin and dentinal tubules to the oral environment. With the refinement of foodstuffs, severe *attrition* is not as common as before. On the other hand, *abrasion*, particularly as a result of tooth-brushing, is becoming a more serious problem. *Erosion* leading to exposure of dentin was traditionally seen in individuals employed in certain chemical industries. Presently it has become a serious problem in the young generation from excessive intake of sweet and acid soft drinks. Nevertheless, it is periodontal disease and the extensive treatment of this disease that today particularly leads to exposure of dentin. Gingival recession is commonly seen in these patients and the root cementum and peripheral layers of the

root dentin are being removed during scaling and root planing. It has also been shown that the so-called enamel cracks that are present in most teeth do not necessarily end at the enamel–dentin junction, but rather extend deep into the dentin (**Fig. 1.30**). These cracks are filled with plaque and microorganisms, and sometimes defects reminiscent of carious lesions are seen at the bottom of such cracks. Since the cracks usually run at an angle to the dentinal tubules, a large number of tubules may become exposed to the oral environment by a single crack.

Irritants from the plaque and saliva may reach the pulp through the exposed dentinal tubules. This is shown by the fact that mineralized deposits are laid down in the exposed tubules. The intratubular deposits are characterized by the large, needle-like hydroxyapatite crystals and the rhomboidal whitlockite crystals seen peripherially in the tubules of carious lesions (**Fig. 1.28**). However, only occasionally are exposed tubules fully occluded as seen in age-changed root dentin and in the sclerotic dentin of carious teeth (see **Fig. 1.6**). Secondary dentin forms as a result of external irritation in all teeth with exposed dentin. The secondary dentin is usually more regular than in carious teeth, but is still characterized by morphological irregularities with a varying number of tubules and with inclusions of functioning blood vessels and strings of soft tissue (**Fig. 1.31**). Pulp stones may be observed in the coronal pulp of these teeth as well, which have possibly developed as a result of external irritation.

In spite of the mineral deposits in the tubules of the primary dentin and formation of often large amounts of secondary dentin, the exposed dentin remains as a rule partially open to the mouth and does not fully protect the pulp from exogenous irritants. In the pulp of these teeth the odontoblastic layer is reduced or missing (**Fig. 1.31**). Circulatory disturbances are evidenced by hemorrhages and disintegrating erythrocytes, and the blood vessels are few and prominent. The most conspicuous finding in teeth with long-standing exposed dentin is a fibrosis of the pulp (**Fig. 1.32**). Large bundles of collagenous fibers are seen in the affected area of the pulp, often in continuity with the secondary dentin. Frequently, fiber bundles may be mineralized.

Connective tissue cells, and sometimes lymphocytes, macrophages, and plasma cells are seen between the fiber bundles. However, a possible in-

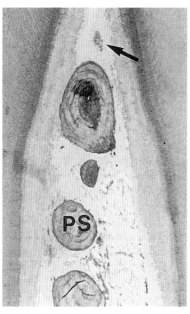
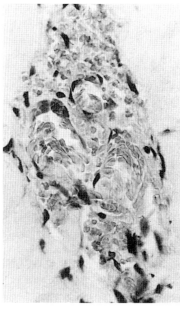

a

b

Fig. 1.31
a Pulp horn from a tooth with exposed dentin. Large amounts of secondary dentin as well as pulp stones (PS) are present. Functioning blood vessels are seen deep inside the secondary dentin (arrow).
b Higher magnification of blood vessels in secondary dentin (hematoxylin-eosin).

flammatory reaction is mild and will not lead to pulp necrosis. The exception lies in teeth with severe periodontal disease and pocket formation to the foraminal areas of the roots. In such teeth a retrograde pulpitis may develop (**Fig. 1.33**). In a single-rooted tooth this condition will lead to disturbances in the blood supply to the pulp relatively quickly, resulting in total pulp necrosis. In teeth with multiple roots, a retrograde pulpitis in one root will spread slowly in a coronal direction, and it may take a long time before the entire pulp becomes necrotic.

Traumatic Injuries

Traumatic injuries to the teeth and jaws will often result in pulpitis and pulp necrosis. A *complicated crown fracture* with pulp exposure will result in an infectious inflammation of the pulp. The actual crown fracture invariably leads to a hemorrhage in the pulp subjacent to the exposure. The blood clot is an excellent substrate for bacterial growth, and the microorganisms of the plaque accumulating on the fractured surface will readily invade the pulp. A local inflammation is seen in the tissue near the exposure after 2–3 days, and total pulp necrosis in such teeth has been observed as early as 7 days after the injury (**Fig. 1.34**). However, in some instances it may take weeks before total necrosis is seen.

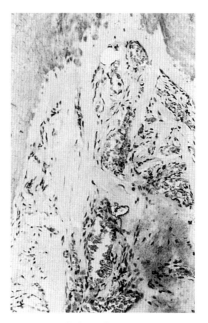

Fig. 1.32 Pulp horn from a tooth with exposed dentin. Large fiber bundles, few and dilated vessels as well as a calcified area are seen in the pulp tissue (hematoxylin-eosin).

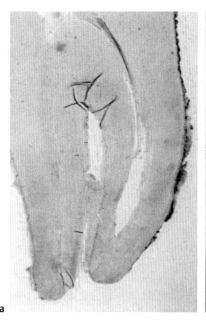

a

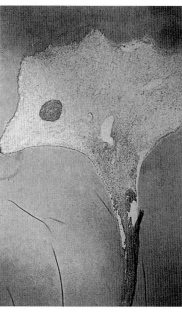

b

Fig. 1.33 Mandibular molar with severe periodontal disease.
a Section showing bacterial plaque to the apex of the mesial root (Brown–Brenn stain).
b Neighboring section showing retrograde pulpitis reaching the coronal pulp (hematoxylin-eosin).

In *root-fractured* teeth, the tissue injuries at the fracture line will cause an inflammatory reaction. The pulpal injury is characterized by ruptured vessels and bleeding into the tissue followed by circulatory stasis in the injured area. If the fracture line is in communication with the oral cavity, bacteria will invade the injured tissues (blood clot), and an infectious pulpitis will develop and cause pulp necrosis as described above for teeth with complicated crown fractures. If, on the other hand, a true intra-alveolar fracture is diagnosed, no foreign irritants will be present at the site of injury. Only a mild inflammatory reaction will then follow, clearing up and removing extravasated erythrocytes and tissue breakdown products. Complete pulpal repair will occur in about 80% of such teeth. The remaining 20% are usually teeth with displacement of the coronal fragment during the injury, resulting in severence of the pulpal blood vessels at the fracture site. The pulp tissue of the coronal fragment will then undergo ischemic necrosis (see p.25). Experience has shown that over time, usually in a few weeks, the ischemic pulp tissue will become infected by way of exposed dentinal tubules and enamel–dentin cracks. Endodontic treatment will then become necessary. However, in the pulp tissue of the apical fragment of the root-fractured teeth, repair usually takes place and the endodontic treatment may be confined to the coronal fragment of the tooth (see p.123).

About 25% of *subluxated teeth* end up with necrosis of the pulp. The sequence of events leading to this end result is not fully understood. By definition, subluxated teeth are loosened, but not displaced. This means that the pulpal blood vessels are not severed at the apex of the tooth. Rather the injury is characterized by ruptures of intrapulpal blood vessels, bleeding into the tissue, and subsequent infection of blood clots through exposed dentin and cracks as described above.

Luxated teeth by definition are displaced by the injury. Consequently, the pulpal blood vessels of these teeth are severed at the apical foramen and the pulp undergoes ischemic necrosis. Repair is possible in incompletely formed teeth with open apices through recanaliculization and revascularization of the pulp (see p.27). However, in most instances, the ischemic pulp tissue becomes infected, necessitating endodontic treatment of the teeth.

Iatrogenic Factors
Operative and restorative procedures may lead to pulpal inflammation. The inflammation is mainly caused by dessication or dehydration of the dentin, by toxic influences from materials and cements, and by leakage along the margins of a restoration.

Dehydration of the dentin may result from the heat caused by cavity or crown preparation without water, from the use of thermoplastic impression materials that are too warm, and from a prolonged and continuous blast of air to exposed dentin. As a result of dehydration, tissue fluids from the pulp will flow into the dentinal tubules toward the dentin surface. This fluid flow causes mechanical disturbances in the pulp. The odontoblasts and sometimes other cells may be sucked into the dentinal tubules, and there is an immediate increase in the bloodflow to the area of the pulp subjacent to the dehydrated dentin (**Fig. 1.35**). There is also an increase in the number of functioning capillaries in the injured area. The injuries result in a mild chemotactic activity and after a few hours, scattered neutrophilic leukocytes are seen in the tissue. The inflammatory reaction to dentin dehydration is generally mild, and it has not been possible to show experimentally that this type of pulpal injury leads to pulp necrosis. However, the inflammation often results in dental hypersensitivity and considerable postoperative discomfort for the patient. There is also some clinical evidence that preparation without water and careless use of thermoplastic impression materials may cause a long-standing chronic inflammation in the pulp with internal root resorption and eventually total pulp necrosis. It is important to understand that it is not the heat itself that causes the pulp reaction, but the dehydration of the dentin. True, it has been shown that a temperature increase of 10 °C in the pulp may cause inflammation. The dentin, however, is an excellent insulator and, for instance, dry cavity preparation gives a temperature increase of only 2–3 °C in the pulp tissue. Thus, cooling of the bur with cold or tempered air will not prevent preparation damage, but rather make it worse. Use of water on the other hand, will prevent dehydration of the dentin and thereby prevent a pulp reaction in an effective and reliable manner.

The *placing of a restoration* may be harmful to the pulp as well. A good example of this is the insertion of cohesive gold fillings (**Fig. 1.36**). The "hammering" which is necessary for this technique, the heating of the gold foil, and the prolonged period of dehydration of the dentin in the cavity usually cause a severe pulp reaction characterized by intrapulpal bleeding and inflammation. This pulp reaction may be irreversible.

Cements and filling materials used in dentistry

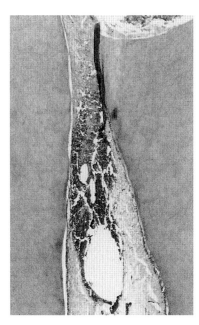

Fig. 1.34 Pulp horn in a monkey tooth with traumatic pulp exposure (complicated crown fracture). On day 7 after the injury there is evidence of severe hemorrhage in the tissue and the pulp is necrotic (hematoxylin-eosin).

may contain components that are irritating to the pulp (**Fig. 1.37**). Especially the tooth-colored materials are of interest in this regard; examples of toxic components are fluorides in silicate and glass ionomer cements and chemically active ingredients to influence the setting reaction or improve the color stability of composite resins. Thus, different brands of the same material may have different biological properties depending on the additives the various manufacturers have included in their products. An example of this is seen when the antibacterial effect of commercially available filling materials based on Bowen's resin is studied, in that it varies from no effect to a strong effect. *Clinically, the rule should be that a tooth-colored material should be used with a base to protect the pulp* (see p. 86).

Marginal leakage will occur to a greater or lesser extent with most restorations, and plaque and microorganisms may be found in the gap between the restoration and the cavity wall (**Fig. 1.38**). Marginal leakage may cause an inflammatory reaction in the pulp. Apparently, the etiological factors are infectious–toxic in nature, but

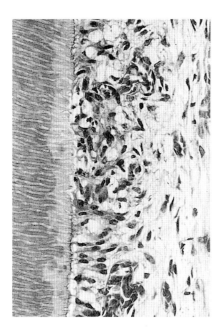

Fig. 1.35 Area of the pulp of a monkey tooth subjacent to a cavity prepared without water. Filled capillaries and a few neutrophilic leukocytes are seen in the odontoblast layer after 1 day (hematoxylin-eosin).

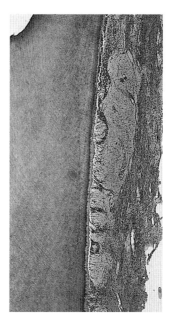

Fig. 1.36 Area of the pulp of a monkey tooth subjacent to a cavity restored with gold foil. A severe inflammatory reaction is seen in the pulp subjacent to the cavity after 30 days (hematoxylin-eosin).

the mechanism is presently not well understood. For example, an amalgam restoration will not seal a cavity any better after 1 week in the mouth than a methyl methacrylate resin filling. Still, under the amalgam restoration no or only a negligible reaction will be observed in the pulp, whereas under the resin restoration usually a severe inflammatory reaction, often with abscess formation, is seen (**Fig. 1.37e**). It might appear that reactions occur between bacterial and plaque components and components leaking out of the resin restoration, resulting in substances with strong immunogenic properties. This may explain why marginal leakage is more detrimental in conjunction with some filling materials than with others. Finally, it should be remembered that the gap between a restoration and the cavity wall represents a definite risk for the development of secondary caries.

Therapeutic irradiation of the head and neck region may damage the pulp. The odontoblasts are especially sensitive cells, and as a result of irradiation, may elaborate abnormal dentin, sometimes filling large parts of the pulpal cavity. Circulatory disturbances and inflammation may result as well. However, the effect of irradiation on the sali-

vary glands, resulting in a decrease in salivary flow, is of much more profound clinical importance. The teeth become more prone to decay, and especially in the cervical area, caries is rampant, often leading to fracture of the teeth, exposure of the pulp, and gradually to irreversible pulpal inflammation. It is important to note that teeth with pulp involvement in irradiated patients should be treated endodontically rather than by extraction, since extraction may result in radionecrosis of the surrounding bone.

During *orthodontic treatment* the teeth can be exposed to forces that are strong enough to cause pulp damage. A recent study shows that orthodontic patients 5 years after completion of the treatment have significantly more nonvital incisors than individuals who have not undergone orthodontic treatment. It is not immediately clear how the pulp is injured. Two possibilities appear to exist. Intrapulpal vessels may rupture as a result of the treatment, resulting in internal bleeding. The blood clot may become infected as discussed above, and an infectious pulpitis will lead to pulp necrosis. In some instances the pulpal blood vessels conceivably may be pinched off at

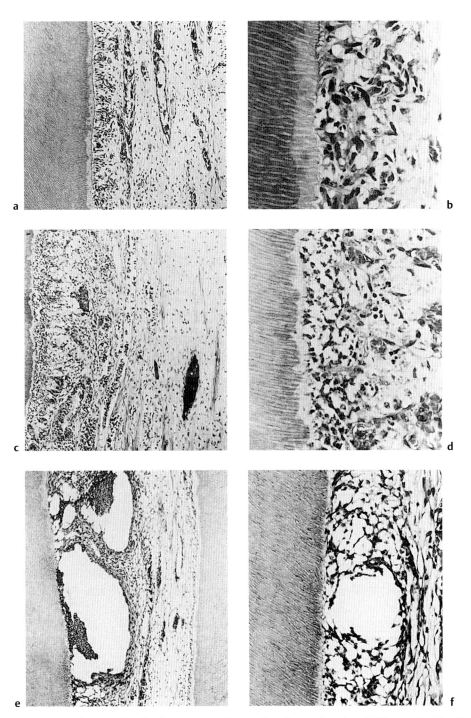

Fig. 1.37 a–f Examples of pulp reactions observed under tooth-colored filling materials after 8 days: mild in **a, b** and severe in **e, f** (hematoxylin-eosin).

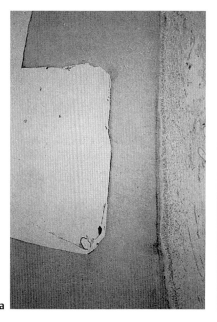
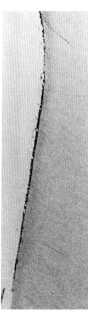

Fig. 1.38
a **Cavity in a dog tooth filled with glass ionomer cement for 60 days.** A bacterial plaque is present between the filling material and the cavity walls (Brown–Brenn stain).
b Higher magnification of bacterial plaque on the cavity floor and bacteria in dentinal tubules (Brown–Brenn stain).

a

b

the apex of the tooth, resulting in ischemic pulp necrosis.

Internal and especially external root resorption are also known complications following orthodontic treatment. In addition to these irreversible changes, orthodontic treatment may lead to dental hyposensitivity or hypersensitivity, that is, an increase or decrease in the pain threshold of the teeth. The pulp reaction in these teeth is not known, but in most instances these conditions appear to be reversible.

Oral and maxillofacial surgery may cause pulp injury and pulp necrosis by severing blood vessels and interrupting the blood supply to the pulp. In instances where this is suspected, it should be remembered that absence of sensitivity does not always mean that the tooth is nonvital. It could be the nerve supply, which lacks reserve lines, that is damaged. The blood vessels of the face and jaws, on the other hand, have anastomoses and the necessary blood supply could be secured in spite of the surgical operation.

Cumulative Effect of Irritants
With the high prevalence of dental disease and the extensive dental treatment in the last two generations, the teeth of most adult and older individuals have been exposed to a wide variety of irritants. Many teeth have suffered from multiple

carious attacks over the years. Most teeth will have exposed dentin because of attrition, abrasion, erosion, enamel–dentin cracks, gingival recession, and the treatment of periodontal disease, and most teeth have multiple restorations that in many instances have had to be renewed several times. The various external irritants that have affected the teeth over time conceivably have a cumulative effect, and if the pulp has not become necrotic, it generally will have this appearance: the odontoblast layer is partially or fully destroyed; secondary dentin and intrapulpal hard tissue fill most of the original pulp chamber; functioning vessels and inclusions of soft tissue are present in the secondary dentin; the soft tissue is rich in fibers and poor in cells; the vessels are few and prominent. The severity of these changes will vary with the degree of external irritation a tooth has suffered and with the type and effectiveness of the treatment rendered.

Systemic Influences
There is considerable experimental evidence that *nutritional deficiencies* may adversely affect the endodontium. Thus, deficiencies of vitamins A, C, and D may interfere with the formation of intercellular substances, dentin matrix formation, and mineralization. Excessive amounts of vitamin D can cause defective dentin formation and calcifi-

cation of the pulp. Connective tissues are also affected by hormones, and in one study it was shown that high dosages of parathyroid extract produced hypomineralization of newly formed dentin matrix. However, it should be noted that these findings derive from experiments in small animals, often performed under extreme conditions, and it appears unlikely that the artificial imbalances created experimentally occur in humans. Clinically, therefore, these findings are probably of minor importance.

Metastases or direct extension of malignant tumors into the pulp have been reported. A case of leukemia is known in which the patient's first signs and symptoms were a loss of sensitivity, but not of the vitality, of the pulp of several teeth and development of periapical radiolucencies on the teeth (**Fig. 1.39**). However, it may be concluded that systemic diseases appear to play a very small part in pulpal pathoses.

Pulp Necrosis

Necrosis means local death of cells. The cellular changes characteristic of necrosis are changes which the cell undergoes after it has died while still remaining in the body. The causes of cell death are the same that cause inflammation. The reaction in the tissue depends to a great extent on the concentration of the irritant. If the irritant is weak, inflammation is produced; if strong, the result may be necrosis.

Necrosis of the pulp is caused by bacteria and bacterial products or by the loss of blood supply. The infectious agents cause liquefaction necrosis, whereas the loss of blood supply leads to ischemia of the tissue and coagulation necrosis.

Liquefaction Necrosis

Autolysis plays an important part in producing liquefaction necrosis. The process is caused by a complex system of intracellular enzymes which, when the cell dies, stop to take part in the metabolism of nutrients brought to the cell and turn their energies on the framework of the cell itself. The products of autolysis are readily diffusable so that they pass into the surrounding fluids and eventually the cell disappears. Clinically, this is readily recognized. When a tooth with a necrotic pulp due to caries is opened, the root canal is near empty, and only scant tissue remnants are found.

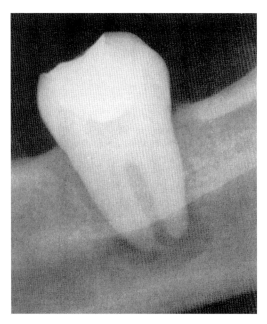

Fig. 1.39 Radiograph of a vital mandibular molar with periapical radiolucency in a 15-year-old. Similar radiolucencies developed on other vital teeth without obvious reasons. The patient was soon diagnosed as having leukemia.

Ischemic Necrosis

When the blood supply to the pulp is cut off, for instance, in conjunction with a luxation injury, the cells undergo necrosis. The reason for the cell death in this instance is a lack of oxygen and nutrients and not the presence of exogenous irritants in the tissue. Cell metabolism will, therefore, not cease immediately after the blood supply is discontinued, but continue in the pulp at a steadily decreasing rate for at least 4–5 days. The plasma of the ischemic tissue contains substances which prevent autolysis of the cells. The intracellular enzymes, rather, cause a coagulation of the cytoplasm, and the nuclear material is often condensed into a small, deeply staining mass (pyknosis). To some extent this process is similar to coagulation of blood. Considerable cellular detail is lost in the ischemic tissue, but the general architectural outlines of the pulp may be recognized for long periods of time. Clinically, a pulp that has undergone ischemic necrosis can readily be recognized when it is extirpated, sometimes weeks and months after a displacement injury of the tooth. The pulp tissue will look whitish in color, but otherwise will not be visibly broken down.

The ischemic pulp tissue may be referred to as an *infarct* since the reaction in the pulp is similar to that occurring in other tissues which lose their primary and collateral circulation. However, the ischemic tissue will become infected sooner or later through ingrowth of bacteria through cracks and exposed dentinal tubules. The coagulated tissue will then break down, mainly because of the action of bacterial proteolytic enzymes, and liquefaction will occur.

Repair in the Pulp

As discussed above, the pulp is an end organ lacking in collateral circulation, and under the influence of strong and persisting exogenous irritants, it will often become necrotic. Still the repair potentials of the pulp are considerable and clinically well recognized. *Thus, when reparative dentistry is in fact possible, it is because pulpal inflammation heals when external irritants, for instance, from a carious lesion are removed, and the resultant cavity*

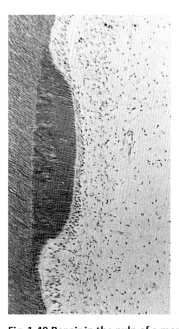

Fig. 1.40 Repair in the pulp of a monkey tooth 60 days after a mild local inflammation was induced. The formation of secondary dentin in the affected area of the pulp is evidence that a reaction has occurred. Otherwise the repair is complete with a normal pulp (van Gieson stain).

is treated with a well-sealing restoration. The tissue reactions during pulpal repair are known from experimental studies.

Local Repair

The tissue reactions characterizing pulpal repair are generally similar to those in other connective tissues, and to a considerable extent depend on the severity of the injury. One characteristic difference is that the odontoblasts of the pulp may form secondary dentin in response to external irritants (**Fig. 1.40**). The secondary dentin formation is looked upon by many as an aspect of pulpal repair, and a commonly used name for this tissue is *reparative dentin*. However, it should be understood that *the secondary dentin forms during the period of external irritation and tissue destruction and not during the period of repair.* It is, therefore, not self-evident that the secondary dentin formation should be regarded as a repair mechanism in the pulp, especially since the stronger the irritants, the more irregular and less protective the tissue becomes. On the whole it is well established that secondary dentin as such offers only limited protection of the pulp. If a carious lesion has reached the secondary dentin, the subjacent pulp will always be inflamed. However, if a large number of odontoblasts are destroyed by the external irritants, the interface between primary and secondary dentin may inadvertently give some protection because of a discontinuity of some tubules of the primary dentin. Thus, rather than look upon the secondary dentin as a sign of pulpal repair it should be regarded as evidence of previous pulpal irritation (**Fig. 1.40**). Presence or absence of secondary dentin will have little bearing on the repair process.

When external irritants have been removed, pulpal repair may occur. If the inflammatory reaction is mild, there will be complete regeneration of the pulp tissue. The only evidence that a local reaction has taken place may be the presence of secondary dentin formed in response to the external irritation and possibly a reduced odontoblastic layer (**Fig. 1.40**). However, if the inflammation is severe, there may be extensive and irreversible tissue changes in the pulp when the repair process is completed (**Fig. 1.41**). The inflamed tissue may be replaced by a fibrous tissue with only a few cells. The odontoblast layer may be completely destroyed in the area of reaction, and cell-containing hard tissue may line the dentin wall where arrested resorption lacunae may be present. As would be expected, the root pulp is usually unaffected by even severe tissue reactions in the coronal pulp (see **Fig. 1.16**).

As mentioned above, abscesses are often present in the pulp of carious teeth. Clearly, surgical drainage of the pus cannot be accomplished in the unexposed pulp, and an abscess is often said to be a sign of irreversible pulpal inflammation. This may not necessarily be so. All repair is fundamentally the same, whether in an open wound or in an enclosed abscess. If the exogenous irritants are removed, attempts at repair will begin. If the abscess cavity is small (which it often is in the pulp), it may become filled with a granulation tissue and then by a fibrous tissue or it may become calcified.

The local repair of the exposed pulp will be discussed in Chapter 5 (under Pulp Capping, p.88).

Revascularization

Pulpal repair may also occur in teeth with ischemic necrosis, notably in immature teeth with large apical foramina. On rare occasions a *recanaliculization* of the pulpal blood vessels may occur after the repositioning of a displaced, immature tooth in its socket. This means that the blood vessels in the pulp reunite with blood vessels in the periodontal ligament so that the blood may start flowing again in the original vasculary network of the pulp. If this occurs, the original pulp cells will survive, since they can tolerate a limited period of ischemia.

A more predictable reaction in immature teeth with ischemic necrosis is a *revascularization* of the pulp. When this occurs, new vessels start growing into the necrotic pulp tissue after about 4 days (**Fig. 1.42**). After 10 days the apical half of the pulp is revascularized, and after 30 days the new vessels have reached the coronal pulp and the pulp horns. With enzyme histochemical techniques it is shown that the oxidoreductase activity of the pulp cells diminishes gradually during the first week after the blood supply is cut off. After 10 days enzyme activity can again be demonstrated, especially along the new vessels that have grown into the necrotic tissue, and after 30 days there is strong oxidoreductase activity in the entire pulp. Histologically, the cellular phase of the repair process can be followed. New fibroblasts are seen in the pulp closely following the proliferation of the blood vessels, and macrophages, sometimes in large numbers, are seen as well.

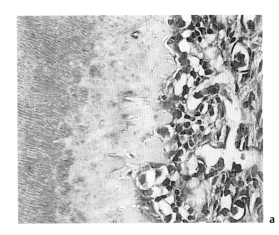

a

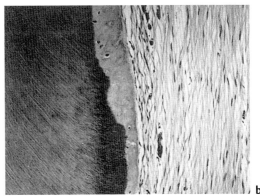

b

Fig. 1.41 Repair in the pulp of monkey teeth after severe local inflammation was induced.

a After 8 days, the odontoblasts are destroyed. A cellular hard tissue forms on the dentin wall and a chronic inflammation can be seen in the pulp.

b After 90 days, the repair is complete. The cellular hard tissue can be seen on the dentin wall. No odontoblasts are present and a fibrous tissue can be seen in the affected area of the pulp (van Gieson stain).

Thus, after 30 days the root canal and pulp chamber again contain vital, cell-rich connective tissue. Naturally, this tissue is not pulp tissue, but periodontal tissue grown into the pulp space from the periodontal ligament. As such it contains the normal bone-forming and cementum-forming cells of the periodontium (see Chapter 2), and gradually over a period of a few months to a year, bone- and cementum-like tissue will form in the new pulp (**Fig. 1.43**). The hard tissue appears to form as a metaplasia of the soft tissue throughout the pulpal cavity. Obviously there are no odonto-

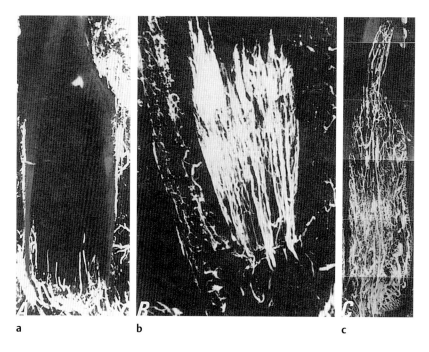

a   b   c

Fig. 1.42 Microangiographs showing revascularization of extracted and replanted dog teeth.

a Four days after replantation, blood vessels start to grow into the ischemic pulp tissue.

b On day 10, the apical half of the pulp is revascularized.

c After 30 days, blood vessels have reached the pulp horns and the entire pulp is revascularized.

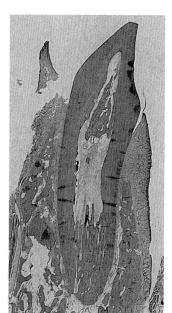

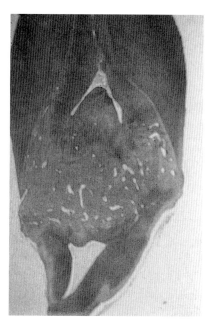

Fig. 1.43 Hard-tissue formation in the pulp of a revascularized dog tooth 180 days after replantation. The hard tissue forms as a metaplasia of the soft tissue throughout the pulpal cavity (hematoxylin-eosin).

Fig. 1.44 Replanted and revascularized tooth with typical soft tissue–containing hard tissue filling the original pulp cavity. The root end, which has formed apically to this hard tissue, consists of dentin laid down by new odontoblasts induced by a more or less intact Hertwig's root sheath (hematoxylin-eosin).

blasts in the new tissue, so dentin formation will not occur. However, if the Hertwig root sheath has remained vital at the apex of a repositioned or replanted immature tooth, induction of new odontoblasts and dentin formation may occur in this area, sometimes leading to the formation of a more or less complete root tip (**Fig.1.44**).

The hard-tissue formation in revascularized teeth will ultimately lead to a clinically and radiographically complete obliteration of the pulp chamber and root canal space (**Fig.1.45**). However, microscopic inclusions of soft tissue will always be present in the hard tissue throughout the original pulp space (**Fig.1.44**). This is of clinical importance, since preparation of such teeth for crowns will often lead to multiple microscopic pulp exposures followed by pulp necrosis and periapical inflammation.

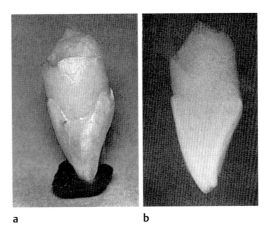

a   b

Fig. 1.45
a Revascularized tooth with pulp space filled with hard tissue.
b Radiograph of tooth in **a**, indicating complete obliteration of the pulp space. However, microscopic remnants of soft tissue are always present in the hard tissue.

Further Reading

Aas JA, Paster BJ, Stokes LN, Olsen I, Dewhirst FE. Defining the normal flora of the oral cavity. J Clin Microbiol 2005;43:5721 – 32.

Aas JA, Griffen AL, Dardis SR, Lee AM, Olsen I, Dewhirst FE, Leys EJ, Paster BJ. Bacteria of dental caries in primary and permanent teeth in children and young adults. J Clin Microbiol 2008;46:1407 – 1417.

Bishop M, Malhotra M. An investigation of lymphatic vessels in the feline dental pulp. Am J Anatomy 1990;187:247 – 253.

Brännström M, Åström A. The hydrodynamics of the dentine; its possible relationship to dentinal pain. Int Dent J 1972;22:219 – 227.

Byers MR. Dental sensory reseptors. Int Rev Neurobiol 1984;25:39 – 94.

Cahen P, Frank RM. Microscopie électronique de la pulpe dentaire humaine normale. Bull Group Int Rech Sci Stomatol 1970;13:421 – 443.

Costerton JW, Stewart PS, Greenberg EP. Bacterial biofilms: a common cause of persistent infections. Science 1999;284:1318 – 1322.

Dahl E, Mjör IA. The fine structure of the vessels in the human dental pulp. Acta Odont Scand 1973;31: 223 – 230.

Frank RM: Etude au microscope électronique de l'odontoblaste et du canalicule dentinaire humain. Arch Oral Biol 1966;11:179 – 199.

Frank RM. Ultrastructural relationship between the odontoblast, its process and the nerve fibre. In Symons NBB, ed: Dentine and Pulp: Their Structure and Reactions. London: Livingstone, 1968, pp 115 – 145.

Hahn C-L, Liewehr FR. Innate immune responses of the dental pulp to caries. J Endod 2007;33:643 – 651.

Heyeraas KJ. Blood flow and vascular pressure in the dental pulp. Acta Odont Scand 1980;38:135 – 144.

Heyeraas KJ. Pulpal hemodynamics and interstitial fluid pressure: balance of transmicrovascular fluid transport. J Endod 1989;15:468 – 472.

Heyeraas KJ, Kvinnsland I. Tissue pressure and blood flow in pulpal inflammation. Proc Finn Dent Soc 1992;88:393 – 401.

Jontell M. Immune defense mechanisms of the dental pulp. Crit Rev Oral Biol Med 1998;9:179 – 200.

Langeland K. Tissue response to dental caries. Endod Dent Traumatol 1987;3:149 – 171.

Langeland K, Dowden WE, Tronstad L, Langeland LK. Human pulp changes of iatrogenic origin. Oral Surg Oral Med Oral Pathol 1971;32:943 – 980.

Mjör IA, Tronstad L. Experimentally induced pulpitis. Oral Med Oral Surg Oral Pathol 1972;34:102 – 108.

Mjör IA, Tronstad L. The healing of experimentally induced pulpitis. Oral Med Oral Surg Oral Pathol 1974;38:115 – 121.

Mjör IA, Sveen OB, Heyeraas KJ. Pulp dentin biology in restorative dentistry. Part I: Normal structure and physiology. Quintessence Int 2001;32:427 – 446.

Skoglund A, Tronstad L, Wallenius K. A microangiographic study of replanted and autotransplanted teeth of young dogs. Oral Med Oral Surg Oral Pathol 1978;45:17 – 28.

Skoglund A, Hasselgren G, Tronstad L. Oxidoreductase activity in the pulp of replanted and autotransplanted teeth in young dogs. Oral Med Oral Surg Oral Pathol 1981;52:205–209.

Skoglund A, Tronstad L. Pulpal changes in replanted and autotransplanted immature teeth of dogs. J Endod 1982;7:309–316.

Stanley HR. The effect of systemic diseases on the human dental pulp. In Siskin M, ed: The Biology of the Human Dental pulp. St Louis: Mosby 1973.

Takehashi K, Kishi Y, Kim S. An electronmicroscopic study of the blood vessels of dog pulps using corrosion casts. J Endod 1982;8:131–135.

Tronstad L. Ultrastructural observations on human coronal dentin. Scand J Dent Res 1973;81:101–111.

Tronstad L. The anatomic and physiologic basis for dentinal sensitivity. Compend Contin Educ Dent 1982;3:99–104.

Tronstad L. Pathology and treatment of diseases of the pulp. In Loe H, Holm-Pedersen B, eds: Geriatric Dentistry. 2nd ed. Copenhagen: Munksgaard, 1996.

Tsatsas BG, Frank RM. Ultrastructure of the dentinal tubular substances near the dentino enamel junction. Calcif Tiss Res 1972;9:238–243.

2
The Apical Periodontium

Structure

The *periodontium* comprises the root cementum, the periodontal ligament, and the alveolar bone. The periodontium attaches the teeth to the bone of the jaws by a fibrous joint, providing a resilient suspensory apparatus resistant to normal functional forces. It should be regarded as an anatomical and functional unit (**Fig.1.9**). The *apical periodontium* is that part of the periodontium which surrounds the root apex.

Composition and Morphology

The cementum and bone are composed of about 65 % inorganic material, mostly in the form of hydroxyapatite. The organic matrix consists of 20 % collagen and 3 % noncollagenous proteins, whereas the remaining 12 % is water.

Cementum covers the root surfaces of the teeth. It is avascular, without innervation and does not normally undergo remodeling. Toward the periodontal ligament the cementum is covered by a zone of precementum about 5 μm wide. Bordering the surface, the cementum-forming cells, the *cementoblasts*, are seen. In the apical periodontium the cementum is cellular with cementocytes in lacunae and canaliculi.

Alveolar bone lines the sockets of the teeth. It is compact and may appear radiographically as a radiopaque narrow zone, the *lamina dura*. The alveolar bone is perforated by a large number of blood vessels, and osteocytes are embedded in lacunae and canaliculi. Toward the periodontal ligament the bone is covered by unmineralized osteoid and the bone-forming cells, the osteoblasts.

The *periodontal ligament* consists of dense, unmineralized connective tissue situated between the cementum and the alveolar bone. It is characterized primarily by a large number of collagen fiber bundles that traverse obliquely from the cementum to the alveolar bone. Apically, these fiber bundles radiate outward from the root surface to insert into the surrounding alveolar bone.

Cells, Fibers, and Ground Substance

The apical periodontium contains several cell types. The *cementoblasts* which form the cementum of the root are highly specialized cells characteristic of the periodontium. Ultrastructurally the cementoblast is similar to the osteoblast and fibroblast of the periodontium and as in the pulp the identity of the various cells is mainly determined by their location.

The major cell type of the periodontium is the *fibroblast*. The fibroblasts form the fibers and the ground substance of the periodontal ligament. In addition, the collagen fibers undergo almost continuous and rapid remodeling, i.e., formation and degradation. Both of these activities are accomplished by the fibroblasts, sometimes simultaneously. As in the pulp, undifferentiated, probably pluripotential cells are found in the periodontium. These cells are thought to be capable of differentiating into any periodontal cell and are therefore important in repair processes after injury and disease. *Mast cells*, which may constitute up to 6 % of the total cell population of the healthy periodontium, develop from the undifferentiated mesenchymal cells as well.

Macrophages are frequently seen in the healthy periodontium. They have a potential for synthesis of a wide range of proteins which influence other cells. The macrophages are present in many stages of development and show phagocytic activity when stimulated.

The *osteoblasts* form the alveolar bone. In addition, together with *osteoclasts*, which are considered normal cells of the periodontium, they are responsible for the continuous remodeling of the alveolar bone.

Also found within the periodontal ligament are *clusters of epithelial cells*. These derive from the Hertwig's root sheath which was active during tooth formation. Cell-to-cell junctions are seen between the epithelial cells, and each cluster of cells is surrounded by a basal lamina separating it from the adjacent connective tissue. In addition, the different epithelial cell clusters are connected by delicate processes, allowing them to function as a syncytium. Their primary function is not known, although it has been suggested that they are reponsible for maintaining the periodontal ligament space by preventing the osteoblasts from migrating to and forming bone on the surface of the root. It is clear that the epithelial cells are viable and metabolically active. Under certain pathological conditions they may begin to proliferate and are seen as larger islands or strings of epithelium in inflamed tissue or as the epithelial lining of radicular cysts (see p. 43).

As mentioned above, the fibers of the periodontal ligament are almost exclusively collagenous in nature. However, as in the pulp, a few elastic fibers are associated with the blood vessels. The cells and fibers of the periodontium are embedded in an amorphous *ground substance* which basically has the same consistency and function as the ground substance of the pulp and connective tissue elsewhere in the body.

Vascular Supply and Innervation
The vascular supply of the periodontal ligament is richly developed (**Fig. 1.11**). The principal supply of blood is provided by the alveolar arteries. Some branches reach the apical periodontium and course coronally, just prior to entering the pulp, whereas gingival arterioles enter the periodontal ligament and course apically. In addition, numerous vessels enter the ligament through the holes of the alveolar bone. Thus, in contrast to the pulp, the apical periodontium has a rich and well-developed collateral blood supply. A rich capillary network is present as well. It is somewhat more developed near the bone than near the root surface. The lymphatic vessels presumably follow the path of the blood vessels and pass to regional lymph nodes.

The nerves of the periodontal ligament follow the path of the blood vessels as well. Both myelinated and unmyelinated nerve fibers are present, and the sensory innervation is of the trigeminal system. The nerve endings are involved with proprioception and pain perception and they react readily to even slight increases in tissue pressure.

Age Changes
The most obvious age change in the apical periodontium is an increase in the thickness of the root cementum. This tissue is deposited continuously throughout life, and its width will triple between 10 and 70 years of age. In other respects, the remodeling of the periodontal ligament and alveolar bone is highly effective throughout life, and these components of the periodontium will be modified more according to external influence than to age. Still, a decrease in the rate of collagen synthesis will occur as well as certain changes in the ground substance. It also appears that tissue repair after inflammation of the apical periodontium in elderly patients may occur by the formation of an unmineralized fibrous tissue rather than the formation of new bone (see p. 52).

Reaction Patterns

Apical Periodontitis
The pulp and the soft tissue of the apical periodontium constitute a continuum via the apical foramina. Untreated pulpal inflammation will, therefore, gradually spread beyond the apex of the tooth. This condition is termed periradicular, periapical, or most commonly *apical periodontitis*. If the inflammation occurs on the side of the root adjacent to a lateral root canal, the term *lateral periodontitis* may be used. At first only the periodontal ligament will be involved in the periapical reaction. However, soon there will be resorption of cementum (and dentin) and alveolar bone so that all tissues of the periodontium will be affected. Thus, *apical periodontitis is a pulpally related inflammation of the attachment apparatus of the tooth*. The inflammatory process may lead to considerable bone loss, sometimes encompassing large areas of the alveolar process. Quite commonly a fistulous tract develops from the inflamed area to a body surface, in most instances to the oral vestibule.

Etiology of Apical Periodontitis
Pulpitis
A local pulpitis in the coronal pulp may occasionally cause inflammatory changes in the apical periodontium. This is recognized clinically by the fact that the tooth becomes tender to biting or percussion. As discussed above, pulpal inflamma-

tion leads to vasodilation and an increase in capillary permeability with filtration of fluids from the blood vessels into the tissue. In most instances lymphatics and blood vessels of the uninflamed areas of the pulp can deal with the increased tissue fluids and transport the fluids away. However, when periapical symptoms arise, this mechanism is apparently flawed or insufficient, and an increase in tissue pressure in the apical periodontium occurs, leading to tenderness of the tooth. Sometimes the tooth is pushed out of its alveolus so that a widened periodontal ligament space appears radiographically. When the increased tissue pressure in the pulp is relieved, either spontaneously or as a result of treatment, the periapical symptoms will disappear as well.

Pulp Necrosis

In teeth with necrotic pulps, the content of the root canal will be dead cells, stagnated tissue fluids, and tissue breakdown products. Many of these tissue components will have a cytotoxic effect and traditionally such breakdown products have been regarded as the main etiological factors for apical periodontitis. However, it is now established that as long as no nonself proteins or other foreign substances are present in the root canal, the periapical response is quite mild, and will not lead to bone resorption and the formation of an apical granuloma (**Fig. 2.1**). The reason for this is that necrotic tissue as such causes only a mild chemotactic activity in serum and has only a slight immunogenic potential. Clinically, the benign nature of the reaction is recognized by the fact that apical periodontitis is not evident radiographically as long as the necrotic tissue of the root canal is not infected with microorganisms.

Infection of the Root Canal

It has been known for a century that bacteria may colonize the root canal. The importance of bacteria as an etiological factor for pulpal and periapical inflammation as expressed in the literature has varied over the years. However, striking evidence for the role of infection came in experiments in the 1960s when it was shown that pulp necrosis and apical periodontitis would not develop in germ-free animals when the pulp was exposed to the oral cavity. In humans it has been shown that an apical periodontitis with bone resorption will develop only if the necrotic pulp becomes infected. Finally, it is known that bacteria

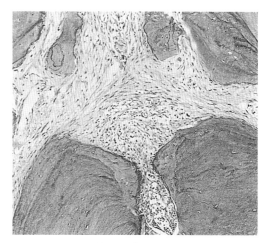

Fig. 2.1 Root tip of a monkey tooth. Pulpal inflammation has reached the apical foramen and involves a small area of the periodontal ligament (hematoxylin-eosin).

which are isolated from root canals of teeth with apical periodontitis will cause an apical periodontitis when inoculated in the root canal of other teeth. When these bacteria are reisolated, it has been shown that they in fact are the inoculated organisms and therefore have the capacity to establish themselves and survive in the root canal and exert pathological influence on periapical tissues.

If a root canal is exposed to the mouth, bacteria will accumulate in the pulp chamber and the canal. The normal plaque/saliva microflora dominated by facultative anaerobic organisms will be present in the root canal. Many strains of obligate anaerobic bacteria will be present as well, but usually in small numbers. If the root canal has a wide opening to the mouth, periapical inflammation with bone destruction will not develop in a predictable manner. However, if the access opening to the root canal is sealed off after the oral flora has been allowed to colonize the root canal system, a selective bacterial growth begins. Already after 7 days, 50% of the flora is anaerobic bacteria, and soon some 90% of the bacteria may be anaerobic. In the apical area of the root canal where the oxygen tension is lowest, the predominance of anaerobic bacteria is even greater than in the main canal. From the root canal the bacteria may enter the tubules of the root dentin (**Fig. 2.2**). One must therefore understand that the term *root canal infection*, which is commonly used, in reality

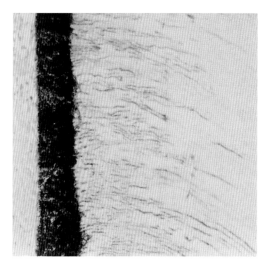

Fig. 2.2 Biofilm on root canal wall in nonvital tooth. Bacteria from the root canal have entered the underlying dentinal tubules (Brown–Brenn stain).

means infection of the root canal system with the main canal, side canals, and apical deltas, as well as infection of the root dentin.

Although it has been estimated that the oral flora consists of more than 700 different bacterial species, usually less than 10 *cultivable* species are recovered from the root canal. However, more than 50% of the oral flora is uncultivable, and only recently have molecular techniques made it possible to obtain a more accurate detection of bacteria and bacterial DNA from clinical samples. Thus, in a recent study, the root canal of 30 teeth with asymptomatic apical periodontitis was evaluated for the presence of 40 commonly occurring microorganisms in endodontic and periodontal infections using whole genomic DNA probes and DNA-DNA hybridization. The DNA of 35 bacteria was detected with a range of 5–31 species (**Table 2.1**). Five probes were negative for all root canals. For the sake of comparison, bacterial samples from the root canal of the same teeth were cultured aerobically and anaerobically and 42 microorganisms with the "normal" range of 0–6 species per canal were recovered. Clearly, there will have to be more uncultivable bacteria than were uncovered with our 40 probes. Thus, a reasonable estimate at present might be that an infected root canal contains, not less than 10, but rather between 10 and 50 bacterial species. Interestingly, this coincides well with the number of microorganisms

found in biofilms in the healthy oral cavity and subgingivally in patients with active periodontal disease.

Considering the large number of microorganisms in the oral cavity, the microbial composition of the root canal flora will have to vary. However, given the results of the molecular study mentioned above it becomes clear that the microbiota of the root canal is very similar to the microbiota of the periodontal pocket *in patients with active periodontal disease.* Thus, *Tannerella forsythia, Campylobacter showae, Fusobacterium nucleatum* ssp. *vincentii,* and *Aggregatibacter actinomycetemcomitans* were present in more than 90% of the root canals. Other designated periodontopathogens like *Porphyromonas gingivalis* (60%), *Campylobacter rectus* (80%), *Prevotella intermedia* (50%), *Selenomonas noxia* (60%), *Peptostreptococcus micros* (70%), *Treponema socranskii* (70%), and *Treponema denticola* (40%) were commonly present as well. The "red complex" bacteria *T. forsythia, P. gingivalis,* and *T. denticola,* which are known to have a decisive influence on the progression of disease in patients with active marginal periodontitis, were together present in 40% of the root canals.

Porphyromonas endodontalis, which in combination with other root canal bacteria is known to cause transmissible infection in guinea pigs, was recovered from 30% of the canals. Interestingly, combinations of the same endodontic bacteria, but without *P. endodontalis,* did not cause transmissible infection in the same experiments. Still, these and other noninfective bacteria may play an important role in maintaining the root canal infection by providing growth factors for the principal pathogens and by synthesizing and degrading extracellular materials in the biofilm.

The associations of bacteria in a mixed infection is not random. With regard to oral bacteria, this is best known from studies on dental plaque where six closely associated groups or complexes of bacterial species are recognized. The red complex mentioned above is one of the groups. An "orange" complex including *Campylobacter rectus, C. showae, Eubacterium nodatum, Fusobacterium nucleatum, P. intermedia, P. micros,* and *P. nigrescens* is important for disease progression as well. A third group includes the *Actinomyces* and a fourth group consists of *Capnocytophaga* species, *A. actinomycetemcomitans, Eikenella corrodens,* and *Campylobacter concisus.* The streptococci make up

Table 2.1 Bar chart of type and frequency of bacteria from the root canal of 30 asymptomatic, nonvital teeth as detected by DNA-DNA hybridization. The length of the bars indicates the percentage of the canals colonized

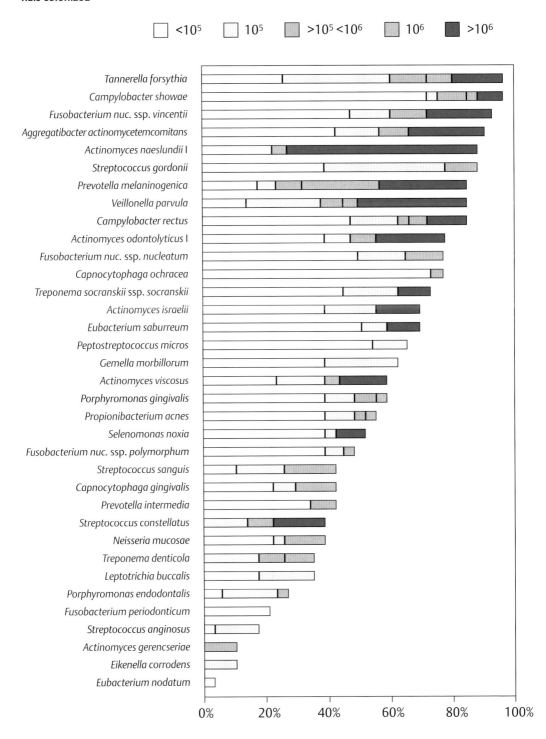

the fifth group and the sixth group comprises *Veillonella parvula* and *Actinomyces odontolyticus*.

Clearly, the root canal is different from the periodontal pocket, and at present it is not known whether the findings in plaque are totally valid in endodontic infections. However, in established root canal infections where Gram-negative species are numerically important, *Fusobacterium nucleatum* plays a dominating role. This species congregates with most oral bacteria, including strains of *P. gingivalis, T. denticola, A. actinomycetemcomitans, P. intermedia, Eubacterium* species, *Selenomonas* species, and *Actinomyces* species. The important red and orange complexes contain most of these coaggregating species.

Microorganisms are also frequently found in the root canal of root filled teeth with apical periodontitis, i.e., in root filled teeth where the treatment has failed. However, in these teeth the flora is different from the flora of untreated nonvital teeth in that it is heavily dominated by facultative anaerobic species. Enterococci, streptococci, and staphylococci are frequently isolated organisms under these conditions. Clinically, this is important in that a different antimicrobial regime might be called for in the retreatment of the failed cases than would normally be used in primary treatment of root canal infections.

Portal of Entry of Bacteria

The *crown of the tooth* is the main portal of entry for bacteria into the pulp and root canal space. This is readily understood in teeth with pulp exposures or in teeth with carious lesions. At first it may be somewhat more difficult to see how the bacteria can reach the pulp through an intact crown. However, in reality there is rarely such a thing as an "intact" crown. Teeth have dentin exposed by attrition or abrasion, or by scaling and root planing during prophylaxis and treatment of periodontal disease. Enamel–dentin cracks filled with plaque and bacteria are commonly present in teeth. They are almost bound to run at an angle with the dentinal tubules so that a single crack may lead to exposure of a large number of tubules (**Fig.1.30**).

Another possible pathway of infection of the necrotic pulp and root canal space is the apical foramina and accessory canals through a hematogenous spreading of the bacteria. However, the evidence for this is presently inconclusive. Still, it is known that oral bacteria that readily enter the bloodstream following dental treatment and prophylactic measures may settle down at sites where there is tissue damage, conceivably also in necrotic tissue of the root canal. The fact that the bacteria isolated from the root canal are also found in the periodontal pocket has been regarded as a strong indication that a hematogenous spreading of bacteria to the root canal indeed occurs. However, exposed dentin is especially prevalent in the cervical area of the teeth adjacent to the periodontal pocket, and infection of the pulp by periodontal bacteria via a direct route through the dentinal tubules seems entirely possible (**Fig.2.2**).

Infection of the Periapical Lesion

Traditionally it has been held that in teeth with asymptomatic apical periodontitis the microorganisms are in biofilms in the root canal system and in tubules of the root dentin, whereas the periapical lesion is free of bacteria. Probably, the defense systems mobilized by periapical inflammation at first will eliminate the bacteria from the root canal that invade the periapex. However, in long-standing infections with a more or less permanently established microflora in the root canal, the host defenses are less effective, and microbial invasion of the periapical lesion may take place.The evidence for this comes from studies of surgically removed periapical lesions using traditional culturing as well as molecular microbiological techniques.

Of interest in this regard are also recent findings suggesting the involvement of herpes viruses in the etiopathogenesis of apical periodontitis. The viruses may cause the release of tissue-destructive cytokines and the initiation of cytotoxic and immunopathologic events. The immune impairment and tissue changes resulting from the virus infection may then aid bacteria in invading and surviving in the periapical lesion.

As in the root canal the infection of the periapical lesion is characterized by a wide variety of combinations of bacteria. Some 20–30 bacterial species are recovered from a granuloma and about half to two thirds are anaerobes (**Table 2.2**). As in the root canal *Fusobacterium, Porphyromonas, Prevotella, Campylobacter*, and *Treponema* species are commonly isolated. In one study, the "red complex" bacteria *Tannerella forsythia, Porphyromonas gingivalis*, and *Treponema denticola* were present in 70% of the lesions and *Porphyromonas* *endodontalis* was present in 50%. Of Gram-positive anaerobes, *Actinomyces, Propionibacterium, Peptostreptococcus*, and *Eubacterium* species are frequently present. In addition, facultative *Actinomyces, Streptococcus, Enterococcus*, and *Staphylococcus* species are recovered.

Recently, a fluorescence in-situ hybridization method has been developed whereby bacteria may be observed and even identified in the tissue of their natural environment. With this technique it has been possible to visualize bacteria directly within periapical lesions of asymptomatic root-filled teeth (**Fig. 2.3**). The bacteria were present in localized areas of the lesions, whereas other areas were free of bacteria. A variety of bacterial morphotypes were seen: cocci, rods, spiral- and spindle-shaped. Organisms with different morphologies were seen to coaggregate forming small ecosystems, possibly biofilm in the tissue. In some areas looser groups of bacteria were present, and single organisms, especially spirochete-like bacteria were seen spread out among fibers and cells. Motility and chemotaxis are major virulence factors of these organisms and they are highly invasive in host tissue. Oral treponemes have been shown to carry several putative virulence factors identical or similar to invasive organisms such as *Treponema pallidum*, the causative organism of syphilis. Probably the importance of treponemes in endodontic infections is highly underestimated.

In periapical lesions *refractory to endodontic therapy*, the periapical flora is highly dominated (80%) by Gram-positive organisms and is clearly different from the root canal flora that normally responds to treatment. In one study, 75% of the refractory lesions contained *Streptococcus, Staphylococcus, Bacillus, Pseudomonas, Stenotrophomonas, Sphingomonas, Enterococcus, Enterobacter, or Candida* species, and typically the organisms persisted in five of eight patients who had taken antibiotics systemically before sampling. Several of these microorganisms have adapted over time to live in many different environments. They may be surrounded by extracellular materials in a biofilm-like structure (**Fig. 6.15**), or the bacterial aggregates may have the form of biofilm granules with diameters up to 3–4 mm (**Fig. 2.4**). These granules often have a bright, yellow color, and because of this in older literature are referred to as *sulfur granules*. One or more *Actinomyces* species is as a rule recognized in the granules, but in addition a wide spectrum of other bacteria like *Propionibac-*

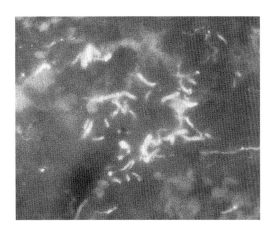

Fig. 2.3 Section from periapical endodontic lesion. Clinical diagnosis: Asymptomatic apical periodontitis. A probe specific for the domain *Bacteria*, EUB 338, has been used to visualize the bacteria in the granulation tissue.

terium, Staphylococcus, Peptostreptococcus, Pseudomonas, and *Treponema* species are recovered from the granules. Most of the organisms in the biofilm granules are simultaneously present in the periapical lesions.

In cases where the endodontic treatment has been incorrect or grossly inadequate, for instance, after repeated but inadequate antibiotic treatment, often in conjunction with multiple openings and closings of the root canal or incorrect and unsuccessful periapical surgical treatment, the presence of enteric and environmental bacteria and yeast is especially conspicuous. In such instances organisms like *Escherichia coli, Bacteroides fragilis, Pseudomonas aeruginosa, Enterobacter, Clostridium, Proteus*, and *Klebsiella* species and yeast are recovered. The presence of these and other mainly nonoral microorganisms suggest that blood-born infection of the periapical lesion may have taken place.

As appears from the above, endodontic infections are polymicrobial in nature and, interestingly, the flora is very similar to the flora of the periodontal pocket in patients with active periodontal disease. The red and orange complexes of bacteria regarded as important for the progression of periodontal disease apparently are important pathogens also in endodontic infections. No single pathogen of special importance has been identified. Still, the role of *Actinomyces* needs to be discussed. Traditionally, *Actinomyces* species, especially *A. israelii*, have been regarded as specific

Table 2.2 Bar chart of type and frequency of bacteria as detected with DNA-DNA hybridization in 17 periapical lesions of asymptomatic teeth following submarginal incision and sampling from the lesions. The length of the bars indicates the percentage of lesions colonized

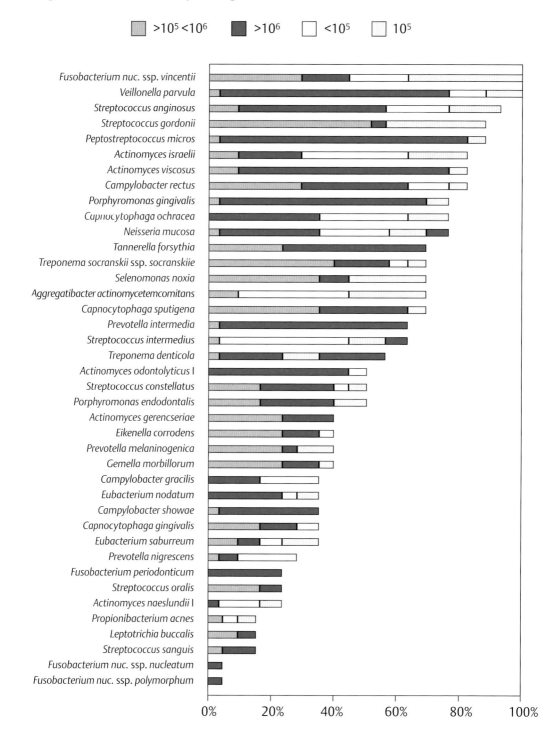

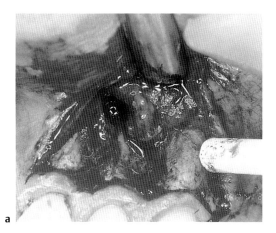

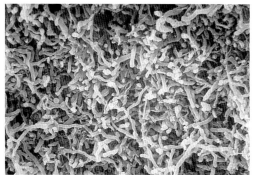

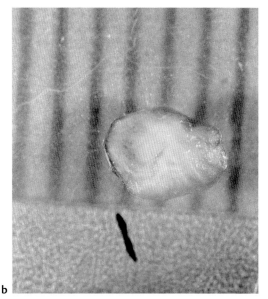

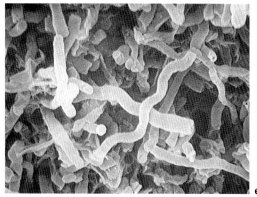

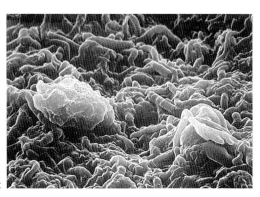

Fig. 2.4

a Surgical treatment of refractory apical periodontitis.

b Three granules of diameters between 2 and 4 mm of a bright yellow color (so-called sulfur granules) are recovered from the periapical lesion.

c Scanning electron micrograph of surface area of sulfur granule seen in **b.** Microorganisms that are tightly packed and glued together make up the outer boundary of the granule. Two macrophages are seen engulfing bacteria.

d Cut surface of granule showing an abundance of bacteria. Rod-like organisms are prominent and spiral-formed bacteria can be seen.

e From cut surface of granule. In addition to spiral-formed and rod-like bacteria, an amorphous material can be seen.

pathogens causing the infectious disease Actinomycosis in a similar manner to *Treponema pallidum* causing syphilis and *Mycobacterium tuberculosis* causing tuberculosis. This may be incorrect. In periodontal research it has been shown that *Actinomyces* are important colonizers and scaffold builders in dental plaque both in health and disease, but also that there is a significant decrease in the *Actinomyces* species and an increase in the proportion of members of the red and orange complexes in patients with active periodontal disease. In the biofilm granules observed in periapical lesions, *Actinomyces* species are never isolated as the sole organism, but with other known pathogens normally found in endodontic and periodontal infections. Thus, so-called actinomycotic infections appear to be polymicrobial in nature. It is well established that *Actinomyces* may survive under harsh conditions and that they have special surface structures enabling them to attach to a variety of surfaces. Thus, their role may well be to create such conditions that other bacteria (the real pathogens) are attracted to the site and may establish themselves there.

Iatrogenic Factors

Periapical inflammation may be caused by iatrogenic factors, i.e., instruments, medicaments, and materials used in endodontic treatment. However, bacteria may be present in the root canal or may be introduced inadvertently during endodontic treatment, and there is little doubt that many clinical reactions that in the past have been ascribed to iatrogenic factors are in fact due to infection.

Still it is clear that when a pulp is extirpated, a *soft-tissue* wound is created near the apical foramen of the tooth. The wound, which represents tissue injury, will cause an inflammatory response as the first phase of tissue repair. If no further irritants are present, repair will occur in 3–4 weeks. The severity of the tissue response to instrumentation will depend on the degree of tissue injury, and vigorous over-instrumentation with laceration and removal of periapical tissue may cause an acute apical periodontitis, sometimes with slight bone resorption so that a periapical radiolucency may be seen. However, in the absence of bacteria, repair will occur uneventfully. *In the presence of bacteria, on the other hand, over-instrumentation is an effective way to spread the infection.* The contaminated endodontic instruments will cause puncture wounds in the periapi-

cal tissues, and the bacteria readily survive and multiply in the damaged and dead tissue. Under such conditions over-instrumentation may lead to proliferation of epithelial cells in the periodontal ligament and possibly to apical cyst formation.

Antiseptics are used in the root canal for irrigation during instrumentation and as intracanal medicaments to obtain a bacteria-free canal. By definition these medicaments have an antibacterial effect, but they also have a toxic effect on human cells. All the antiseptics used in endodontics, especially phenolic and aldehyde compounds, are potent tissue irritants (**Fig. 2.5**). Thus, the intracanal medicaments may cause periapical cell death. Clinically, this is recognized as exudation from the periapex into the root canal. Sometimes it may be difficult to distinguish between exudate from an infectious and a chemical inflammation. However, if no bacteria are present, discontinuation in the use of the cytotoxic medicament will result in rapid repair.

Possibly all root canal sealers which are used today have a certain tissue-irritating effect, especially in the freshly mixed state. However, if a sealer is confined to the root canal space, the tissue–material interface is small and the inflammatory reaction in the contacting tissue will be mild. After a few weeks when the setting reaction of the materials is completed, the materials generally have no further biological effect, and in the absence of bacteria, tissue repair will occur. If the root canal is overfilled so that material is forced into the periapical tissues, the tissue–material interface is larger and the tissue irritation more severe. Also, when a material is forced into a tissue, it will have a rough, uneven surface that will cause tissue irritation and inflammation mechanically. Thus, a radiolucent zone may develop surrounding a material in the periapical tissues. Macrophages will be activated and gradually the uneven surface of the material will become smooth. A fibrous capsule will then form around the material and the repair process is completed. However, depending on the type and consistency of the material, it may also be completely removed, either by phagocytes, by dissolution in the tissue fluids, or by both.

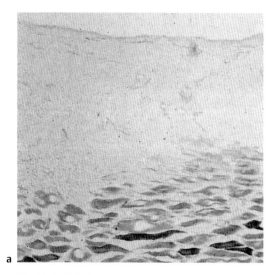

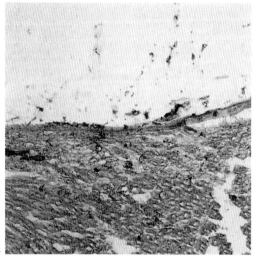

Fig. 2.5
a **Nonepithelialized tissue exposed to 10 % formalin for 15 min incubated for the demonstration of succinate dehydrogenase.** No oxidative enzyme activity is evident in the surface area of the affected tissue, demonstrating the cytotoxic effect of formalin.
b Control section not exposed to formalin showing oxidative enzyme activity to the surface.

Pathogenesis of Apical Periodontitis
Action of Bacteria

Apical periodontitis may be acute and symptomatic or chronic and asymptomatic. A chronic course of development is by far the most com-

mon, and periapical inflammation is of an insidious character where near-balanced conditions exist between the defense mechanisms of the body and the bacteria causing the inflammation. *The unique feature to be handled by the host defense in this situation is that the bacteria situated in biofilms in the root canal and the root dentin are protected by the tooth from the cells of the periapical tissues.* The bacteria will survive and multiply inside the tooth practically unaffected by the inflammation and immune response they cause in the tissues outside the tooth. This explains why bacteria of generally low-grade virulence may induce and sustain an apical periodontitis. Morever, the periapical tissue response will be similar to the response elsewhere in the body when bacteria are able to survive the body's defense reactions, and a *granuloma* will develop.

The role of the various endodontic bacteria in the pathogenesis of periapical granulomas is extremely complex and far from understood. Some bacteria may have a direct toxic effect on the tissues through proteolytic enzymes, cytotoxins, and hemolysins. A good example is the *leukotoxin produced by Aggregatibacter actinomycetemcomitans.* This leukotoxin is very potent and kills neutrophilic leukocytes and monocytes, including macrophages, and suppresses lymphocytes. It may effectively compromise a tissue's ability to eliminate or control invading bacteria or bacterial products. *A. actinomycetemcomitans* also produces collagenase, strong alkaline and acid phosphatases, a fibroblast-inhibiting factor, a potent lipopolysaccharide, and an additional bone resorption–inducing toxin.

Porphyromonas gingivalis and to a varying degree other *Porphyromonas* and *Prevotella* species also have known tissue-toxic properties. They produce proteases, alkaline and acid phosphatases, and other enzymes that may initiate bone resorption, a fibroblast-inhibiting factor, and toxic substances like volatile sulfur compounds and others. *Capnocytophaga* species have strong aminopeptidase activity, produce a trypsin-like enzyme, strong alkaline, and acid phosphatases which may act on alveolar bone, and a fibroblast-inhibiting factor. A fibroblast-inhibiting factor is also produced by *Fusobacterium nucleatum.* With the exception of *A. actinomycetemcomitans* endodontopathic bacteria have endotoxins that are only weakly toxic and propably without an appreciable direct cytotoxic effect.

When bacterial enzymes and toxins cause cell death, breakdown products that attract phagocytes will be released. However, much more important in the pathogenesis of apical periodontitis are *bacterial antigens,* which are not necessarily toxic, but which react with lymphocytes and macrophages to cause an activation of the immune system. Intact bacteria are highly antigenic, as are soluble bacterial components including cell-wall structures, lipopolysaccharides, and toxins, and may cause specific immune responses by the host. Specific responses are characterized by the activation of T and B lymphocytes that bear antigen-binding receptors for the bacterial antigens. Examples of such responses are proliferation of and mediator production by T lymphocytes, T cell regulated microphage activation, and antibody production by B lymphocytes.

In addition, nonspecific responses contribute to the pathogenicity of apical periodontitis. For example, lipopolysaccharide can activate B lymphocytes to proliferate and secrete antibodies of diverse specificity. Moreover, lipopolysaccharide is a potent stimulator of macrophages, inducing them to produce several bone-resorptive mediators. Neutrophilic leukocytes are attracted to sites of infection by a number of bacteria-driven chemoattractants and also undergo migration in response to complement components which are generated following complement acivation by antigen–antibody complexes. Antigen–antibody complexes placed within the root canal have been shown to induce bone resorption, probably via a neutrophilic leukocyte-mediated mechanism. However, the host defense is rather effective. This is convincingly demonstrated by the fact that a periapical granuloma in most instances progresses at a slow pace and effectively prevents the spread of the infection outside the periapical area.

Periapical Granuloma

The granulomas may be divided according to the causal agent into *infective granulomas and foreign body granulomas.* It is not known whether foreign bodies, for instance, root filling materials in the periodontal ligament, may cause a granulomatous inflammation, and for all practical purposes the periapical granuloma may be regarded as an infective granuloma due to bacteria.

Thus, apical periodontitis is characterized by the formation of granulation tissue at the apex of the tooth (**Fig.2.6**). A normally well-developed capsule consisting of collagenous fibers forms around the granulation tissue and attaches to the root surface. If the tooth is extracted, the entire granuloma may accompany the tooth as a hat-shaped formation over the apex (**Fig.2.7**). It is important to understand that the apical granuloma is not primarily a bony lesion (oste-itis), but an inflammatory reaction of the attachment apparatus of the tooth comprising both the root cementum (and root dentin), the periodontal ligament, and the alveolar bone. Thus, as the size of the granuloma slowly increases, resorption of the bone, and to a lesser degree of the root end, occurs.

Clearly, bacteria are the etiological agents of periapical granuloma formation and, clearly, bone resorption is an active process carried out by osteoclasts. However, the intermediate pathways linking the infection with the resorption are poorly understood. Bacterial components, especially lipopolysaccharides, can themselves stimulate osteoclastic resorption, but are of relatively

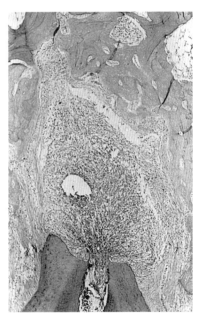

Fig. 2.6 Monkey tooth with a periapical granuloma. The periapical granuloma is an inflammatory reaction of the attachment apparatus of the tooth comprising root cementum and root dentin, the periodontal ligament, and the alveolar bone. It is surrounded by a fibrous capsule and there is no inflammation in the bone outside this capsule (hematoxylin-eosin).

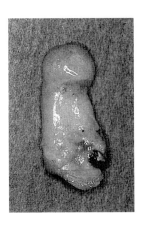

Fig. 2.7 Extracted tooth with a periapical granuloma. Note the shiny surface of the granuloma due to the surrounding fibrous capsule.

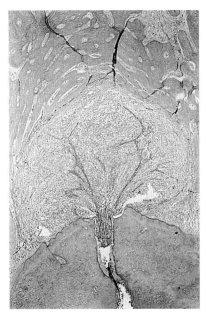

Fig. 2.8 Monkey tooth with a periapical granuloma containing strings of epithelium in all likelihood because of proliferation of epithelial rests of Malassez (hematoxylin-eosin).

low potency. Products of arachidonic acid metabolism, most notably prostaglandin E_2, have also been implicated in the process of inflammatory resorption. The chronic inflammatory cells present in large numbers in periapical granulomas produce several highly potent cytokines that cause bone resorption. These include macrophage-derived interleukin-1 and tumor necrosis factor, and the lymphocyte product lymphotoxin.

Histologically, the established granuloma consists of about 50% fibroblasts, endothelial cells, and capillaries, and 50% inflammatory cells. The dominating inflammatory cells are macrophages, followed by T and B lymphocytes, plasma cells, and neutrophilic leukocytes. These cells can potentially mediate the entire spectrum of immunological phenomena, including, delayed-type hypersensitivity, and immune complex reactivity (IgM, IgG). Of the lymphocytes present, T cells are generally more numerous than B cells, indicating an ongoing, specifically antibacterial reactivity. T helper and T suppressor cells are represented in approximately equal numbers in chronic lesions. However, in actively developing lesions, T helper cells (CD4+) outnumber the T suppressor cells (CD8+), whereas T suppressor cells predominate when the lesion size stabilizes. This suggests that T helper cells play a key role in the development of an apical granuloma, whereas T suppressor cells may dampen excessive immune reactivity, leading to cessation of lesion growth. T helper cells possess several mechanisms by which they can mediate bone lysis. Besides stimulating B cells to produce antibodies, they produce the resorptive cytokine lymphotoxin, a macrophage migration-inhibiting factor, and interferon-γ, which together

attract and activate macrophages. Activated macrophages in turn elaborate the bone-resorptive cytokines interleukin-1 and tumor necrosis factor, as well as prostaglandin E_2.

Sometimes Malassez epithelial rests will proliferate in the granulation tissue, forming islands and strings of epithelium throughout the granuloma (**Fig. 2.8**).

Periapical Cyst
By definition a cyst is a liquid-containing, epithelium-lined cavity. In some instances a cyst develops from within a periapical granuloma (**Fig. 2.9**). These cysts are termed *apical, periapical, or radicular cysts* and are characterized by the fact that they are always and without exception attached to the root of the tooth in the same way as the granuloma. If the irritants in the root canal are persistent and strong enough, the granulation tissue of a granuloma may break down and become necrotic. This tissue breakdown will occur most often adjacent to the apical foramen where the irritants enter the tissue. As was discussed above, the cells of the epithelial rests of Malassez are often known to proliferate in periapical granulo-

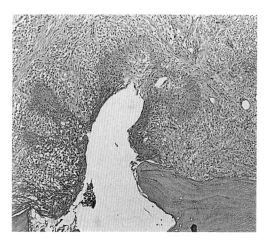

Fig. 2.9 Monkey tooth with a small cyst within a periapical granuloma. Note that the cyst has formed adjacent to the apical foramen. The epithelial lining of the cyst cavity should be regarded as a defense measure on behalf of the body (hematoxylin-eosin).

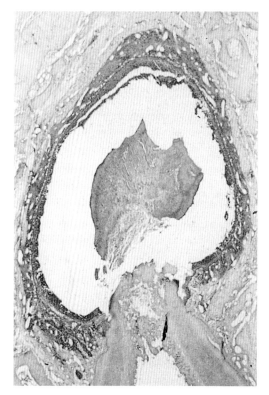

Fig. 2.10 Large periapical cyst where the epithelial lining of the cyst cavity is brought in close contact with the fibrous capsule of the granuloma (hematoxylin-eosin).

mas. When granulation tissue necrotizes, the proliferation of epithelium occurs rather predictably in the tissue bordering the necrotic area. Gradually, a fairly complete epithelial lining is formed, the necrotic tissue liquefies, and a cyst cavity has developed inside the granuloma (**Fig. 2.9**).

The proliferation of the epithelium and the formation of the epithelial cyst lining should be regarded as a defense measure on behalf of the body, similar to what occurs in periodontal disease when a deepened periodontal pocket is lined by epithelium. At first the cyst cavity encompasses only a small area of the granuloma adjacent to the apical foramen. However, the epithelial lining is now the first line of defense, so that gradually and with continuing tissue irritation the cyst cavity will increase in size until the epithelial lining is brought in close proximity with the fibrous capsule of the granuloma (**Fig. 2.10**). The entire lesion may then continue to develop and increase in size and it may reach impressive dimensions, sometimes filling the larger part of a quadrant of the maxilla or the mandible (**Fig. 2.11**).

Similar to the granuloma, the development of the periapical cyst appears to be mediated by immunological reactions. This is suggested by the observation of immunocompetent cells in the proliferating epithelial layer and the presence of immunoglobulins in the cyst fluid. Many studies have been performed to determine the frequency of cyst formation in periapical granulomas and figures between 6% and 43% have been reported. However, none of these studies is conclusive. Still, it might appear that a frequency of 6% is reasonably close to the factual situation.

Lateral Periodontitis and Furcation Lesions
As is known, accessory root canals occasionally reach the periodontal ligament laterally on the root surface or in the furcation area of multirooted teeth (**Figs. 2.12, 2.13**). Granulomatous lesions may then develop adjacent to these canals in the same manner as discussed for the apical granuloma. Because of their location in the periodontium, the lateral and interradicular lesions sometimes may be difficult to differentiate from periodontal disease or from endo–perio lesions.

Endo–Perio Lesions
An "endo–perio" lesion may be defined as a combined lesion that must be treated both endodontically and periodontally in order to heal.

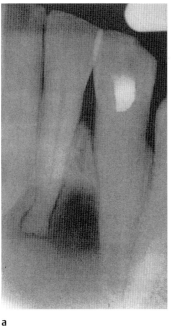
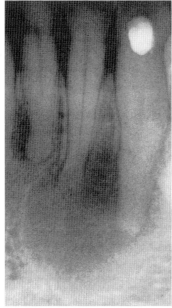
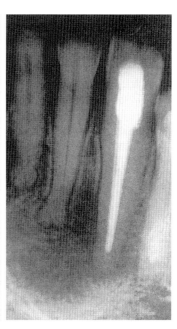

a   b   c

Fig. 2.11
a Radiograph of a large periapical radiolucent lesion from a mandibular canine. Large quantities of a clear exudate possibly indicate a cystic lesion.

b After 6 months of calcium hydroxide treatment (see Chapter 6), the lesion has filled in nicely with new bone. **c** Postoperative radiograph with root canal filling.

Etiologically, an endo–perio lesion may develop from an endodontic lesion as well as from periodontal disease. In the first instance, the lesion is usually caused by a long-standing fistula to the sulcular area of the tooth that destroys the attachment of the periodontium to the root surface so that a periodontal pocket lined with epithelium develops (**Fig. 2.14**). Endodontic treatment of the tooth is of course necessary, but the lesion as it now has developed will not fully respond to this treatment. Periodontal treatment is required as well and, if successful, the lesion will heal with an epithelial attachment to the root surface.

In the second instance, the endo–perio lesion is due to periodontal disease with pocket formation all the way to the foraminal areas of the root so that a retrograde pulpitis develops (**Fig. 2.15**). In this situation as well, both endodontic and periodontal treatment is necessary and the success of the treatment will usually depend on the effectiveness of the periodontal treatment and on whether or not an epithelial attachment to the root surface can be established.

In addition to the combined lesions, *lesions that have the clinical and/or radiographic appearance of a combined lesion are often referred to as endo–perio lesions.* A typical example of such a situation is an endodontic lesion with a fistula along the root that has led to radiographically visible bone resorption, giving the appearance of marginal breakdown (**Fig. 2.16**). However, it takes considerable time before a fistula that ends in the sulcular area has caused denudation of the root

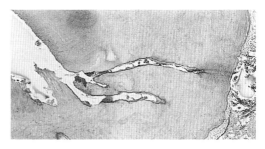

Fig. 2.12 Monkey tooth with lateral root canal and lateral periodontitis (hematoxylin-eosin).

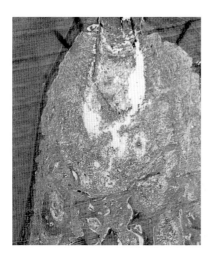

Fig. 2.13 Dog tooth with interradicular periodontitis (furcation lesion; hematoxylin-eosin).

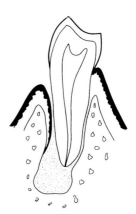

Fig. 2.14 Diagram illustrating a tooth with apical periodontitis and a long-standing fistula to the sulcular area. The fistula has led to exposure of the root surface and the formation of a periodontal pocket. Both endodontic and periodontal treatment are necessary, and the lateral lesion can only heal with an epithelial attachment to the root surface.

surface and pocket formation (**Fig. 2.17**). As long as the cementum is protected by a layer of healthy periodontal tissue, however thin, the lesion, including the lateral and marginal components, will heal completely following endodontic treatment (**Figs. 2.16**, **2.17**). *Periodontal treatment in this situation should not be initiated since scaling will result in removal of the delicate healthy tissue on the root surface and a periodontal pocket will form. Repair can then only occur with an epithelial attachment.* Similarly, periodontal disease may sometimes give the appearance of an endo–perio lesion with combined marginal and periapical loss of bone (**Fig. 2.18**). A positive sensitivity response from the tooth then suggests that there is no endodontic component of the lesion, and *endodontic treatment should not be initiated and would not contribute to the healing of the lesion.*

Condensing Apical Periodontitis

Areas with increased radiopacity are often seen in the bone at the apex of the teeth (osteoclerosis, **Fig. 2.19**). Occasionally the sclerosis is pulpally related and is then referred to as *condensing apical periodontitis* (**Fig. 2.20**). A periapical granuloma is mainly a productive lesion. This aspect of periapical inflammation appears to be enhanced in instances with condensing apical periodontitis when irregular masses of bone trabeculae with few and small marrow spaces as well as fibrous

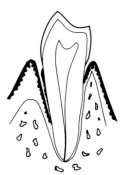
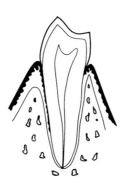

Fig. 2.15 Diagram illustrating a tooth with a periodontal pocket to foraminal areas of the root. If a retrograde pulpitis develops, endodontic treatment will be necessary. The lateral lesion may heal with an epithelial attachment following periodontal treatment.

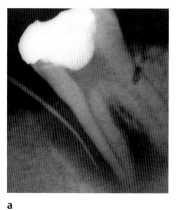
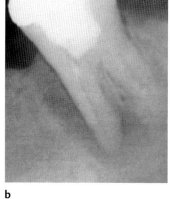
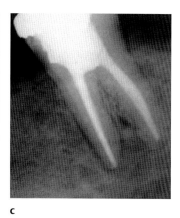

a   b   c

Fig. 2.16
a Radiograph of a mandibular molar with apical, lateral, and interradicular radiolucency. The tooth was loose and scheduled for extraction. However, after renewed examination it was concluded that the radiolucency along the mesial root

might be an endodontic fistula, and endodontic treatment was begun.
b Radiograph after 2 months with calcium hydroxide in the root canals. The tooth is clinically firm and the radiolucency is dramatically reduced. **c** Radiograph at 20-month control showing complete healing.

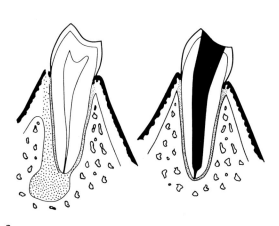
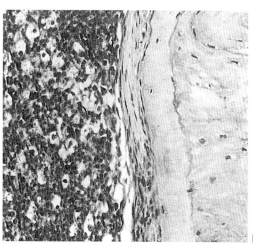

a   b

Fig. 2.17
a Diagram illustrating a tooth with apical periodontitis and a fistula alongside the root, where the root surface is still covered by healthy periodontal tissue (left). In this instance, complete healing with reestablishment of a normal periodontium will follow endodontic treatment (right).

b Area from the root of a monkey tooth with a fistula alongside the root. Note that healthy periodontal tissue comprising a few cell layers protects the root surface from the pus (hematoxylin-eosin).

tissue are seen in the granulation tissue. The process appears to be a reaction to a long-standing, low-grade irritation since the periapical radiopacity may appear before the pulp is totally necrotic.

However, complete breakdown of the pulp will soon follow. When the irritants are removed, the radiographic density of the involved bone often returns partially or fully to normal (**Fig. 2.20**).

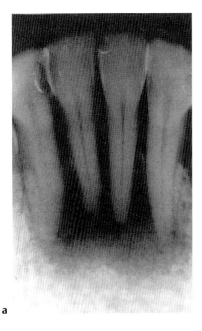
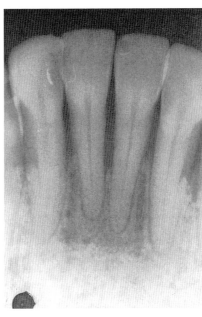

a

b

Fig. 2.18
a **Radiograph of mandibular incisors with a large, apparent periapical lesion.** The teeth give a positive sensitivity response.
b Radiograph following periodontal treatment shows complete healing.

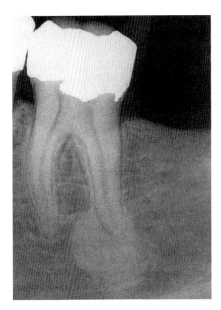

Fig. 2.19 Radiograph of a mandibular molar with periapical osteosclerosis at the distal root. The sclerotic lesion is not endodontically related. The pulp is vital and a normal periodontal ligament space is seen at the apex of the distal root.

Symptomatic Apical Periodontitis

Apical periodontitis may start out with an acute episode. In these instances there is no radiographic evidence of inflammation or periapical bone resorption, and the diagnosis is based solely on clinical signs and symptoms such as *pain, negative sensitivity, and always tenderness to percussion.* However, in by far the most instances, a symptomatic apical periodontitis is *an exacerbation of an already existing chronic inflammation.* The symptoms are the same, primarily pain and tenderness to percussion, but *in these instances the diagnosis of apical periodontitis can be verified radiographically.*

The reason for the symptoms is a quantitative and/or qualitative increase in the toxicity and especially the antigenicity of the irritants reaching the periodontium, or a decrease in the resistance of the patient, or both. Basically what this means is that bacteria from the root canal must have the ability to enter and invade the periapex, and they have to be in sufficient numbers and have the capacity to overwhelm the local host defenses. The presence of *Porphyromonas* and *Prevotella* species and certain other bacteria in the root canal may be important in this regard. Iatrogenic factors are extremely important, in that infected material as well as live bacteria from the canal may be brought into the periapex during root canal instrumentation. Overinstrumentation and overfill-

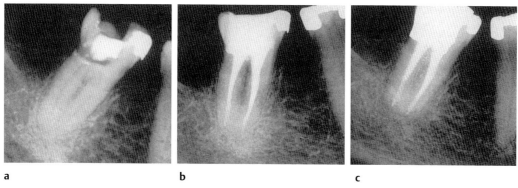

a   b   c

Fig. 2.20
a Radiograph of a nonvital tooth with condensing apical periodontitis.

b Tooth is treated endodontically.
c Follow-up radiograph after 1 year. The periapical area has regained its normal radiographic density.

ing of the root canal may lead to tissue damage and release of inflammatory mediators even in the abscence of bacteria. In addition, in sensitized patients, an acute antigen–antibody complex reaction may be caused by medicaments and materials. This is well known from clinical endodontics when, for instance, iodine compounds have been used as intracanal medicaments in patients who proved to be allergic to iodine. Acute reactions have also been observed after root canal filling with certain materials.

During the symptomatic phase of periapical inflammation, the cell picture is dominated by neu-

trophilic leukocytes. Proteolytic enzymes from these and other cells cause tissue breakdown. This results in accumulation of pus, abscess formation, and an increase in tissue pressure in the area. Inflammatory mediators released during the suppuration process initiate bone resorption and the resorptive process will advance, usually in the direction of least resistance. An especially painful period is experienced if the pus breaks through the bone and is situated underneath the periosteum. Gradually, the periosteum will also be broken through so that the abscess assumes a submucosal or subcutaneous position (**Fig. 2.21**). The

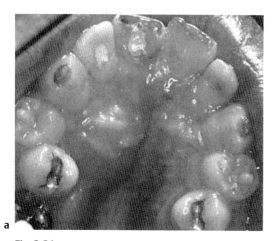

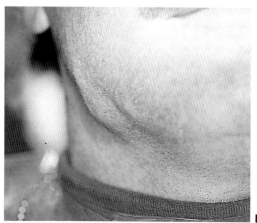

a   b

Fig. 2.21
a Submucosal palatal abscess from a nonvital right maxillary central incisor.
b Subcutanous abscess from a mandibular first molar

with apical periodontitis. The flora of the periapical lesion and of the pus from the abscess was dominated by *Actinomyces* species (Periapical actinomycosis).

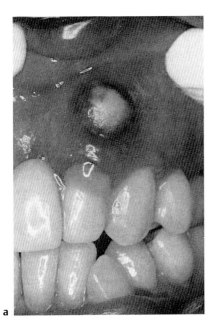

a

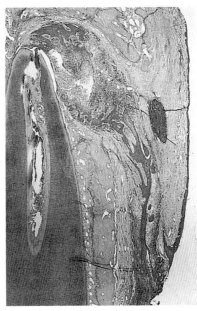

b

Fig. 2.22
a **Pus from an abscess in the oral vestibule** spontaneously breaking through in the sulcular area of the lateral incisor.
b Nonvital monkey tooth with an epithelialized fistula to the oral vestibule.

pressure is now greatly relieved and the pain usually subsides although the swelling may be considerable. Eventually the pus usually breaks through to a surface (**Fig. 2.22**).

The direction of the breakthrough of the abscess is generally determined by the shortest route, but is influenced by the anatomy of the area. Most commonly the drainage will occur in the oral vestibule (**Fig. 2.23**). In the maxilla, palatal drainage may occur from the lateral incisors and from the palatal roots of the molars. Moreover, abscesses from maxillary teeth may empty into the sinus and the nose. A spread to the brain is also possible, and it has been claimed that about 10% of brain abscesses which are diagnosed are of dental origin.

Fistula

The passage or tract leading from an abscess to a body surface is called a fistula. As discussed above, a fistula often forms as a result of an acute episode or an exacerbation of an apical periodontitis. However, it should be emphasized that a fistula forms just as readily without symptoms and is often diagnosed in the dentist's chair without the patient having noticed it. When pus has drained, the orifice of the fistula may close and epithelialize only to open up again when pressure builds up periapically. This may occur without symptoms as well and without the patient's

knowledge. In many instances the fistulous tract becomes epithelialized (**Fig. 2.22**). If the periapical inflammation responds to treatment, the fistula will heal and the epithelium disintegrate. Only a slight scar may remain on the mucosa or the skin where the opening was.

As appears from the above, the opening of the fistula is usually located on the mucosa adjacent to the tooth from which it originates. However, occasionally the fistula may end quite far from the diseased tooth. Diagnostic mistakes may then be made, often leading to irreversible treatment of a healthy tooth (**Fig. 2.25**). *A fistula should, therefore, always be traced with a radiopaque object, for instance, a gutta-percha point, to determine the tooth of origin radiographically.*

Bacteremia

Bacteria may be translocated to the bloodstream during endodontic treatment of infected teeth. If the instrumentation of the root canal ends inside the apical foramen, the frequency of bacteremia appears to be less than if the root canal is over-instrumented. Thus, in one study 31% of the patients where the instrumentation ended 1 mm short of the apical foramen yielded cultivable bacteria in the blood; 54% of the patients had bacteria in their blood when the instruments were introduced beyond the apical foramen.

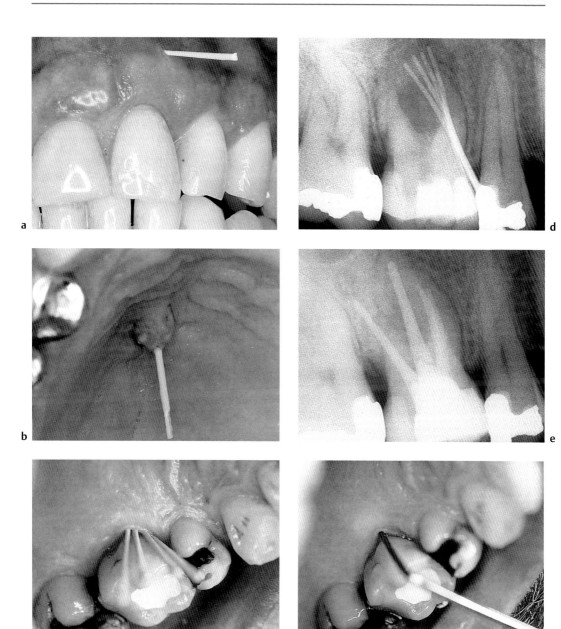

Fig. 2.23
a **Fistula in oral vestibule.**
b Palatal fistula.
c Four gutta-percha points in periodontal defect.
d Radiograph of points reaching to the apex of tooth with apical radiolucency. Question: Is periodontal defect due to endodontic fistula alongside the root or periodontal pocket to the apex? Tooth is nonvital, therefore endodontic treatment first.
e Radiograph showing periapical healing following endodontic treatment.
f Probing depth normal. Periodontal defect has healed following endodontic treatment Buccal drainage of an abscess is most common in the mandible as well. However, lingual drainage from premolars and molars occurs usually under the mylohyoid muscle. Lingual drainage is a serious condition, and cooperation with a specialist should be considered as these abscesses may continue to spread into the throat, resulting in life-threatening complications. Abscesses may also break through extraorally, most often on the chin or beneath the mandible (**Fig. 2.24**).

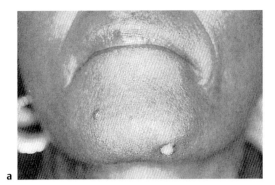

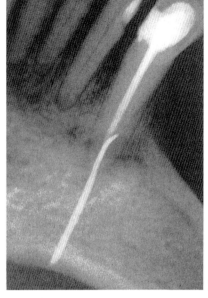

Fig. 2.24
a Extraoral fistula on patient's chin.
b By means of a gutta-percha point, the fistula is traced radiographically to an endodontically treated canine.

The microorganisms that gain entrance to the blood circulate throughout the body, but are usually eliminated by the reticuloendothelial system within minutes (transient bacteremia). As a rule a transient bacteremia leads to no other clinical symptoms than possibly a slight increase in body temperature. However, if the circulating microorganisms find favorable conditions, they may settle at a given site and after a certain time lag start to multiply (**Fig. 2.26**). Thus, in compromized patients, bacteremia may be a potential danger, leading to disease away from the oral cavity. Oral bacteria have been isolated from abscesses in internal organs and the brain, from heart valves with infective endocarditis or stenosis, from coronary arteries of bypass and transplant patients, and generally from atheromas in patients with cardiovascular disease (**Fig. 2.26**). Studies using biochemical tests as well as genetic methods have confirmed that bacteria recovered from brain abscesses and atheromas may have identical characteristics as organisms isolated from sites of infection in the oral cavity, strongly suggesting that the bacteria originated in the oral cavity.

According to classic textbook information, the viridans streptococci have been regarded as especially important in bacteremia-related diseases (e.g., infective endocarditis). However, anaerobic infections are often overlooked, mostly due to lack

of necessary laboratory equipment and identification techniques. In spite of the fact that blood is a highly oxygenated medium, anaerobic organisms survive well in blood. For instance, many of the organisms have enzymes that are protective against toxic oxygen-reaction products, and several facultative species work in concert with anaerobes, promoting their survival. Recent and ongoing research clearly shows that oral anaerobes are more prevalent in nonoral infections than has so far been anticipated.

Repair in the Apical Periodontium
If the etiological factors causing the development of apical periodontitis are removed by endodontic treatment, healing may occur. Macrophages and other phagocytes remove breakdown products, including disintegrating epithelium from cyst walls and fistulas. Macrophages and lymphocytes produce factors chemotactic for fibroblasts, bringing these cells to the inflamed area. Moreover, they produce fibroblast-activating factors which cause these cells to proliferate and produce collagen to replace the fibers lost during the destructive phase of the disease. New cementoblasts are differentiated and cementum is laid down in resorptive areas of the root. Osteoblasts will form new bone to replace the bone that was resorbed and the apical periodontium is gradually restored.

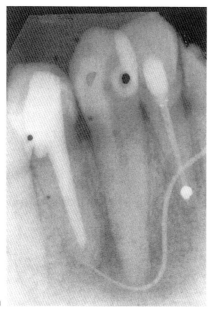
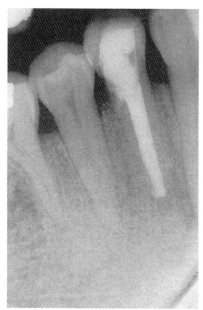

a

b

Fig. 2.25

a Radiograph of the right mandibular canine area. The patient has had a fistula opening up to the vestibule adjacent to the lateral incisor for 6 years. The lateral incisor has been treated endodontically without success. Then an apicoectomy with retrograde filling was performed with the same lack of

success. Upon referral of the patient, the fistulous tract was carefully traced to the endodontically treated first premolar.

b Following retreatment of the premolar, the fistula immediately closed and periapical healing was observed.

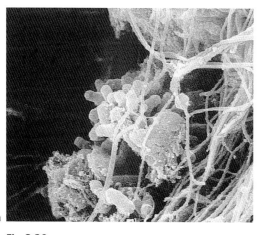
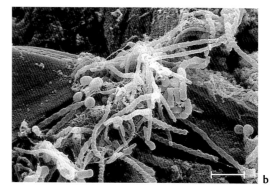

a

b

Fig. 2.26

a Scanning electron micrograph from aortic aneurysm. Circulating bacteria seemingly have been "caught" in a net of fibrils in area of vessel wall.

b Scanning electron micrograph from stenotic lesion of aortic valve. Coaggregating microorganisms with different morphologies are seen. Oral bacteria have been recovered from lesions in the heart.

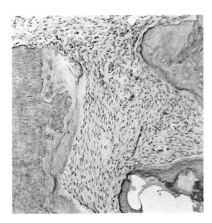

Fig. 2.27 Apical end of a nonvital tooth after successful endodontic treatment. Cemental repair of areas in the root which have undergone resorption is evident (hematoxylin-eosin).

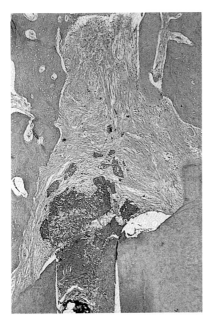

Fig. 2.28 Monkey tooth showing fibrous periapical healing following endodontic treatment of apical periodontitis. A dentin chips plug is present in the apical end of the root canal (hematoxylin-eosin).

Only an irregular shape of the root end (since resorbed dentin is not replaced) may suggest that an apical periodontitis has existed in the area (**Fig. 2.27**).

In some instances, especially in elderly patients and after surgical removal of a periapical granuloma or cyst, the area of bone resorption may not fill in completely with new bone, but with an unmineralized fibrous tissue (**Fig. 2.28**). Obviously, this is of no consequence for the patient, but occasionally may cause diagnostic difficulties in that the scar tissue cannot always be differentiated from granulation tissue in radiographs.

Apical periodontitis does not always heal following endodontic treatment. In most instances this is a result of inadequacies of the treatment. However, as discussed above, in long-standing lesions, an infection may be established in the tissues outside the root. The extraradicular bacteria may survive the treatment and sustain the periapical inflammation.

Radiographic Appearance and Differential Diagnosis

Periapical inflammatory processes cause changes in periapical bone, mainly bone loss, which will appear as *periapical radiolucencies* in radiographs. Thus, the radiograph is an extremely important diagnostic aid in endodontic diagnostics. However, the radiolucency is not pathognomonic for apical periodontitis.

On the contrary, several local and systemic processes may have similar radiographic manifestations.

Changes in bone texture are the earliest radiographic signs of apical periodontitis. However, these changes may be difficult to assess, and a widening of the periodontal ligament space in the periapical region is usually considered as the most reliable initial sign (**Fig. 2.29**). On occasion, symptomatic apical periodontitis with abscess formation may cause rapid and widespread demineralization of bone, and radiographs taken during the acute phase may reveal extensive radiolucent areas with indefinite borders. Once the acute phase has subsided, a large portion of the bone may return to normal radiopacity, leaving a periapical radiolucency of smaller size which is well demarcated against surrounding bone.

Periapical Granulomas and Cysts

Radiographically, a periapical granuloma or periapical cyst is seen as a round or oval radiolucency that extends away from the apical portion of the root of the tooth (**Fig. 2.30**). Variation in the position of the radiolucency usually indicates the presence of a major lateral canal (**Fig. 2.12**). The borders of the lesion are most often fairly well circumscribed, but in many instances the lesion has a fuzzy appearance (**Fig. 2.30**). Traditionally, it has been held that the radiographic appearance of a periapical lesion is suggestive of whether the lesion is a granuloma or a cyst, in that a cyst is allegedly more sharply defined and has a central portion which is more radiolucent than a granuloma. This is a misconception. A cyst cavity more often than not comprises only a small part of a granuloma so that the border zone of a lesion in both instances will consist of granulation tissue surrounded by a fibrous capsule. In computed tomography (CT) scans, however, the density of the content of a cyst cavity can be distinguished from that of granulation tissue and fibrous tissue (**Fig. 2.31**). Otherwise, a definite diagnosis of periapical granuloma or cyst can be arrived at only after microscopic examination of biopsy material. Clinically, the inability to differentiate radiographically between a granuloma and a cyst is of only minor importance in that the treatment is the same in both instances. Failure of a periapical lesion to respond to treatment may depend more on whether or not it is infected than on the nature of the lesion.

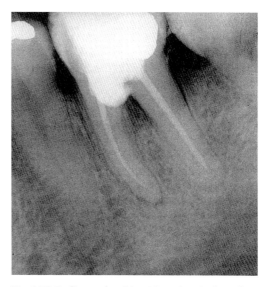

Fig. 2.29 Radiograph with widened periodontal ligament space at the apex of the mesial root, probably because of inadequate instrumentation and disinfection of the root canal.

Foramina and Other Structures
Because of their radiographic appearance and location, some anatomical landmarks may be mistaken for inflammatory periapical lesions. The *incisive canal* is often seen in radiographs. It varies

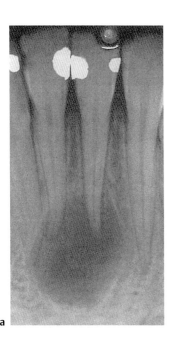

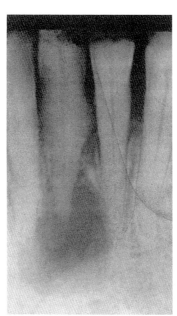

Fig. 2.30
a **Radiograph showing a periapical lesion of pulpal origin.** The lesion has sharp borders, but from the radiograph it cannot be determined whether it is a granuloma or a cyst.
b Radiograph showing a periapical lesion of pulpal origin with fuzzy borders. It cannot be determined from the radiograph whether the lesion is a cyst or a granuloma.

a

b

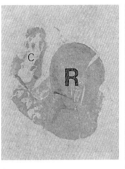 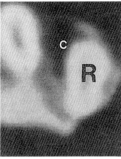

a   b

Fig. 2.31
a Histological section of a root end with a periapical lesion with a small cyst cavity (C).
b In a CT scan of the jaw at this level, the cyst cavity (C) clearly has a lower density than adjacent granulomatous tissue (root = R).

greatly in width and length and may appear as a periapical lesion associated with a maxillary central incisor. However, by using different projection angles, the root end as a rule may be projected free from the incisive canal. The *mental foramen* appears as an oval or round radiolucent area in the mandibular premolar region (**Fig. 2.32**). Its location varies in relation to the roots of the teeth, and its image may be seen inferior to, at the same

level as, or superior to the apex of the root. Its image may also be superimposed onto the apex of a tooth, usually the second premolar, and be mistaken for a periapical lesion. The nasal fossae are sometimes abnormally large and may encroach upon the roots of the central incisors. Moreover, the *dental papilla* of a developing tooth, especially if it is superimposed on the mandibular canal, may produce an area of marked radiolucency that may be mistaken for a periapical lesion.

Periodontal Disease
Periodontal disease frequently has radiographic manifestations that may be mistaken for apical periodontitis. As described for the periapical abscess, a periodontal abscess may cause widespread periradicular destruction of bone involving the periapical area as well (**Fig. 2.18**). A positive sensitivity response of the tooth will aid in the differential diagnosis. In periodontal disease, the pattern of bone destruction is often vertical along the root, and in advanced cases, the bone loss may progress beyond the apex of the tooth (**Fig. 2.33**). The resulting radiographic lesion can be mistaken for a lesion of pulpal origin, especially if the periodontal pocket is situated on the buccal or lingual aspect of the tooth. A consequence of periodontal disease is commonly an increased mobility of the teeth. This, in turn, may lead to a widening of the

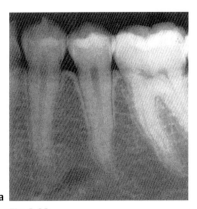

a

Fig. 2.32
a Radiograph showing a radiolucent area between mandibular premolars readily diagnosed as mental foramen.
b Radiograph of same premolars taken from a different angle. Mental foramen is "distorted" and might mistakenly be diagnosed as apical periodontitis emanating from the second premolar.

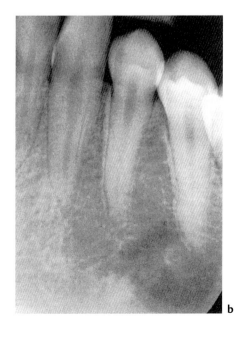

b

periodontal ligament at the root end, giving the radiographic appearance of a periradicular radiolocency.

Vertical Fracture

A vertical fracture of a tooth may result in communication between the gingival sulcus (oral cavity) and the apical periodontium. The fracture line will be a portal of entry for bacteria from the mouth into the tissues, causing inflammation and bone destruction. A periapical lesion often forms which may have the appearance radiographically of a pulpally related lesion (**Fig. 2.34**). Since a vertical fracture may be incomplete, its diagnosis in many instances is extremely difficult. Sometimes it is recognized clinically because a periodontal pocket forms along the fracture line and in other instances a simple exploratory surgical procedure may aid in establishing the correct diagnosis.

Cysts of the Jaws

Cysts of the jaws and some cyst-like conditions have radiographic features and sometimes a location that may make them appear to be periapical lesions of pulpal origin. In most instances, these cysts are *periodontal cysts*. They may develop from retained root tips of primary teeth or epithelial remnants once associated with the periodontal ligament of primary teeth. They may also develop in the periodontal ligament of permanent teeth away from the apex and unattached to the root or they may be residual periapical cysts that remain in the jaw after the tooth from which they originated has been extracted (**Fig. 2.35**). Moreover, the dentigerous cyst which develops in association with the crown of unerupted or supernumerary teeth may sometimes have an extension that makes a correct diagnosis difficult.

Of the nonodontogenic cysts, the incisive canal cyst and the globulomaxillary cyst are the most important from a differential diagnostic point of view. The incisive canal cyst is in most instances situated in the midline extending laterally to both sides. However, it may extend laterally to one side only and may then be located over the apex of a central incisor. The globulomaxillary cyst is situated between the maxillary lateral incisor and the canine (**Fig. 2.36**). It usually extends toward the marginal crest of the bone, and as it increases in size may cause divergence of the roots of the adjacent teeth, or it may cover the apices of neighboring teeth. Both the incisive canal cyst and the

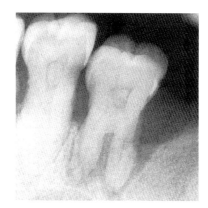

Fig. 2.33 Radiograph of a mandibular molar with severe periodontal disease. Note radiolucent zones alongside the roots. The tooth reacted positively to sensitivity testing.

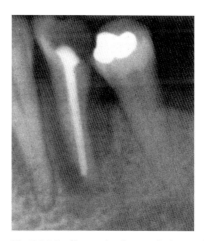

Fig. 2.34 Radiograph of an endodontically treated mandibular premolar with radiolucent areas alongside the root. This pattern of bone resorption is strongly indicative of a vertical fracture in that noxious agents reach the fracture line from the oral cavity and are released laterally to the periodontium, causing bone resorption. The clinical examination confirmed the tentative diagnosis.

globulomaxillary cyst may become infected and cause pain, tenderness, and abscess formation with sometimes considerable swelling.

Traumatic bone cysts occur most commonly in the mandible (**Fig. 2.37**). Radiographically their borders are usually not as well defined and more irregular than those of periapical granulomas and cysts. Their content is characterized by a blood-

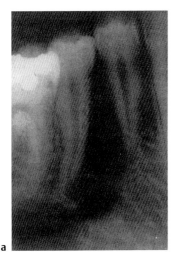
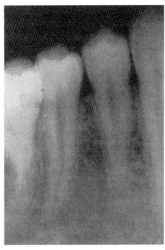

a   b

Fig. 2.35
a Radiograph of a mandibular premolar with a lateral periodontal cyst. The teeth all react positively to sensitivity tests.
b The cyst was removed surgically. This radiograph shows complete healing 6 months postoperatively.

colored viscous fluid which may be visualized by aspiration. However, with this lesion, as with all cysts and cyst-like lesions in the jaw, sensitivity testing remains the most important differential diagnostic aid.

Periradicular Osteosclerosis

Sclerotic bone is frequently seen in the periapical area of teeth (**Fig. 2.19**). Traditionally, this condition was regarded indiscriminately as condensing apical periodontitis, and if the tooth showed a positive sensitivity reaction, the lesion was assumed to be due to low-grade irritation from a chronic inflammation in the pulp. Currently it is understood that only few of the periapical sclerotic lesions are pulpally related (**Fig. 2.20**). The etiology of the remaining lesions which should be diagnosed simply as *periradicular osteosclerosis* is not clear, although it has been claimed that they are the result of a local disturbance in the osteogenic–osteolytic balance in bone metabolism. In rare instances periradicular sclerotic lesions may cause slight root resorption, but other than from a differential-diagnostic point of view, they are without clinical interest.

Tumors of the Jaws

A wide variety of tumors may have a radiographic appearance similar to periapical lesions of pulpal origin. Of the *odontogenic tumors*, ameloblastomas, cementomas, and odontogenic fibromas occur most frequently.

The *ameloblastoma* is a true neoplasm that is radiographically described as a multilocular cyst-

like lesion of the jaw with a honeycomb or soap bubble-like configuration (**Fig. 2.38**). However, in some instances the ameloblastoma may occupy a single or monocystic cavity, making the radiographic diagnosis difficult. An important observation is that the ameloblastoma as a rule produces more extensive apical root resorption of the teeth it comes in contact with than lesions of pulpal origin. The ameloblastoma occurs most frequently in

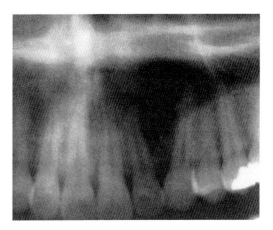

Fig. 2.36 Area of a panoramic radiograph showing a radiolucent lesion between the maxillary left lateral incisor and canine. The teeth in the area have intact crowns and react positively to sensitivity testing. Note deviation of the roots of the lateral incisor and canine teeth. Tentative diagnosis: Globulomaxillary cyst.

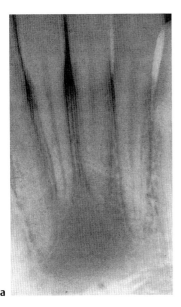

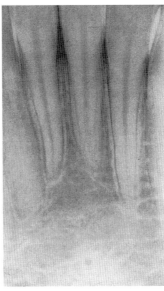

a   b

Fig. 2.37
a **Radiograph of mandibular incisors with a radiolucent lesion over their roots.** The teeth have intact crowns and react positively to sensitivity tests. Tentative diagnosis: Traumatic bone cyst.
b Radiograph taken after 3 years. The radiolucent lesion has resolved without treatment.

the posterior regions of the mandible, but is seen in all areas of the jaws. It has a potential for malignancy and should always be removed surgically.

The *cementoma* results from proliferation of the tissues of the periodontal ligament. It remains continuous with the ligament and attached to the root end of the tooth (**Fig. 2.39**). Cementomas occur far more frequently in the mandible than in the maxilla, especially in the mandibular anterior region and between the roots of the mandibular first molar. The radiographic appearance depends on the stage of development. In the first stage, when the lesion consists of unmineralized fibrous tissue, it appears as a well-demarcated, round, and radiolucent area quite similar to a lesion of pulpal origin. It is at this stage that most diagnostic mistakes are made. In the second stage, mineralized areas are seen within the radiolucent lesion. This radiographic appearance is typical for the cementoma, and at this stage the lesion should not be mistaken for a granulomatous or cystic lesion. The same applies for the third stage of development, when the cementoma may be completely mineralized. A cementoma never causes resorption of the root of the tooth with which it is in contact and over time will resolve without treatment (**Fig. 2.40**).

An *odontogenic fibroma* is a benign tumor arising from the periodontal ligament (**Fig. 2.41**). The tumor is composed of fibrous or fully developed connective tissue, and as it increases in size, it causes periradicular bone resorption. Radiographically, therefore, a radiolucent area will be seen in conjunction with the tooth from which the tumor developed. Clinically, the tumor will be firm and not tender to palpation and quite different from a swelling that is inflammatory in nature.

Two *benign nonodontogenic tumors*, the giant cell granuloma and the hemangioma, should be considered. The *giant cell granuloma* may be designated as peripheral or central in origin. It is the

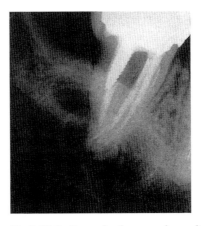

Fig. 2.38 **Radiograph of a second mandibular molar with periapical radiolucent, multilocular lesion.** Tentative diagnosis: Ameloblastoma.

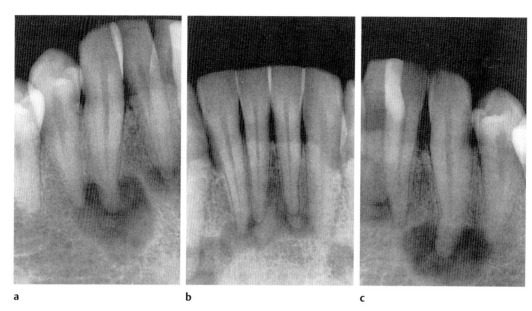

a   b   c

Fig. 2.39 Radiographs of the mandibular teeth of a patient with multiple cementomas. The radiographic appearance may vary from radiolucent (**a**), radiolucent with radiopaque areas (**b**), to mostly radiopaque (**c**).

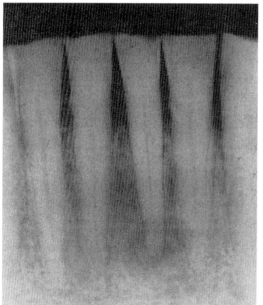

a

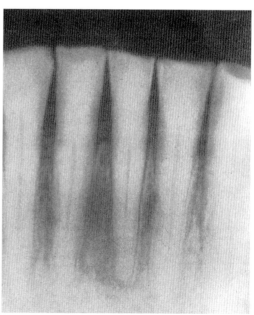

b

Fig. 2.40
a Radiograph of a mandibular incisor with a cementoma.

b After 2 years the lesion has resolved without treatment.

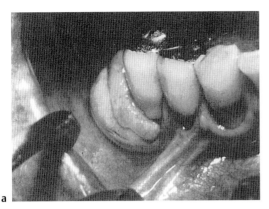

a

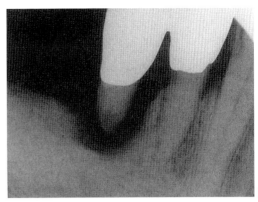

b

Fig. 2.41
a Firm swelling suggestive of tumorous growth in the region of a mandibular second premolar.

b Radiographically, a periradicular radiolucency can be seen. The tumor was removed and the microscopic diagnosis was odontogenic fibroma.

central tumor that affects the alveolar bone, most often in children and young adults and twice as frequently in the mandible as in the maxilla. Radiographically, the central tumor demonstrates two variations. The first is a homogenous, osteolytic, and monolocular lesion. The second type exhibits multiple osteolytic foci and bone trabeculae within the tumor. With both types, malpositioning of teeth and resorption of the roots of the teeth with which the lesion comes in contact are common findings. The monolocular variation of the giant cell granuloma may have an appearance rather similar to a periapical lesion of pulpal origin. The multilocular type, on the other hand, is so different that a diagnostic mistake would be unlikely.

Hemangiomas are rather uncommon and are not routinely considered in the differential diagnosis of the lytic lesions of the jaws. However, they may have a radiolucent appearance and may be located near the apices of the teeth. In case of the slightest suspicion that a lesion might be a hemangioma, needle aspiration of the content should be used to verify the diagnosis and to prevent profuse bleeding that can be difficult to control.

Carcinomas and sarcomas of various types are found in the jaws, either as primary or metastatic tumors. In most instances the tumors have a clinical and radiographic appearance that sets them apart from lesions of pulpal origin. However, a *carcinoma* of the gingiva may look like apical periodontitis, and metastatic carcinoma of the jaws may cause periapical radiolucencies (**Fig. 2.42**). A

sarcoma will cause early bone changes that may be either sclerotic or lytic. *Leukemia* may debut with loss of sensitivity of the pulp and development of multiple periapical radiolucencies. Also, *malignant lymphomas* have been observed in conjunction with teeth. This tumor may cause loss of

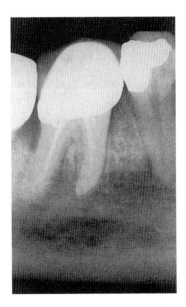

Fig. 2.42 Radiograph of a mandibular molar with technically inadequate root canal filling and a periapical radiolucency. The extension and form of the radiolucent lesion is not typical of a lesion of endodontic origin. Microscopic examination following biopsy produced the diagnosis of carcinoma.

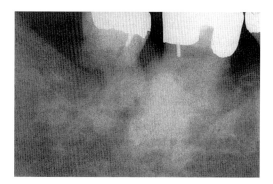

Fig. 2.43 Radiograph of mandibular molars with the cotton wool-like osteosclerosis typical of Paget's disease. Note the resorption of the distal root of the second molar.

alveolar bone and swelling so that both clinically and radiographically pulpal or periodontal disease may be suspected.

There are many reports in the literature of malignant tumors mistakenly being diagnosed as apical periodontitis and treated endodontically. Since these conditions fortunately occur rather infrequently, we do not gain much diagnostic experience and mistakes are bound to happen. However, we need to be alert and not push strange and unusual findings under the carpet if we do not understand them. If in doubt, we clearly owe it to our patients to refer them to a specialist for further examination and evaluation.

Systemic Diseases

A wide variety of systemic disorders like hormone and vitamin deficiencies and developmental disturbances may cause oral manifestations with dental and osseous anomalies.

However, in most instances the changes are generalized and not readily mistaken for lesions of pulpal origin, although endodontic pathosis is frequently seen in these patients. An exception may be *histiocytosis X*, which may occur as *eosinophilic granuloma* in the form of solitary, radiolucent bony lesions in the periapical area of teeth. This disease may cause extensive destruction of alveolar bone and swelling and loosening of the teeth. Thorough curettage may suffice to eliminate the lesion.

Paget's disease, or *osteitis deformans*, which is a skeletal disease with oral manifestations of unknown etiology should also be mentioned. In the early stages of Paget's disease, osteolytic lesions occur in the bone immediately surrounding the roots of the teeth and resorption of the roots may occur (**Fig. 2.43**). As the disease progresses, apposition of bone exceeds resorption, and a generalized cotton wool-like osteosclerosis is seen. At this stage the disease is readily differentiated from periapical lesions of pulpal origin.

Further Reading

Barnett F, Duran C, Hasselgren G, Tronstad L. Tissue response to anodyne medicaments. Oral Surg Oral Med Oral Pathol 1984;58:605 – 609.

Barnett F, Schwartzben L, Tronstad L. Extensive periapical lesion with inconsistent radiographic findings. J Endod 1984;10:26 – 27.

Beertsen W, McCulloch CAG, Sodek J. The periodontal ligament: a unique, multifunctional connective tissue. Periodontology 2000 1997;13:20 – 30.

Charon NW, Goldstein SF. Genetics of motility and chemotaxis of a fascinating group of bacteria. The spirochetes. Ann Rev Gen 2002;36:47 – 73.

Dahle UR, Sunde PT, Tronstad L. Treponemes and endodontic infections. Endod Topics 2003;6:160 – 170.

Dahle UR, Tronstad L, Olsen I. Characterization of new periodontal and endodontic isolates of treponemes. Eur J Oral Sci 1996;104:41 – 47.

Dahle UR, Tronstad L, Olsen I. Spirochaetes in oral infections. Endod Dent Traumatol 1993;9:87 – 94.

da Silva RM, Camargo SC, Debelian G, Eribe ER, Tronstad L, Olsen I. DNA-DNA hybridization demonstrates a diverse endodontic microflora. Int Union Microbiol Soc, Paris: Proc World Congress, 2002, p. 33.

da Silva RM, Lingaas PS, Geiran O, Tronstad L, Olsen I. Multiple bacteria in aortic aneurysms. J Vasc Surg 2003;38:1384 – 1389.

Debelian GJ, Eribe ER, Olsen I, Tronstad L. Ribotyping of bacteria from root canal and blood of patients receiving endodontic therapy. Anaerobe 1997;3:237 – 243.

Debelian GJ, Olsen I, Tronstad L. Anaerobic bacteremia and fungemia in patients undergoing endodontic therapy: an overview. Ann Periodontol 1998;3: 281 – 287.

Debelian GJ, Olsen I, Tronstad L. Bacteremia in conjunction with endodontic therapy. Endod Dent Traumatol 1995;11:142 – 149.

de Paz LC. Redefining the persistent infection in root canals: possible role of biofilm communities. J Endod 2007;33:652 – 662.

Gatti JJ, Dobeck JM, Smith C, White RR, Socransky S, Skobe Z. Bacteria of asymptomatic periradicular endodontic lesions identified by DNA-DNA hybridization. Endod Dent Traumatol 2000;16:197–204.

Gomes BPFA, Lilley JD, Drucker DB. Associations of endodontic symptoms and signs with particular combinations of specific bacteria. Int Endod J 1996;29: 69–75.

Happonen RP, Söderling E, Viander M, Linko-Kettunen L, Pelliniemi LJ. Immunocytochemical demonstration of *Actinomyces* species and *Arachnia propionica* in periapical infections. J Oral Pathol 1985;14:405–413.

Harasztky VI, Zambon JJ, Trevisan M, Zeid M, Genco RJ. Identification of periodontal pathogens in atheromatous plaques. J Periodontol 2000;71:1554–1560.

Hornhef MH, Wick MJ, Rehn M, Nomark S. Bacterial strategies for overcoming host innate and adaptive immune responses. Nature Immunol 2002;3:1033–1040.

Kakehashi S, Stanley HR, Fitzgerald RJ. The effect of surgical exposures of dental pulps in germ-free and conventional laboratory rats. Oral Med Oral Surg Oral Pathol 1965;20:340–349.

Katz JO, Underhill TE. Multilocular radiolucencies. Dent Clin North Am 1994;38:63–81.

Kolltveit KM, Geiran O, Tronstad L, Olsen I. Multiple bacteria in calcific aortic valve stenosis. Microb Ecol Health Dis 2002; 14: 110–117.

Koppang HS, Koppang R, Stölen SO. Identification of common foreign material in postendodontic granulomas and cysts. J Dent Ass S Africa 1992;47:210–216.

Lin LM, Huang GT-J, Rosenberg PA. Proliferation of epithelial cell rests, formation of apical cysts, and regression of apical cysts after periapical wound healing. J Endod 2007;33:652–662.

Munson MA, Pitt-Ford T, Chong B, Weightman A, Wade WG. Molecular and cultural analysis of the microflora associated with endodontic infections. J Dent Res 2002;81:761–766.

Paster BJ, Olsen I, Aas JA, Dewhirst FE. The breadth of bacterial diversity in the human periodontal pocket and other oral sites. Periodontol 2000 2006;42:1–8.

Roças IN, Siqueira JF, Santos KR, Coelho AM. "Red complex" (*Bacteroides forsythus, Porphyromonas gingivalis*, and *Treponema denticola*) in endodontic infections: a molecular approach. Oral Surg Oral Med Oral Pathol 2001;91:468–471.

Rolph HJ, Lennon A, Riggio MP et al. Molecular identification of microorganisms from endodontic infections. J Clin Microbiol 2001;39:3282–3289.

Selliseth NJ, Selvig KA. The vasculature of the periodontal ligament: a scanning electron microscopic study using corrosion casts in the rat. J Periodontol 1994; 65:1079–1087.

Siqueira JF, Roças IN. PCR based identification of *Treponema maltiphilum, T. amylovorum, T. medium* and *T. lecithinolyticum* in primary root can infections. Archs Oral Biol 2003;48:495–502.

Slots J, Hames HS. Herpesvirus in periapical pathosis: an etiopathogenic relationship? Oral Surg Oral Med Oral Pathol 2003;96:327–331.

Socransky SS, Haffajee AD, Cugini MA, Smith C, Kent RL Jr. Microbial complexes in subgingival plaque. J Clin Periodontol 1998;25:134–144.

Socransky SS, Haffajee AD. Dental biofilms: difficult therapeutic targets. Periodontol 2000 2002;28:12–55.

Stashenko P, Wang CY, Tani-Ishii N, Yu SM. Pathogenesis of induced rat periapical lesions. Oral Med Oral Surg Oral Pathol 1994;78:494–502.

Stashenko P, Yu SM. T helper and T suppressor cell reversal during the development of induced rat periapical lesions. J Dent Res 1989;68:830–834.

Stashenko P. Role of immune cytokines in the pathogenesis of periapical lesions. Endod Dent Traumatol 1990;6:89–96.

Stern HM, Dreizen S, Mackler BF, Selbst AG, Levy BM. Quantitative analysis of cellular composition of human periapical granulomas. J Endod 1981;7:117–122.

Sunde PT, Olsen I, Debelian GJ, Tronstad L. Microbiota of periapical lesions refractory to endodontic therapy. J Endod 2002.

Sunde PT, Olsen I, Göbel UB, Theegarten D, Winter S, Debelian G, Tronstad L, Moter A. Fluorescence in situ hybridization (FISH) for direct visualization of bacteria in periapical lesions of asymptomatic root-filled teeth. Microbiol 2003;149:1095–1102.

Sunde PT, Olsen I, Lind PO, Tronstad L. Extraradicular infection: a methodological study. Endod Dent Traumatol 2000:16:84–90.

Sunde PT, Tronstad L, Eribe ER, Lind PO, Olsen I. Assesment of periradicular microbiota by DNA-DNA hybridization. Endod Dent Traumatol 2000;16:191–196.

Sundqvist G, Eckerbom MI, Larsson AP, Sjögren IT. Capacity of anaerobic bacteria from necrotic dental pulps to induce purulent infections. Infection and Immunity 1979;25:685–693.

Sundqvist G. Assosiations between microbial species in dental root canal infections. Oral Microbiol Immunol 1992;7:257–272.

Torabinejad M, Kriger RD. Experimentally induced alterations in periapical tissues of the cat. J Dent Res 1980;59:87–96.

Tronstad L, Barnett F, Cervone F. Periapical bacterial plaque in teeth refractory to endodontic treatment. Endod Dent Traumatol 1990;6:73–77.

Tronstad L, Barnett F, Riso K, Slots J. Extraradicular endodontic infections. Endod Dent Traumatol 1987;3: 86–90.

Tronstad L, Kreshtool D, Barnett F. Microbiological monitoring and results of treatment of extraradicular endodontic infection. Endod Dent Traumatol 1990;6:129–135.

Tronstad L, Sunde PT. The evolving new understanding of endodontic infections. Endod Topics 2003;6:57–77.

Trope M, Pettigrew J, Petras J, Barnett F, Tronstad L. Differentiation of radicular cyst and granulomas using computerized tomography. Endod Dent Traumatol 1989;5:67–72.

Trope M, Tronstad L, Rosenberg ES, Listgarten M. Dark field microscopy as a diagnostic aid in differentiating exudates from endodontic and periodontal abscesses. J Endod 1988;14:35–38.

Wang CY, Stashenko P. Characterization of bone resorbing activity in human periapical lesions. J Endod 1993;19:107–111.

Ximenes-Fyvie LA, Haffajee AD, Socransky SS. Comparison of the microbiota of supra- and subgingival plaque in subjects in health and periodontitis. J Clin Periodontol 2000;27:648–657.

Young D, Hussel T, Dougan G. Chronic bacterial infection: living with unwanted guests. Nature Immunol 2002;3:1026–1032.

3
Endodontic Symptomatology

Advanced toothache is commonly described as the most intolerable pain and is often considered more unbearable than pain at childbirth or pain caused by kidney or gallbladder stones. Still, pain is a subjective experience and although the transfer of pain impulses occurs in the same way in all individuals, the reaction to pain is subjective and to a great extent depends on psychological phenomena. This fact makes it difficult to perform an objective examination of the physiology of pain.

A variety of pain conditions can be diagnosed in the oral and perioral regions. In this context, pain of endodontic origin is common, and as many as 90% of patients with a maxillofacial pain condition need to be examined endodontically (**Fig. 3.1**). About 60% of the patients will actually have pain of endodontic origin and will be in need of endodontic treatment.

Commonly, endodontic symptoms are considered to be of dentinal, pulpal, and periapical origin. However, since dentinal pain is mediated by pulpal nerves, we will consider endodontic symptoms as being either of pulpal or periapical origin.

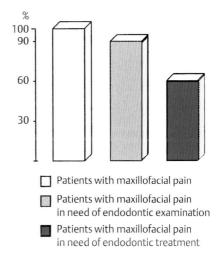

Fig. 3.1 Endodontic diseases are important and common etiological factors for maxillofacial pain.

Pulpal Pain

Dental Hypersensitivity
The teeth are normally sensitive to irritants, for instance, to temperature changes. Over the years, wear and tear, caries, periodontal disease, and the treatment of these diseases may have altered the pain threshold of the teeth and they may have become hypersensitive to external irritation. In most instances hypersensitivity is due to the fact that an area of dentin has become exposed to the mouth so that there is communication between the oral cavity and the pulp via the dentinal tubules. Extreme hypersensitivity may be seen after periodontal surgery with extensive scaling and root planing and in conjunction with abrasion or erosion defects in the cervical areas of the teeth. Carious lesions may cause a hypersensitive reaction, and hypersensitivity is often seen in teeth

after the excavation of caries and restoration of a cavity with a filling material, either because of thermal conductivity of the material used or because of leakage along the margins of the restoration. *The pulp of a hypersensitive tooth is in most instances healthy and free of inflammation.* However, an inflammatory reaction in the pulp, which is not necessarily symptomatic in itself, may alter the responsiveness of pulpal nerves so that stimuli which would normally elicit no symptoms or a normal reaction may instead cause a hypersensitive reaction of the tooth. Dental hypersensitivity, therefore, may be an indication of pulpal pathosis.

The anatomical basis for dental hypersensitivity is the sensory nerves in the peripheral pulp with unmyelinated nerve endings between and in close contact with the odontoblasts in the pulp and the dentinal tubules. There is at present little evidence that the more peripheral parts of the dentin are innervated so that a mechanism may have to exist whereby stimuli are transferred from the root surface to afferent nerves in the inner dentin and the pulp. This mechanism is not fully understood. It has been suggested that the odontoblasts with their pro-cesses might transfer sensory impulses to the nerves in the pulp, and the relationship that exists between nerve endings and odontoblasts may in fact be comparable to cell interactions in other sensitive areas of the organism, for instance, in taste buds and certain areas of the skin. However, the close contact between the two cells might also exist simply because the odontoblast has a metabolic function. The *odontoblast-receptor theory* has lost support in recent years and appears unlikely for several reasons, primarily because odontoblastic processes are not observed in the peripheral parts of the dentin. Also, there is evidence that a dental hypersensitivity reaction will not subside in teeth where the odontoblasts have been destroyed.

Current research appears to support the *hydrodynamic theory*, which explains dental hypersensitivity on the basis of mechanical stimulation of nerves in the circumpulpal dentin and peripheral pulp, resulting from rapid fluid flow in the dentinal tubules caused by pain-provoking irritants. It is known that under certain conditions tissue fluids from the dentinal tubules may seep onto an exposed dentinal surface. The lost fluids in the dentinal tubules will then be replaced by fluids from the pulp. Allegedly, this fluid movement may occur with considerable speed (2–4 mm/s), so that if the dentinal tubules were emptied, they would fill up again in about 1 second. A number of experiments have been carried out to determine whether fluid movement actually occurs in the dentinal tubules as a result of pain stimuli. A stream of air onto exposed dentin, for instance, will lead to an outward fluid movement in the exposed tubules; it has been calculated that the content of the tubules at the dentin–pulp border will move 5–10 µm during the first second of the air blast. Similar results are observed when hypertonic solutions such as sugar are applied to exposed dentin, and an outward movement occurs when blotting paper or certain materials known to cause pain are applied to the dentin. Application of cold, either to exposed dentin or to an intact tooth, causes the same fluid movement, presumably because the contents of the tubules contract and the tubules fill up with fluids from the pulp. A lowering of the temperature at the tooth surface of 20 °C results in a fluid movement at the pulp–dentin border of the same magnitude as is caused by a 1-second air blast. The influence of heat is apparently more complicated. Applying dry heat to exposed dentin causes evaporation of fluid on the surface and an outward fluid movement. On the other hand, if warm water is applied to exposed dentin or to an intact tooth, it causes the content of the dentinal tubules to expand, resulting in a fluid movement in the tubules toward the pulp.

Thus, many stimuli known to elicit pulpal pain appear to cause movement of the fluids in the dentinal tubules, and if rapid enough, the fluid movement will mechanically stimulate nerve endings. This theory offers a simple and understandable mechanism for the elicitation of pain, and it appears physiologically acceptable. However, the evidence supporting the theory is still inconclusive. For instance, it has not been possible to show that mechanical irritation of exposed dentin, like probing with an explorer, which may cause excruciating pain, results in fluid movement in the dentinal tubules.

The symptoms due to dental hypersensitivity are usually sharp and lancinating and they quickly subside when the external irritation has stopped. This means that episodes of pain due to dental hypersensitivity as a rule are of short duration. However, if, for instance, a sucrose-containing food somehow remains in a carious lesion of a tooth for a period of time, a pain reaction may persist until the sugar has dissolved or been removed. In such instances, pain due to dental hypersensitivity may mistakenly be diagnosed as being due to a symptomatic pulpitis and endodontic treatment or, worse, extraction of the tooth may be carried out.

Symptomatic Pulpitis

As a rule, pulpal inflammation is asymptomatic (**Fig. 3.2**). It may persist as a painless local reaction in the coronal pulp for considerable time, sometimes for years if the external irritation is mild. However, if untreated, the inflammation will spread in an apical direction, and the pulp may become totally necrotic and an apical periodontitis may develop without any sensation on the part of the patient at any time during the progression of the disease. *Clinically, therefore, pulpal pathosis in most instances is diagnosed during routine dental examinations and not as a result of episodes of symptomatic pulpitis.*

Thus, it is not possible to determine the type and severity of pulpal damage by the absence or presence of clinical symptoms. The first condition for becoming a good diagnostician, therefore, is to accept that endodontic symptomatology usually plays only a minor role in making a correct clinical diagnosis. Adequate knowledge about etiology and pathogenesis of inflammation in the pulp and adjacent tissues is in most instances far more important. For example, if a child has suffered an injury and presents with a complicated crown fracture *within half an hour* of the accident, the pulp of the traumatized tooth will not be inflamed, regardless of the presence or absence of pain. It is equally definite that if this patient presents *1 week* after the pulp was exposed, the pulp will be inflamed or even necrotic, regardless of whether symptoms are present or not. In these instances we arrive at different clinical diagnoses and choose radically different therapies (pulp capping in the first instance; pulpectomy or root canal treatment in the second), without letting the presence or abscence of symptoms influence us at all.

However, symptoms are sometimes the only reason that pulpal pathosis is detected, and it is important to understand as much as possible what different symptoms may mean. This understanding is especially important when it is difficult to locate an aching tooth. In such instances it may be possible with certain examination methods to get the involved tooth to react differently from its neighboring teeth, and thereby arrive at the correct clinical diagnosis.

Symptomatic pulpitis may be an acute pulpitis, but most often it is an *exacerbation of a chronic inflammation* in the pulp. Whereas dental hypersensitivity is generally due to stimulation of rapid-responding A-fibers in the pulp, a symptomatic pulpitis is associated with slower-reacting C-fiber activity as well. The symptoms are not caused by the presence of inflammatory cells per se, and it is not understood why a long-standing asymptomatic pulpitis all of a sudden and often without apparent provocation may begin to elicit pain. Also, it is not known why the pain from a pulpitis is usually not continuous, but may disappear as suddenly as it began. An increase in local

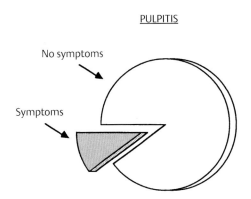

PULPITIS

No symptoms

Symptoms

Fig. 3.2 Pulpal pain is commonly described as intolerable and unbearable. However, in by far the most instances, pulpitis persists and progresses without pain or other symptoms.

pressure is probably necessary for eliciting pain in pulpitis. This may be provoked by external irritation or by intrapulpal changes causing vasoactive agents to produce additional vascular permeability. When a clinical exacerbation is a reality, pain-producing inflammatory mediators may have both a direct effect on the nerve endings causing pain, and an indirect effect, lowering the pain threshold and increasing the pain from external stimuli. A recent finding is that bacterial activity as such may cause pain. Thus, it is known that *Porphyromonas gingivalis* releases potent proteases which may cause the release of bradykinin in the tissue.

Clinically, patients may characterize pulpal pain as sharp, dull, heavy, intermittent, continuous, throbbing, diffuse, or grinding. In other words, pulpal pain may be felt in many different ways. Many attempts have been made to relate the type of pain to the degree of tissue damage in the pulp. Histopathological and clinical nomenclature have, therefore, been combined, resulting in a number of descriptions and diagnoses. The diagnosis *acute serous pulpitis*, for example, has traditionally meant that the patient had pain (acute), that the pulp is inflamed (pulpitis), and that as yet no abscesses have formed in the pulp (serous). Clinically, it has been assumed that this condition is present when a tooth is especially sensitive to cold and when the pain persists for some time after the cold stimulus is removed. Similarly, *acute suppurative pulpitis* meant that an abscess has formed in the pulp. Clinically, heat would sup-

Table 3.1 Evaluation of clinical diagnosis by histologic evidence (Baume 1970)

Presumptive clinical diagnosis	No. of cases	Histopathologic condition					Con-firmed diagnosis (%)
		Initial inflammation (Vascular changes only)	Acute inflamm.	Chronic inflamm.	Abscess forma-tion	Necrotic chances	
Hyperemia	26	6	6		14		23
Serous pulpitis	51	14	10	1	22	4	20
Chronic pulpitis	9		2	1	6		11
Suppurative pulpitis	20		8	2	6	4	30
Total	106	20	26	4	48	8	22

posedly increase the pain in a tooth with this diagnosis and cold would cause relief. Numerous studies have shown that the alleged relationships between symptoms and the actual state of the pulp at best exist in about 20% of the teeth (**Table 3.1**). Such a diagnostic system, therefore, is meaningless and confusing and should not be used. *The only way to determine the actual state of the pulp is to examine the tissue in the laboratory after extirpation of the pulp or extraction of the tooth.*

Still, if the goal is somewhat less ambitious, pulpal pain may provide important information, often decisively determining diagnosis and treatment of a tooth. *Four features of pulpal pain are especially important: the intensity of the pain, its duration, whether it occurs after stimulation (provoked) or spontaneously (unprovoked), and whether it occurs repeatedly.* Thus, severe, irreversible inflammation should be suspected when a patient has intense and continuous pain. Similarly, spontaneous pain usually indicates the presence of severe and irreversible pulp pathosis. Anamnestic information about repeated attacks of pain over a long period of time will also give reason to suspect serious pulp damage. Thus, intense, long-lasting pulpal pain that has occurred repeatedly over a period of time is a rather definite indication of severe, irreversible pulpal inflammation. In addition, the tissue damage in the pulp is considered to be severe if the pain is provoked by heat only rather than by hot and cold stimuli or by cold only.

This fairly imprecise knowledge about the meaning of pulpal symptoms may be used with advantage in diagnostic tests (see p. 77). If a tooth reacts to a thermal stimulus and the pain disappears when the stimulus is removed, the pulp may be inflamed, but the pain may also be due to a hypersensitivity reaction. However, if the pain persists for some time after the stimulation, there would be more reason to suspect pulpal inflammation. Only remember that the severity of the damage to the pulp cannot be determined with such tests and, most importantly, that in by far the most instances even severe irreversible pulpitis is free of symptoms.

Periapical Pain

Symptomatic Apical Periodontitis

Like pulpal inflammation, *apical periodontitis as a rule is asymptomatic* (**Fig. 3.3**). When symptoms occur, they may be caused by acute inflammation, but more often are due to an exacerbation of a chronic apical periodontitis. The most dramatic symptom is pain which starts spontaneously, initially mildly, and then gradually increases. The pain is continuous, and may be heavy and grinding. Especially at first, it may be difficult or even impossible to differentiate between pulpal and periapical pain. The diagnosis must then be made based on other clinical findings, first and foremost on whether or not the pulp is vital.

Tenderness of the tooth is usually the patient's first complaint. The tooth feels high and tender to biting or percussion because edema in the periodontal ligament presses the tooth out of its socket. The edema may also cause abnormal mobility of the tooth, and, over time, tenderness and swelling (collateral edema) in the mucosa over the apex of the tooth. Also, the regional lymph glands may be swollen and tender.

If the acute episode or exacerbation is severe, a purulent breakdown of the periapical tissues may occur. The pain is strong and intense as long as the pus is enclosed in the periodontium and bone, and the very strongest when the exudate is located subperiostally because of the rich innervation of the periosteum. The breakthrough of the periosteum by the purulent exudate in most regions is recognized by a dramatic relief of pain. Now the patient may see a dentist because of a swollen face and not so much because of the pain. The swelling is most often due to edema of the loose connective tissues of the maxillofacial region. If the infection spreads further, a purulent inflammation of the tissues may develop. This condition is commonly referred to as *cellulitis* (**Fig. 3.4**) and is frequently combined with general symptoms of illness. A fever of 102–104 °F (39–40 °C) is not uncommon.

As with symptomatic pulpitis, the actual trigger mechanism of acute apical periodontitis or a symptomatic episode of a chronic periapical inflammation is not known. In general terms it may be inferred that the symptoms are due to a change in the quantity or quality of the irritants or a decrease in the patient's resistance to the irritants, or any combination thereof. There is some evidence to tie the presence of certain bacteria to the occurrence of periapical symptoms. Especially *Porphyromonas* and *Prevotella* species are of interest in this regard, but also *Peptostreptococcus* and other organisms have been associated with painful apical periodontitis. However, since it has also been shown that these bacteria may be present in asymptomatic periapical lesions, a clear-cut rela-

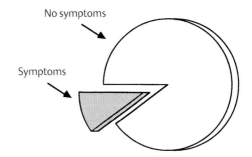

APICAL PERIODONTITIS

No symptoms

Symptoms

Fig. 3.3 Apical periodontitis is as a rule asymptomatic. When symptoms occur, they may be caused by acute inflammation or, most often, by an exacerbation of a chronic apical periodontitis.

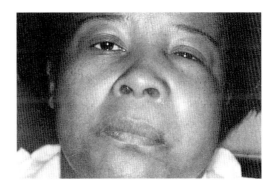

Fig. 3.4 Patient with facial swelling of endodontic origin. The local pain had largely subsided, but the patient felt sick and her body temperature was elevated.

tionship between the presence of specific bacteria and periapical symptoms is not obvious at this time.

Oral and Perioral Pain of Endodontic Interest

A wide variety of pain conditions in the oral and perioral region are of endodontic interest from a differential-diagnostic point of view. Most of these conditions are rare and the dentist cannot be expected to have detailed knowledge about many of them. The most commonly occurring diseases are discussed in the following sections.

Periodontal Diseases

Inflammation of the gingiva and the marginal periodontium, apart from a possible localized soreness, is symptomless, probably because of a continuous drainage through the sulcus. However, occasionally an abscess develops from a periodontal pocket. Usually this abscess is localized in the marginal area of the periodontium and is readily recognized (**Fig. 3.5**). However, on occasion the exudate is more widespread, so that the swelling

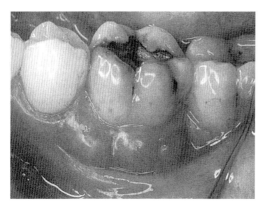

Fig. 3.5 Abscess in marginal area of the periodontium.

takes on the appearance of an abscess that might have originated in the apical periodontium. Conversely, a periapical abscess may sometimes drain alongside the root with a fistula ending in the sulcular area. This situation may remind one of severe periodontal disease in that the fistula may mimic a deepened pocket (see p. 45).

Sensitivity testing of the tooth is the most important procedure for arriving at the correct diagnosis in these instances. If the pulp is vital, we have a periodontal abscess. On the other hand, if the pulp is necrotic, chances are that the abscess is of endodontic origin (**Fig. 3.6**). Endodontic treatment should then precede any periodontal treatment and it will be clinically evident fairly soon whether or not the diagnosis is correct. Thus, a fistula may close, the gingival tissues will tighten up, and probing depth and tooth mobility may decrease. A difficult diagnostic problem sometimes exists when a periodontal abscess, usually in the furcation area of a multi-rooted tooth, is superimposed on an asymptomatic apical periodontitis in that the symptoms may suggest an exacerbation of the periapical inflammation (**Fig. 3.7**). Although endodontic treatment of the tooth is indicated, it will obviously have no effect on the symptoms from the periodontal abscess. A correct diagnosis is, as always, a prerequisite for correct treatment.

Recently it has been shown that the bacterial flora of endodontic and periodontal abscesses differ in certain respects. Thus, in an endodontic abscess, the number of spirochetes is between 0 and 10%, whereas in a periodontal abscess the spirochete count is about 40%. This difference can be readily detected in the dark field microscope and

can be used with advantage for differential-diagnostic purposes.

Other diseases of the periodontium that should be mentioned are *acute necrotizing ulcerative gingivitis* (Vincent's infection) and pericoronitis. In addition to general symptoms of illness, Vincent's infection is characterized by necrosis and ulceration of the papillae and marginal gingiva and is rather readily recognized. Pericoronitis is an inflammatory condition that most often occurs in conjunction with complicated eruption of the third molars of the mandible. The pain may be excruciating and is commonly accompanied by trismus.

Infection of Cysts and Salivary Glands

The *cysts of the jaws* like periodontal cysts, dentigerous cysts, incisive canal cysts, and globulomaxillary cysts may become infected with resultant abscess formation and swelling. These conditions may appear to be of endodontic origin. The most important differential-diagnostic test is to determine the vitality of the teeth in the involved area.

Swelling of the major salivary glands may sometimes be mistaken for cellulitis of endodontic origin (**Fig. 3.8**). The swelling may be due to accumulation of saliva because of an obstruction of the duct, usually by salivary stones. This type of swelling occurs especially at meal times and may or may not be associated with pain. Continued obstruction of the duct will lead to inflammation of the gland because of invasion of bacteria. Exacerbations of the inflammation with purulent breakdown, abscess formation, and swelling will occur at certain intervals. This condition may be mistaken for an endodontic infection, but careful examination of the teeth and surrounding areas with sensitivity and percussion tests should rule this out and point one in the right direction.

Sinusitis

Sinusitis, especially *maxillary sinusitis*, is probably the most common extraoral cause of pain in patients seeing a dentist. The patient normally complains about toothache in several or all teeth that have roots in contact with the sinus floor. The pain is constant, often relatively mild, but irritating, and may on occasion become extremely severe. The patient will usually indicate that the teeth are too long and painful when biting. The teeth may be sensitive to percussion and, most importantly, *hypersensitive to cold*. Sometimes it is

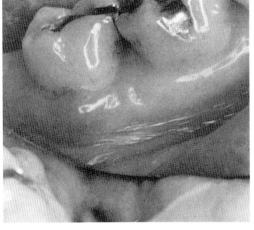

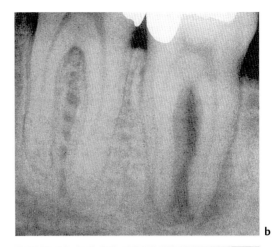

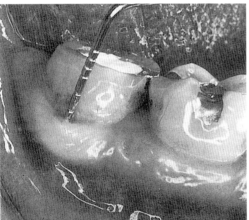

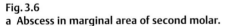

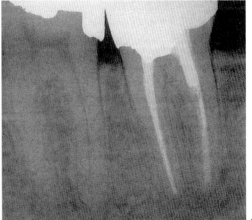

Fig. 3.6
a Abscess in marginal area of second molar.
b Radiograph of tooth in **a** with apical and interradicular periodontitis.
c Two weeks following initiation of endodontic therapy with complete debridement of root canals and

calcium hydroxide trestment. The periodontal abscess has resolved.
d After 3 months with calcium hydroxide treatment and obturation of root canals, complete healing is observed.

difficult to differentiate between pain from a sinusitis and pulpal pain. It is then important to remember that in patients with sinusitis almost without exception several adjacent teeth are involved. In addition, there are often extraoral symptoms such as tenderness in the bone above the sinus, increased pain when leaning forward quickly, and headache from the frontal sinuses.

Temporomandibular Joint Dysfunction Syndrome

The symptoms associated with this syndrome vary considerably. However, they are of a regional nature and patients with temporomandibular joint (TMJ) problems may persistently claim that the pain they are experiencing is coming from the teeth. TMJ pain is always localized to the upper jaw. It is not as intense as advanced pulpalgia or pain from periapical inflammation, but has a chronic, long-standing character and is, therefore, quite irritating. *Soreness and edema in the area of*

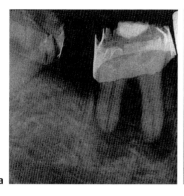
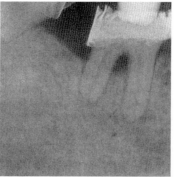

a   b

Fig. 3.7
a Radiograph of a mandibular first molar extremely tender to percussion. Based on the clinical and radiographic findings, symptomatic apical periodentitis was diagnosed. Endodontic instrumentation provided no relief, and an additional examination revealed a periodontal abscess in the furcation area superimposed on the large endodontic lesion. Drainage of the furcation provided immediate relief.
b Radiograph after 6 months of calcium hydroxide treatment. At this time with complete periapical healing, the furcation lesion of periodontal origin is visualized.

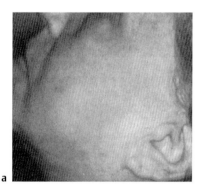
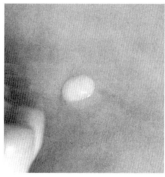

a   b

Fig. 3.8
a Patient with facial swelling because of an infection of the parotid gland.
b Intraorally, pus is seen emerging from the salivary duct.

the joint may be evident and frequently movement of the mandible is limited. It is important to remember that most TMJ symptoms are due to stress or stress-related factors. Patients with these problems, therefore, often need medical attention.

Trigeminal Neuritis

Inflammation of the trigeminal nerve may cause pain of low to moderate intensity. The causes of the condition are usually bacterial or viral infections centrally in the nervous system, but local irritation may cause a neuritis as well. An example of the local type is the so-called nonpurulent exacerbation that may occur during endodontic treatment, probably due to over-instrumentation or the use of toxic medicaments, or both. Clinically, this is a rather undramatic condition since no abscess formation or swelling occurs and no exudate is seen in the root canal. However, the pain is continuous and quite intolerable and will last for about 10 days. The treatment can only be palliative, and a moderate analgesic therapy should be instituted.

Herpes zoster neuritis is an infectious viral disease of an extremely painful and incapacitating nature and may involve the face and mouth by infection of the trigeminal nerve. Sometimes the patient localizes the pain to a quadrant of a jaw or even a single tooth. The diagnosis may be difficult since possible vesicles or blisters in the mouth may develop several days after the onset of the pain. If herpes zoster neuritis is suspected, the patient should be referred to a neurologist.

Chronic Neurogenic Pain

The pain conditions discussed above were all normal physiological reactions to injury or disease, i.e., the patients suffered from *acute pain.* Acute pain may be regarded as a warning system of the body to prevent further injury. It is self-limiting and stops when the cause of the pain is removed.

Chronic pain on the other hand, typically persists after removal of the cause of the pain. Chronic pain may be due to intense and long-lasting stimulation of peripheral pain receptors resulting in the development of dysfunction in the nervous system or to central neuroplastic changes without peripheral injury or disease. After a few months, chronic pain will as a rule have a *psychogenic component.* A chronic pain condition is today accepted as a disease in itself.

The dental nerves undergo changes that may lead to the development of chronic neurogenic pain. Thus, the first deafferentation occurs already when the primary teeth are lost. Then there is a relatively stable period, but in midlife most individuals will have alterations/injuries of the dental nerves both peripherally and centrally because of trauma, extraction of wisdom teeth and other teeth, caries and periodontitis (infection), and endodontic treatment. Ten thousand somatosensoric nerve fibres (pain receptors) enter the pulp of a single-rooted tooth through the apical foramina. This means that when a pulpectomy is performed in a maxillary molar, some 30000 nerve fibres are transsected. Moreover, when the pulp of a molar tooth necrotizes, some 30000 nerve endings become necrotic. Logically, these peripheral insults to the nerve should have an effect more centrally in the nervous system, and animal experiments have shown that the corresponding central neuron shows an increase in activity and receptive area up to 1 year following endodontic treatment. In clinical follow-up studies it has been found that as many as 5% of patients receiving endodontic treatment may develop a chronic neurogenic pain condition.

Chronic neurogenic pain may be paroxysmal (neuralgia) or continuous. Patients suffering from *trigeminal neuralgia* may see a dentist because the pain is felt in the jaws, especially the maxilla, in spite of the fact that it derives from intracranial causes. Often the pain appears to be localized in one tooth or several teeth, or, typically, the pain may be released by touching the skin or mucosa in the vicinity of a tooth (*trigger zone*). Typical for the symptoms associated with trigeminal neuralgia are attacks of pain with a duration from 10s to 2–3min. The pain reaches a maximum intensity instantly and decreases after 20–30s. After an attack, there is a pain-free period when a new pain attack cannot be released (*refractory period*). This phenomenon is an important differential-diagnostic criterion and quite characteristic for the condition. Patients who are suspected of suffering from trigeminal neuralgia should be referred to a neurologist.

The continuous neurogenic pain is commonly referred to as *neuropathic pain.* Neuropathic pain occurs when a multireceptive neuron lowers its threshold for activation, either spontaneously or after long-lasting and intense pain stimulation. The neuron loses its ability to differentiate between different stimuli like pressure, touch, temperature, and pain, and all stimulation will be interpreted as pain. The pain will then be sustained by the normal tone of the nerve fibers. As appears from the above, *trigeminal neuropathic pain* may begin spontaneously in central neurons without peripheral stimulation. Still the pain may be projected to a definite area of the mouth, most often a tooth, and although a thorough clinical and radiographic examination shows no signs of disease in the painful area, the patient will be absolutely convinced that the pain is coming from that area. Even though irreversible therapy should not be carried out based on a diagnosis of pain only, the actual situation may become so unclear and difficult that pulp extirpation or extraction of a tooth is carried out. This type of treatment will intensify the central neuroplastic changes and lead to an increase in the size of the peripheral receptive area so that neighboring teeth may hurt as well. A pathological interaction with the autonomous nervous system may occur and give symptoms like redness, swelling, tears, stuffy nose, etc. that easily may be misinterpreted as signs of local inflammation. The hunt for a peripheral cause of the pain may then continue.

However, local, peripheral injury or disease as well as treatment of the peripheral condition with long-lasting nociseptive pain may also give rise to neuroplastic changes that again may lead to chronic neuropathic pain. It is then important to understand that the pain will persist even if the original, peripheral cause of the pain is removed. Repeated endodontic and surgical interventions may only make the situation worse.

The symptoms in patients with trigeminal neuropathic pain may offer difficult differential-diagnostic problems, even if one is familiar with the condition. Also, it is difficult or downright impossible for these patients to accept that no invasive therapy can correct their problem. They regularly develop into "doctor hoppers" in an attempt to get relief. As a result they become amazingly familiar with professional terminology, the symptomatology of oral diseases, and likely therapeutic measures. After a while, therefore, it is difficult to get a reliable history from patients with neuropathic pain, and many times useless irreversible therapy is performed because the patient is able to fool the dentist. Patients with chronic neurogenic pain should be referred to a neurologist or preferably to a clinic specializing in the treatment of chronic pain.

Referred pain

In some instances pain may be localized to an area from which it does not originate. This is called *referred pain.* There are many such projection areas in the mouth and face, probably due to the fact that the trigeminal, facial, glossopharyngeal, and vagus nerves pass closely together.

Referred pain is commonly seen in the teeth. Typically, a well-developed pulpalgia may fail to localize in the offending tooth, but instead radiate to other teeth, often in the opposite jaw, or to various areas in the head and neck. A well-known example is pain originating in a mandibular molar which is referred to the ear.

The teeth are sites for referred pain from infections and tumors as well as many vascular and muscular conditions in the head and neck. Thus, certain forms of *migraine* can give projections that cover part of the face and therefore can be suspected to be of dental origin. However, the history usually gives information that points to the correct etiology. Characteristically, migraine pain begins suddenly and lasts for a few hours. As a rule, the patient will not be able to see a dentist until the pain attack is over.

On occasion *thoracic viscera such as the heart* may refer pain to the teeth. The pain is usually associated with *angina pectoris* and the patients will normally have other symptoms which may aid in the diagnosis such as chest pain and pain in the left arm. However, cases have been reported in which pain that was diagnosed as being of pulpal origin was the first and only symptom of an impending heart attack. Usually the pain referred from the heart affects teeth of the lower left mandible. However, the pain may also be referred to the maxilla and even to teeth on the patient's right side. Thus, if other symptoms of angina pectoris are not obvious, these patients present with an extremely difficult diagnostic problem. Our reward if we are able to arrive at the correct diagnosis is that we may be instrumental in saving the patient's life.

Further Reading

Avery JK, Rapp R. Pain condition in human dental tissues. Dent Clin North Am 1959, pp 489 – 501.

Baume L. Dental pulp conditions in relation to carious lesions. Int Dent J 1970;20:308 – 321.

Brännström M, Åström A. The hydrodynamics of the dentine; its possible relationship to dentinal pain. Int Dent J 1972;22:219 – 227.

Cooper SA. The relative efficacy of ibuprofen in dental pain. Compen Contin Educ Dent 1986;8:578 – 597.

Dubner R, Hargreaves KM. The neurobiology of pain and its modulation. Clin J Pain 1989;5:Suppl 2, 51 – 56.

Fearnhead RW. Histological evidence for the innervation of human dentine. J Anat [London] 1959;91: 267 – 277.

Frank RM, Sauvage L, Frank P. Morphological basis of dental sensitivity. Int Dent J 1972;22:1 – 19.

Hargreaves KM, Dionne RA. Endogenous pain pathways: application to pain control in dental practice. Compend Contin Educ Dent 1982;3:161 – 216.

Klausen B, Helbo M, Dabelsteen E. A differential diagnostic approach to the symptomatology of acute dental pain. Oral Surg Oral Med Oral Pathol 1985; 59:297 – 301.

Law AS, Lilleg JP. Trigeminal neuralgia mimicking odontogenic pain. Oral Surg Oral Med Oral Pathol 1995;80:96 – 100.

Natkin E, Harrington GW, Mandel MA. Anginal pain referred to the teeth. Oral Surg Oral Med Oral Pathol 1973;40:678 – 680.

Owatz CB, Khan AA, Schindler WG, Schwartz SA, Keiser K, Hargreaves KM. The incidence of mechanical allodynia in patients with irreversible pulpitis. J Endod 2007;33:552–558.

Sessle BJ. Acute and chronic craniofacial pain: brainstem mechanisms of nociceptive transmission and neuroplasticity, and their clinical correlates. Crit Rev Oral Biol Med 2000;11:57–91.

Sessle BJ. The neural basis of temporomandibular joint and masticatory muscle pain. J Orofac Pain 1999;13:238–245.

Sigurdsson A, Jacoway JR. Herpes zoster infection presenting as an acute pulpitis. Oral Surg Oral Med Oral Pathol 1995;80:92–95.

Tanaka TT. Facial pain disorders commonly confused with TMJ dysfunction. J Can Dent Ass 1985;13:56–61.

Tronstad L. The anatomic and physiologic basis for dentinal sensitivity. Compend Contin Educ Dent 1982;3:99–104.

Tsatsas BG, Frank RM. Ultrastructure of the dentinal tubular substances near the dentinoenamel junction. Calcif Tiss Res 1972; 9: 238–242.

4

Endodontic Examination and Diagnosis

As was mentioned above, as many as 90% of patients with oral or maxillofacial pain should be examined for endodontic diseases. A correct diagnosis is arrived at by combining information from the patient and sometimes the patient's physician with the actual clinical findings. Although the diagnosis may often appear obvious and straightforward, the clinical examination should always be thorough and systematic. Only then can the dentist's knowledge and clinical experience be fully utilized. A good chart system is invaluable in this regard.

History

Taking the history is an important part of the clinical examination, often giving information that immediately points to the patient's illness. Since there are virtually no systemic contraindications to endodontic treatment, the medical history can normally be short and of a summary nature. However, it is necessary to form a picture of the general health of the patient, and not infrequently this information will contribute directly to the dental diagnosis. The following questions must be included in a medical history:
Do you have heart problems?
Are you allergic to anything?
Are you diabetic?
Have you been infected with hepatitis or HIV?
Are you taking any medication at the moment?
What is your physician's name, address, and phone number?

Depending on the patient's answers, the history will develop in as great a depth as is deemed necessary. Do not hesitate to call the patient's physician for information, and with obviously sick patients it is advisable to treat them with the knowledge of and in cooperation with their physicians.

The *dental history* should identify the reason why the patient is seeking dental care (*chief complaint*). First the patient must be allowed to describe this reason *in his or her own words*. Afterward the dentist asks necessary leading questions to expand on the information given by the patient. During the interview the patient usually remembers additional information and a rather complete picture of the patient's problem will develop.

Clinical Examination

The clinical examination begins with an extraoral inspection while taking the patient's history. The examination is then extended to the area the patient has referred to in the history and to adjacent and contralateral areas. One quick glance may be enough to arrive at the diagnosis and to decide on appropriate therapy. For example, a tooth may be so damaged by caries that a remaining root rest will have to be extracted. Other times visual findings like caries, discolorations, swellings, fistulae, etc. may lead to other considerations. The clinical examination then continues with the aid of a mirror, explorer, periodontal probe, and other instruments and devices as found to be practical or necessary for a general oral/dental examination.

Percussion and Palpation Tests

The percussion test is a simple but extremely useful examination method which is used to ascertain an inflammatory condition in the apical periodontium of a tooth. The handle of a hand instrument, usually a mirror, is used to tap on the teeth in a *vertical direction*. A tooth with symptomatic apical periodontitis will then be more sensitive to the percussion than the contralateral or neighboring teeth. Only remember, healthy teeth may be somewhat sensitive to percussion as well and if the symptoms from an apical periodontitis are weak or uncertain, it is important to test several teeth repeatedly in no special order to ensure consistency in the observations. Pulpal diseases cannot be revealed by means of the percussion test until the apical periodontium is involved. On the other hand, a pe riodontal abscess or even asymptomatic periodontal disease with severe loss of marginal bone may render teeth tender to percussion. However, such teeth will react mostly to *horizontal percussion*, i.e., percussion perpendicular to the long axis of the tooth and less to vertical percussion like endodontically involved teeth. The percussion test is the examination method that will first give *clinical indications* of an apical periodontitis.

Palpation is performed to ascertain tenderness, swelling, fluctuation, hardness, and crepitation in underlying tissues. Here again it is important to make comparative examinations of neighboring and contralateral areas. Intraorally the palpation test preferably is carried out with the tip of an index finger. Sometimes and in special areas like the floor of the mouth it may be practical to use the index finger on both hands. During extraoral palpation of lymph nodes, swellings, sinus, and tempero-mandibular joint areas, etc., two to three fingers on one or both hands are used. The palpation test may be very useful during an endodontic examination and its usefulness will only increase with increasing skill and clinical experience.

Sensitivity Tests

Sensitivity tests are performed in an effort to determine whether the pulp of a tooth is vital or not. This test is often of crucial importance. The sensitivity of a tooth can be tested in many ways. Normally heat, cold, or electrical stimulation are used. With all test methods it is imperative that the tooth to be tested be clean and completely dry so that the possibilities for conduction of the stimulus to nerves of the gingiva and the periodontal ligament are minimized. For a heat test, temporary stopping (gutta-percha) may be used. It is heated over an alcohol flame and with a plastic instrument applied with slight pressure to assure good contact to the incisal edge or to the buccal surface of the tooth away from the gingiva. It is immediately removed if the patient shows a reaction, otherwise it is left in place until it cools off.

A *cold test* can be performed with ice, but more effective are frozen sticks of carbon dioxide ($-78\,°C$). Effective tests can also be carried out with a cotton pellet sprayed with difluorodichloromethane (DDM) ($-50\,°C$), which is *immediately* placed in good contact with the incisal edge or buccal surface of the tooth. The cotton pellet is removed if there is a reaction, or it is left in place until it has lost its effect.

For *electric sensitivity testing* a special apparatus, an electric pulp tester, is required. The electric pulp tester is equipped with an electrode that is placed in contact with the tooth to be tested as described for the thermal tests (**Fig. 4.1**). An electric current can then be supplied to the tooth through the electrode, and the current (or the voltage) is increased manually or automatically until the patient shows a reaction. The electrode is then immediately removed. Otherwise the test

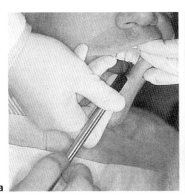
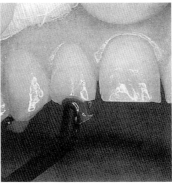

Fig. 4.1
a Electric pulp tester in use. Since the dentist wears rubber gloves, the patient needs to touch the handpiece of the testing device to complete the electric circuit.
b Test electrode in contact with the incisal edge of a tooth. Toothpaste is used to ensure good contact.

a   b

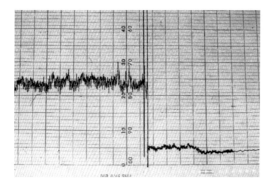

Fig. 4.2 Vitality testing of contralateral teeth with a laser Doppler flowmeter. Curve to the left, vital pulp with blood circulation. Curve to the right, non-vital pulp without blood circulation.

continues until maximum stimulus has been reached.

The *sensitivity tests* are not always reliable and the results of these tests obviously have to be evaluated together with other findings and symptoms. The electric test is considered by many to be the least reliable method. However, this method has many advantages and an electric pulp tester should be part of the armamentarium of every dental office. The main advantage of the electric test is that a specific value is obtained for the reaction threshold of the tooth. This value may then be used for the purpose of comparison between tests of different teeth and between repeated tests of a single tooth over time. This may be especially useful in the follow-up of traumatically injured teeth, but is generally useful in all follow-up examinations of vital teeth. The use of electric pulp testers in patients with pacemakers is contraindicated.

In instances when the noninvasive sensitivity test methods give inconclusive results, it will most often be possible to determine whether the pulp is vital or not by the *preparation of a test cavity* in the crown of the tooth and toward the pulp. The cavity is placed in a location so that it may later become the access cavity for root canal treatment of the tooth if the pulp is found to be necrotic. On the other hand, if there is a vital response from the tooth, the drilling is stopped and the test cavity is restored like any other cavity with a base and a filling material. The test cavity method is especially useful in teeth with crown restorations and the crown margins in contact

with the gingival tissues. It may also be useful in young teeth with incompletely formed roots that respond erratically to all types of sensitivity tests, probably because the nerve supply to the pulp of these teeth is not sufficiently developed.

Recently, efforts have been made to develop test methods which, rather than triggering a nervous response, aim at determining whether or not there is blood circulation in the pulp. Promising results have been obtained, for instance, with laser Doppler flowmetry (**Fig. 4.2**), although its use in dentistry is hampered by a certain lack in reproducibility of the results because of sensitivity of the test electrode to motion, and by the high cost of the apparatus. Pulse oximetry is another noninvasive method widely used in medical practice to evaluate vascular health by measuring blood oxygen saturation. The results of a recent study on teeth are interesting, and suggest that the method may be become useful to determine pulp vitality.

Provocation Tests

Thermal stimulation may be of value in provoking symptoms from teeth with asymptomatic pulpitis. A rather common situation is a patient presenting with a history of toothache at night, often repeatedly over a period of time. At the time of the examination, however, the patient has no pain and no signs or symptoms point to a specific tooth. It may then be possible by thermal stimulation of the teeth in the area of the mouth indicated by the patient to detect the offending tooth. Both cold and heat stimulation may be used, although in most instances heat will be the most effective. The offending tooth may then be recognized because the provoked pain will remain for a period of time after the stimulation of the tooth has been discontinued.

Anesthesia Test

On occasion patients will present with symptoms of pulpitis, sometimes severe, without any signs pointing to the offending tooth. Provocation tests are usually not helpful in this situation since the pain is already strong and continuous. The patient is in agony and expects or even requests that something be done. Selective infiltration of a local anesthetic solution may then be helpful. In recent years *intra-ligament anesthesia* has been used, because with this method small amounts of anesthetic solution can be placed with great accuracy so that it conceivably affects the pulp of only one or two teeth. When the anesthesia test is used, the most distal tooth is anesthetized first and then one tooth at a time in a mesial direction until the pain goes away.

Optical Tests

Optical tests may be performed to determine the presence of cracks and incomplete fractures in the teeth. Coronal cracks may cause a variety of symptoms, depending on their location and extension in the tooth, and they may be very difficult to diagnose. The use of a strong local light source, most conveniently a fiberoptic light, may then be advantageous in that the crack will often effectively stop the penetration of the light through the tooth (**Fig. 4.3**).

Dyes like iodine or plaque-disclosing solutions may also be applied to teeth with suspected incomplete fractures. They should be applied under a rubber dam for a period of 5–6 minutes and as penetration into the crack occurs the crack is vi-

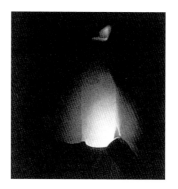

Fig. 4.3 Vertical crack in a tooth visualized by means of strong light. The crack stops most of the light and thereby becomes visible.

sualized. The diagnosis "*cracked*" or "*incompletely fractured tooth*" can then usually be verified by careful selective biting on a semi-hard object like a small wooden stick.

Radiographic Examination

Modern endodontic diagnostics rely heavily on a radiographic examination. Often the radiographic findings determine the diagnosis outright. Remember, therefore, that radiographic findings are not pathognomonic for a special disease or pathological condition. A radiolucent area at the apex of a tooth is normally a sign of apical periodontitis, but it may also be indicative of a cementoma, a giant cell granuloma, various cysts, cancer metastases, and many other pathological and even normal conditions (see p. 54). The radiographic findings must, therefore, always and without exception be evaluated together with the findings of the clinical examination.

Preferably, *a long cone parallelling* technique should be used for periapical examination in order to obtain as true a radiographic orientation of the teeth and their supporting structures as possible. Moreover, a *film holder* that allows periodic-comparable radiographs to be taken should be used. This is especially important in all follow-up examinations when recent radiographs are compared with films taken at previous appointments (**Fig. 4.4**).

The occlusal radiograph is sometimes valuable in endodontic diagnosis (**Fig. 4.5**). It provides a more extensive view of the jaws, especially the maxilla, and it is an invaluable aid in determining the buccolingual extension of large periapical lesions. The occlusal projection may be especially useful in patients with traumatic injuries of their teeth and supporting structures.

Tentative Diagnosis

Sometimes the clinical and radiographic examinations are inconclusive and the patient is in pain. *It is then important not to initiate irreversible treatment without a definite diagnosis.* We still have to do our utmost to get the patient out of pain and the correct procedure is to make a tentative diag-

nosis. Most often this situation occurs in patients who have taken good care of their teeth and have multiple restorations rather than untreated cavities, and most often it has been possible to identify the quadrant with the painful tooth. Guided mainly by the radiographic findings (deepest re-

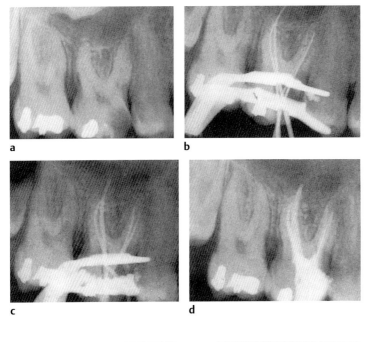

a

b

c

d

Fig. 4.4 Series of radiographs taken with the long cone parallelling technique and a film holder during endodontic treatment of a maxillary molar.
a Preoperative radiograph.
b Tooth length radiograph.
c Master cone trial radiograph.
d Postoperative radiograph. Maxillary molars are the most difficult teeth of which to obtain periodic-comparable radiographs. However, with a good technique, good results can be obtained.

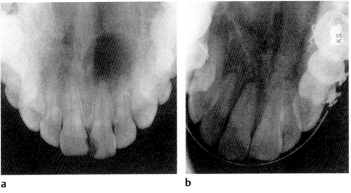

a

b

Fig. 4.5 Occlusal radiographs of maxillary anterior teeth.
a Extension of a periapical lesion from the left central incisor is demonstrated.
b Extrusive and lateral displacement of incisors is visualized.

storation in quadrant, suspicion of carious dentin under restoration, evidence of "sloppy" restorative work, etc.), the tooth from which the pain most likely originates is determined. All restorations in this tooth are then removed in order to inspect the cavity floors. Quite often in such instances, soft carious dentin or an old pulp exposure is found and the diagnosis is clear. However, it may also be that no further clinical observations are made. The cavity is then filled with zinc oxide–eugenol cement, which has an excellent local anesthetic and sedative effect and will relieve even severe pulpal pain effectively (see p. 86). If necessary, one tooth at a time is treated this way until a definite diagnosis has been established and permanent therapy can be performed.

Clinical Diagnosis

As discussed above, in traditional endodontic diagnostic terminology, great efforts were made to relate the actual (microscopic) state of the pulp to clinical signs and symptoms. As a result, traditional endodontic diagnostic systems comprised both histological and clinical terms (Table 4.1).

Today it is accepted that the degree of damage in an inflamed pulp cannot be determined by clinical means, but only after laboratory examinations of the tissue (Table 3.1). Below, a simple and practical clinical diagnostic system that utilizes only *clinical terminology* is presented.

Table 4.1 Clinical diagnostic systems as presented in textbooks on endodontics

	Tronstad	Walton & Torabinejad	Ingle & Beveridge	Cohen & Burns	Grossman
PULPAL DIAGNOSIS	Healthy pulp	Normal	No mention	No mention	Normal
	Asymptomatic pulpitis	Reversible pulpitis	Incipient acute pulpalgia	Reversible pulpitis	Hyperemia Asymptomatic (chronic) Reversible pulpitis Symptomatic (acute)
	Symptomatic pulpitis	Irreversible pulpitis	Moderate & advanced Acute pulpalgia Chronic pulpalgia	Irreversible pulpitis	Irreversible pulpitis Acute Chronic Asymp. with pulp exposure
		Hyperplastic pulpitis	Hyperplastic pulposis		Hyperplastic pulpitis
	Necrotic pulp	Necrosis	Necrosis	Necrosis	Necrosis
PERIAPICAL DIAGNOSIS	Normal	Normal	Normal	Normal	Normal
	Symptomatic apical periodontitis	Acute apical periodontitis	Acute apical periodontitis	Acute apical periodontitis	Acute apical periodontitis (vital and nonvital)
	Asymptomatic apical periodontitis	Chronic apical periodontitis	Chronic apical periodontitis	Chronic apical periodontitis	Granuloma
	Apical periodontitis with abscess	Suppurative apical periodontitis	Suppurative apical periodontitis	Suppurative apical periodontitis	Chronic alveolar Abscess (if fistula is present)
	Apical periodontitis with fistula	Acute apical abscess	Acute apical abscess	Acute apical abscess	Acute alveolar abscess
			Phoenix abscess	Phoenix abscess	
		Apical cyst	Apical cyst	Apical cyst	Cyst
	Condensing apical periodontitis	Condensing osteitis	Apical condensing osteitis	Periapical osteosclerosis	Condensing osteitis

Healthy pulp. This diagnostic term implies that the pulp is *vital* and presumably *free of inflammation*. The diagnosis is used, for example, when endodontic treatment of an intact tooth is indicated for prosthetic or other reasons, or during the first hours after a traumatic injury of a tooth with coronal fracture and pulp exposure.

Pulpitis. This diagnostic term implies that the pulp is *vital* and *inflamed*. The diagnosis says nothing about the degree of damage in the pulp or whether the inflammation is reversible or irreversible since this information cannot be obtained by clinical means. Although it normally has little bearing on the choice of therapy, it can be of value to know if a patient had symptoms or not when the treatment was initiated. It is, therefore, practical to have two clinical diagnoses for the inflamed pulp.

Symptomatic pulpitis. This diagnostic term implies that the pulp is vital, inflamed, and that the patient has *symptoms of pulpitis*. While symptomatic pulpitis can be acute, it is normally an *exacerbation of a chronic inflammation* in the pulp.

Asymptomatic pulpitis. This diagnostic term implies that the pulp is *vital* and *inflamed* and that the patient has no *symptoms*. The diagnosis is made on the basis of our knowledge of the etiology of pulpal inflammation and the reaction pattern of the pulp. A typical example of when this diagnosis should be used would be a vital, asymptomatic tooth with a carious pulp exposure.

Necrotic pulp. This diagnostic term implies that the pulp is *nonvital* or *necrotic*. This condition may be suspected when there is a *negative reaction to sensitivity tests*, but the diagnosis can be made with certainty only after inspection of the root canal space. The pulp necrosis can be partial or total, which can be of significance for the choice of therapy.

Apical periodontitis. This diagnostic term implies a *pulp-related* inflammation in the apical periodontium. The inflammation can be limited to the periodontal ligament, but normally involves the root cementum and dentin and the alveolar bone (*apical granuloma, cyst*).

Symptomatic apical periodontitis. This diagnostic term implies that the periapical inflammation begins with an acute phase or that an *exacerbation of a chronic apical periodontitis* occurs. In instances of acute periapical inflammation, radiographic changes will not be evident.

Asymptomatic apical periodontitis. This diagnostic term implies that the apical periodontitis has developed *without symptoms*. The condition may be suspected when the pulp is necrotic, but the diagnosis can only be made *after radiographic examination* showing a radiolucent (in rare instances radiopaque) area at the apex of the tooth.

Apical periodontitis with abscess. This diagnostic term implies that the periapical inflammation has caused a purulent breakdown of periapical tissues with accumulation of pus and abscess formation in the periodontium, *subperiostally, submucosally, or subcutaneously.*

Apical periodontitis with fistula. This diagnostic term implies that periapical exudate discharges onto a body surface, establishing a fistula with periapical drainage.

The terms *"lateral"* or *"interradicular"* are substituted for "apical" when the periodontitis is on the side of the root or in the furcation area of a multirooted tooth.

Further Reading

Baume LJ. Diagnosis of diseases of the pulp. Oral Surg Oral Med Oral Pathol 1970;29:102–116.

Cooley RL, Robinson SF. Variables associated with electric pulp testing. Oral Surg Oral Med Oral Pathol 1980;50:66–73.

Dummer PMH, Hicks R, Huws D. Clinical signs and symptoms in pulp disease. Int Endod J 1980;13:27–35.

Fuss Z, Trowbridge H, Bender IB, Rickoff B, Sorin S. Assessment of reliability of electrical and thermal pulp testing agents. J Endod 1980;12:301–305.

Gopikrishna V, Tinagupta K, Kaudaswamy D. Evaluation of efficacy of a new custom made pulse oximeter dental probe in comparison with the electrical and thermal tests for assessing pulp vitality. J Endod 2007;33:411–414.

Ingolfson ÆR, Riva CE, Tronstad L. Reliability of laser Doppler flowmetry in testing vitality of human teeth. Endod Dent Traumatol 1994;10:185–188.

Langeland K. Management of the inflamed pulp associated with deep carious lesions. J Endod 1981;7:169–181.

Närhi M. The characteristics of intradental sensory units and their responses to stimulation. J Dent Res 1985;64:564.

Nissan R, Trope M, Zhang CD, Chance B. Dual wavelength spectrophotometry as a diagnostic test of the pulp chamber contents. Oral Surg Oral Med Oral Pathol 1992;74:508–514.

Okesson JP, Falan DA. Nonodontogenic toothache. Dent Clin North Am 1997;41:367–383.

Petersson K, Söderström C, Kiani-Anaraki M, Levy G. Evaluation of the ability of thermal and electric tests to register pulp vitality. Endod Dent Traumatol 1999;15:122–133.

Seltzer S, Bendler IB, Zionitz M. The dynamics of pulp inflammation: correlation between diagnostic data and actual histologic findings in the pulp. Oral Surg Oral Med Oral Pathol 1963;16:846–871.

Sharar Y, Levimer E, Tzukert A, McGrath PA. The spatial distribution, intensity and unpleasantness of acute dental pain. Pain 1984;20:363–370.

Steiman HR. Endodontic diagnostic techniques. Curr Opin Dent 1991;6:723–728.

Trope M, Jaggi J, Barnett F, Tronstad L. Vitality testing of teeth with a radiation probe using 133 xenon radioisotope. Endod Dent Traumatol 1986;2:215–218.

Van Hassel HJ, Harrington GW. Localization of pulpal sensation. Oral Surg Oral Med Oral Pathol 1969;28:573–580.

Yanpiset K, Vongsavan N, Sigurdson A, Trope M. Efficacy of laser Doppler flowmetry for the diagnosis of revascularization of reimplanted immature dog teeth. Dent Traumatol 2001;17:63–70.

5

Treatment of Teeth with Vital Pulp

Endodontic Aspects of Restorative Procedures

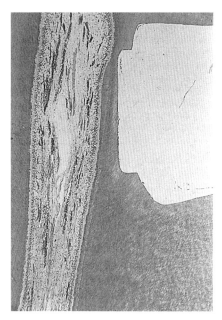

Fig. 5.1 Extremely deep cavity prepared with ultraspeed, low-torque equipment, a sharp bur, and an abundance of water. The cavity was restored with a calcium hydroxide base and amalgam. After 30 days, a healthy pulp and only the slightest amount of secondary dentin formation attest to the innocuousness and safety of the method.

As was discussed in the chapter on the etiology of pulpal inflammation (see p. 20), operative and restorative procedures may have harmful influences on the pulp. The pulpal changes may be irreversible and result in pulp necrosis. Milder iatrogenic irritation may cause symptoms of dental hypersensitivity which can be extremely troublesome for the patient for shorter or longer periods of time.

Postoperative discomfort can most often be prevented if accepted biological principles are adhered to during the treatment of the patient. The measures to prevent pulpal complications are simple and straightforward and can be easily incorporated into routine restorative techniques. In the following sections, simple guidelines are given.

Cavity and Crown Preparation

Cavity and crown preparation should be carried out with ultraspeed (>200 000 rpm), low-torque equipment, sharp burs, and an abundance of water. This technique is amazingly safe and cavities may be prepared to the immediate vicinity of the pulp, virtually without any changes or reaction in the pulp tissue (**Fig. 5.1**). Remember that *it is the use of an adequate water spray that is the key to the safety of the ultraspeed equipment* since only water can prevent a dehydration of the dentin by the otherwise unavoidable friction heat generated during the preparation of the tooth (**Fig. 5.2**). Only at 3000 rpm or lower should a bur be used without water in a dry cavity. This is useful during excavation of soft carious dentin in deep cavities. For this purpose and at this speed it may also be practical to use a high-torque handpiece since, with this equipment, a bur will *excavate* the soft carious dentin rather than cut it as might be the case if used with a low-torque handpiece.

Other than for detail work at *low speed, high-torque handpieces should preferably not be used in the preparation of cavities or crowns*. The high torque inevitably leads to a certain vibration of the bur which again may cause internal bleeding in the pulp. The blood may even flow into the dentinal tubules, coloring part of the crown or the entire crown red (**Fig. 5.3**). It is not clear at this time whether such an injury is reversible or not. However, infection of the blood clot is a likely occurrence, and especially if the tooth in question is to serve as an abutment for a bridge, it is common clinical practice to perform a pulpectomy and root filling on the tooth before the bridge is cemented.

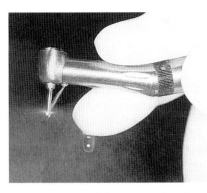

Fig. 5.2 Ultraspeed, low-torque handpiece with a bur running freely at full speed. The water is adjusted to hit the head of the bur. It is then dispersed by the rotation of the bur.

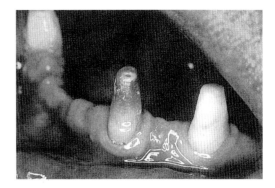

Fig. 5.3 Teeth being prepared as bridge abutments. In the middle tooth the coronal dentin is colored red due to intrapulpal bleeding.

Moreover, a bur may vibrate or rotate eccentrically if it has become bent. This happens quite often, for instance, if care is not taken when a bur is introduced into a friction-grip handpiece. Therefore, even with the use of low-torque equipment one has to check regularly that *the bur runs concentrically.* This is especially important during crown preparation when long, thin, diamond burs that easily bend are often used.

Cavity Cleansing and Drying

Before a cavity is filled or a crown cemented, the dentin surface should be thoroughly cleansed. An effective and biologically sound way to do this is with water or, as is normally done in practice, with a spray of water and air. In other words, *the goal is not to disinfect the dentin, but to clean it* and remove saliva, blood, possible rests of materials, and other extraneous matter.

The clean dentin surface should then be dried with minimal dehydration of the dentin. This can be achieved with blasts of air to remove water from the adjacent mucosa, gingiva, and sulcular area of the tooth. Most of the water in the cavity will also have been removed by this regional drying. The final drying of the cavity is then done carefully with a few short blasts of air and cotton pellets in an effort not to dehydrate the underlying dentin. *It is important to develop a fast, effective, and biologically acceptable technique for the cleansing and drying of prepared dentin surfaces, since this clearly is one of the key factors in preventing patient discomfort and pain following treatment.*

Surface bacteria which might survive the cleansing and drying procedures will die when the cavity is restored or the crown cemented. If bacteria are found in a gap between a restoration and the cavity wall at a later time, they are new bacteria and have come in from the oral cavity as a result of marginal leakage. It is, therefore, inappropriate to use antibacterial drugs for the cleansing of cavities and teeth prepared for crowns.

Impression Methods

As with cavity and crown preparation, the most important factor during the taking of an impression is the prevention of dehydration of the dentin and subsequent pulp reactions. With the modern elastic impression materials this is not a problem if the tooth is not unnecessarily dehydrated prior to the taking of the impression. Even thermoplastic materials may be used if care is taken. The prepared tooth is then sprayed liberally with water and dried off carefully with cotton or gauze, leaving a moist dentin surface. The impression material is heated only to such an extent that it can be manipulated with the fingers, although with some difficulty (i.e., to 50–60 °C). When applied to the tooth, usually in a copper ring, the material is cooled off with water and removed as quickly as the method allows. The tooth is then immediately sprayed liberally with water to counteract the certain amount of dehydration that unavoidably occurs with this method. Obviously, from a preventive–endodontic point of view, thermoplastic impression materials should not be used, and with the improvements in the accuracy of other

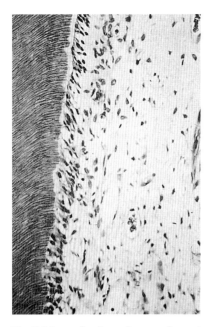

Fig. 5.4 Area of pulp under a cavity restored with a dry zinc oxide–eugenol paste. After 30 days, the pulp is normal. Note that secondary dentin has not formed (hematoxylin-eosin).

biologically more acceptable methods its use should at least be restricted to certain infrequent situations where this method might still appear to give superior results.

Pulp Protection

Materials with desirable biological properties, but which are too weak or otherwise not suitable to be used as restorative materials may be used as base materials in a cavity. There are two reasons for using a base material. The first reason is to protect the pulp from harmful components in a filling material and from marginal leakage. The second reason is to influence the repair processes in the pulp in a beneficial way to enhance healing. There are essentially two types of material available for cavity protection today: zinc oxide–eugenol and calcium hydroxide; most commercially available preparations are based on one of these materials.

A paste of zinc oxide and eugenol provides a bacteria-tight seal of the cavity. This is a very important characteristic of this material and is probably a main reason for its suitability as a base in a cavity. Also, eugenol is a local anesthetic with an

especially good effect on the C-fibers of the pulp, so that when a paste of zinc oxide and eugenol is placed in a cavity, enough eugenol may penetrate to the pulp to temporarily inhibit intradental nerve activity. Zinc oxide–eugenol paste, therefore, has an excellent sedative effect. In addition, eugenol is an antiseptic and, when mixed with zinc oxide, gives the paste a definite antibacterial effect. Eugenol also interferes with prostaglandin production in the pulp, so that a zinc oxide–eugenol cement has an anti-inflammatory effect as well.

The material has a certain toxic effect when tested in vitro. However, when used in a cavity, it has no adverse effect on the pulp (**Fig. 5.4**). On the contrary, the biocompatibility of the material is so well established that it is the accepted material for negative controls in studies on the pulpal effect of dental materials. Thus, zinc oxide and eugenol is exceptionally well suited as a base material, a sedative dressing, a temporary restoration, etc. It is interesting to know that it has been used for such purposes since the time of the pharaohs in ancient Egypt.

Zinc oxide and eugenol may also be used for temporary or semipermanent cementation of crowns. When used for this purpose, it should be remembered that the setting reaction of zinc oxide and eugenol is hydrophilic, which means that the material has a strong affinity for water and needs water to set. *A zinc oxide–eugenol cement, therefore, should be applied on a wet tooth.* Otherwise the material will take up fluids from the dentinal tubules and the pulp, often causing severe hypersensitivity of the tooth.

The use of zinc oxide and eugenol is contraindicated under all resin materials since eugenol interferes with the polymerization of a resin. However, where maximum pulp protection is sought, zinc oxide and eugenol should always be used, at least in the deeper parts of the cavity. If a resin then is used to restore the tooth, the zinc oxide–eugenol material will have to be covered by a second base material which is compatible with the resin restoration.

Calcium hydroxide, when used in a base material, is well tolerated by the pulp (**Fig. 5.1**). It does not have the sedative effect of zinc oxide and eugenol, but has an excellent antibacterial effect, an anti-inflammatory effect, and can be used under all types of restorative materials. Calcium hydroxide cements will usually not provide a lasting bacteria-tight seal of the cavity. Although the materials have been shown to initially block the dentinal tubules quite effectively, it may gradually be washed out of a cavity when there is marginal leakage. Recently, light-cured calcium hydroxide–resin preparations have been brought on the market. These preparations appear to be tolerated by the pulp and are conceivably more stable than the two-component cements. However, the therapeutic effects of calcium hydroxide may be blocked by the cured resins of these products.

The use of resin-based *dentin adhesives* has presently become routine in operative dentistry. As a result, marginal leakage in conjunction with bonded restorations is greatly reduced. However, the use of adhesives has also to a great extent led to a discontinuation in the use of base materials under resin restorations. It is far from established that this is sound clinical practice. Patients commonly suffer from dental hypersensitivity following this type of treatment, and endodontists have noticed an increased number of teeth with resin restorations referred for endodontic treatment since the base materials were abolished. Therefore, it is questionable whether the well-established clinical practice of using a base under a resin restoration should be discontinued at this time. The classical rule that a base should be applied to the *deepest part* of a cavity if the cavity is

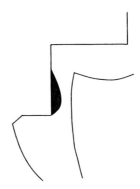

Fig. 5.5 Diagram illustrating a section through a class 2 cavity. The base material, when placed in the deepest part of the cavity, will protect the pulp, but not interfere with the placement of the restoration.

deeper than what is needed for retention purposes still seems to be valid (**Fig. 5.5**). This approach leaves more than enough free enamel and dentin surfaces to be used for bonding a restoration to the tooth.

Marginal Leakage

True adhesive filling materials do not exist at present and marginal leakage is a clinical problem with all types of restorative materials. Marginal leakage cannot be prevented in conjunction with

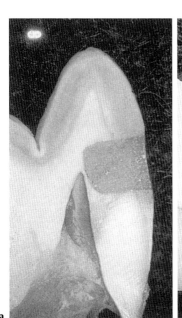
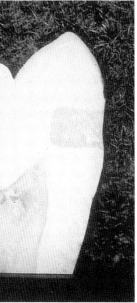

Fig. 5.6
a **Class 5 composite resin restoration placed without acid-etching of cavity walls.** Marginal leakage with penetration of a dye to the pulp can be seen.
b Class 5 composite resin restoration placed after acid-etching of cavity walls. No marginal leakage is evident.

a   b

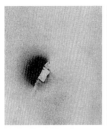 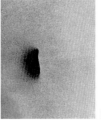

a   b

Fig. 5.7
a Class 5 amalgam restoration. Marginal leakage
 with penetration of a radioactive isotope around
 the restoration is seen.
b Class 5 amalgam restoration. A copal varnish was
 applied to the cavity walls before the amalgam
 was inserted. No marginal leakage is evident.

silicate or *glass ionomer cement fillings* (**Fig. 1.38**).
However, the fluoride released from these materials has a good anticaries effect and secondary caries is generally not a problem with these materials.

With early *resin restorations*, marginal discoloration and secondary caries were major problems,
and clinical use of the composite resins was about
to be discontinued when the acid-etch technique
became available (**Fig. 5.6**). By using the *acid-etch
technique* combined with a good resin-based adhesive system, the clinical problems with marginal leakage in conjunction with composite resin
restorations have been largely overcome.

With *amalgam restorations*, initial marginal
leakage can be prevented effectively by applying
a layer of varnish in the cavity before the amalgam is inserted (**Fig. 5.7**). The cavity varnish will
wash out gradually, but corrosion products from
the amalgam will fill the gap between the restoration and the cavity walls, resulting in a well-
sealed cavity. Since amalgam restorations are
well tolerated by the pulp, the cavity varnish will
provide adequate pulp protection as well in
many instances. However, in deep cavities a base
material is used in the deepest part, as discussed
above, and the varnish is applied to the cavity on
top of the base material in order to prevent marginal leakage. *Thus, a cavity varnish should be
used in conjunction with all amalgam restorations, in shallow and deep cavities, and in vital
and nonvital teeth.*

As can be seen from the above, biologically appropriate restorative treatment can be performed
with simple, routine clinical methods. One only
has to think in terms of prevention and pulp protection, and the number of cases with postoperative pain, iatrogenic pulpitis, and pulp necrosis
will be dramatically reduced.

Pulp Capping

Treatment of the exposed pulp by pulp capping
has a long clinical history. *The purpose of the
treatment is to keep the exposed pulp vital and
functioning in the tooth.* However, it soon became
apparent that pulp wounds have a definite tendency to heal poorly, and that pulp necrosis usually develops in pulp-capped teeth. Thus, in the
1930s the thesis that "the exposed pulp is a lost
organ" was generally accepted. Today, over 70
years later, pulp capping can still be a doubtful
treatment form. On the other hand, a number of
experimental studies have shown that pulp capping may have a success rate near 90% if specific
clinical criteria are met and the treatment is performed correctly. Therefore, an exposed pulp is
not necessarily a lost organ (**Fig. 5.8**).

For pulp capping to be successful, the following
factors are of decisive importance: the condition
of the pulp (preoperative diagnosis), the pulp-capping material, and the accomplishment of a permanent bacteria-tight seal of the pulp cavity.

Indications
The exposed pulp of a tooth to be treated with
pulp capping should be *healthy and free of
inflammation.* Since pulpal inflammation as a rule
is asymptomatic, this presents a problem in *preoperative diagnosis* that is most often unsolvable.
An exposed pulp free of inflammation can with
present methods be diagnosed with certainty only
when the exposure occurs accidentally, for example, as a result of crown preparation of an intact
tooth or, more commonly, as a result of a traumatic injury (complicated crown fracture). However, even if the pulp is healthy at the time of
exposure, it will soon become inflamed if left
exposed to the oral environment. Bacteria will
colonize the wound surface and may invade

super-ficial layers of the pulp since extravasated blood is usually present in the tissue. An accumulation of inflammatory cells may be present in the pulp subjacent to the exposure site already after 48 hours. The pulp capping should, therefore, if at all possible be performed within 2 days after the exposure occurred. If the treatment is then carried out correctly, the prognosis is excellent (approximately 90%).

Accidental pulp exposures constitute only a small portion of the teeth with exposed pulp. More frequently the pulp is exposed during excavation of soft carious dentin. *In these instances it must be assumed that the pulp is inflamed.* If pulp capping is performed in teeth with carious exposures, therefore, the number of failures will increase dramatically and a success rate in the area of 30–40% can be expected.

Thus, with our present knowledge and the materials and methods that are now available to us, the indications for treatment of the exposed pulp with pulp capping are rather narrow. However, in the teeth with healthy pulps where the treatment is indicated, it is an elegant and reliable method. *It is especially useful in the treatment of incompletely formed incisors in children where the preservation of the pulp will allow the development of the teeth to continue, resulting in fully formed, strong teeth that can function for a lifetime.*

Wound Dressing and Tissue Reactions

A vast number of materials and medicaments have been used as pulp-capping agents: gold and silver, different types of cements, antiseptic pastes, chemotherapeutics, ivory powder, dentin chips, plaster of Paris, magnesium oxide, calcium hydroxide, and many others. It is interesting to note that both biologically inert materials like gold and silver and irritating antiseptic preparations like phenolic compounds are equally unsuitable as pulp-capping agents.

The first important progress with this type of therapy was gained in the 1920s with a paste of zinc oxide and eugenol. This material has a mild antiseptic effect and seals the cavity well. Healing of the exposed pulp *without hard-tissue bridging* of the pulp wound was observed. An attempt was made at obtaining hard-tissue formation at the exposure site by covering the pulp wound with dentin chips or ivory powder under the zinc oxide and eugenol paste. This approach showed some promise, but it was not until the late 1930s when calcium hydroxide was introduced as the wound dressing that pulp capping as a clinical treatment method started to be taken seriously. With calcium hydroxide it became possible for the first time on a routine basis to obtain a healthy pulp, free of inflammation, covered by a hard-tissue barrier, a *dentin bridge*, at the exposure site (**Fig. 5.8**).

Calcium hydroxide is a white powder that can be mixed with physiological saline to a paste. The paste is highly alkaline with a pH of 12.5 and its application to the pulp results in *necrosis of the pulp tissue contacting the paste*. The necrotic area of the pulp is sharply limited and the subjacent vital pulp tissue shows no or only a mild inflammatory reaction (**Fig. 5.9**).

In the transition zone between the necrotic and the vital tissue, a relatively structureless "demarcation zone" is observed after a few days. This zone is rich in collagen and gradually becomes mineralized. It represents the beginning of the formation of the mineralized barrier. This first formed hard tissue contains no dentinal tubules, but after approximately 10 days odontoblasts which have differentiated from cells in the pulp are seen lining up along the pulpal aspect of the

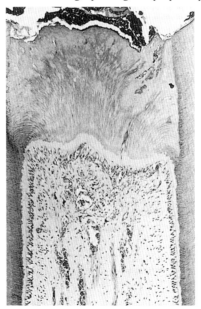

Fig. 5.8 Successful pulp capping in a monkey tooth. A dentin bridge has walled off the exposed pulp following calcium hydroxide treatment. The pulp is healthy and free of inflammation (hematoxylin-eosin).

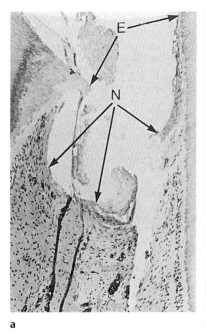
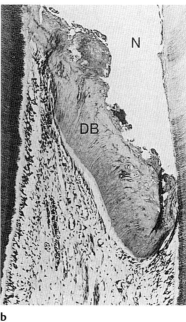

a   b

Fig. 5.9 Pulp capping of monkey teeth with exposed, healthy pulps (hematoxylin-eosin).
a After 8 days, an area of the pulp (N) subjacent to the calcium hydroxide paste placed on the pulp exposure (E) has become necrotic. The adjacent pulp tissue is free of inflammation.
b After 90 days, a dentin bridge (DB) has formed in the pulp adjacent to the necrotic tissue (N). The underlying pulp tissue is healthy and free of inflammation.

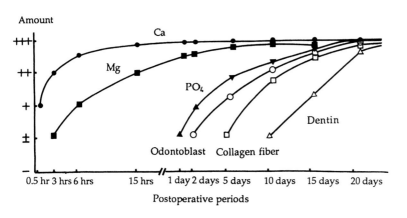

Fig. 5.10 Diagram showing the sequence of events during the formation of a dentin bridge following pulp capping of healthy pulp with calcium hydroxide.

hard tissue, and formation of tubular dentin onto the atubular tissue begins (**Fig. 5.10**). The dentin formation goes on until the bridge has reached a certain thickness and then stops, usually after about 60 days. The pulp is now again completely surrounded by hard tissue, and in successful cases will be healthy and free of inflammation.

This sequence of events represents the typical reaction of the *exposed, uninflamed pulp* to calcium hydroxide. However, as pointed out above, in some instances the reaction may take a different course and the treatment may not be successful. In particular, it must be understood that the

dentin bridge formation in itself is no guarantee of pulpal repair; the pulp may become necrotic after the dentin bridge formation has started (**Fig. 5.11**). When other materials such as magnesium oxide are used as a pulp capping agent, it is routinely observed that pulp necrosis follows dentin bridge formation.

Pulpal Seal

In addition to the preoperative status of the pulp and the choice of wound dressing, it is of crucial importance for the outcome of the treatment that the pulp cavity be sealed bacteria-tight until the dentin bridge has formed and pulpal repair is completed. If the pulp exposure occurs within a cavity, this presents no great problem. The calcium hydroxide is applied to the pulp wound and the cavity is filled with zinc oxide and eugenol which gives the necessary seal. However, if the pulp wound is located on a fractured dentin surface, it is very difficult to obtain a reliable seal. Traditionally, calcium hydroxide paste was applied to the wound in such instances and a temporary crown was cemented with zinc oxide and eugenol cement. However, due to the awkward shape of a fractured tooth, its smooth enamel surfaces, and the unavoidable biting on the temporary crown, leakage between the cement and the tooth surface readily occurred, causing the treatment to fail.

A reliable method of achieving the necessary bacteria-tight seal of the pulp cavity is to perform what might be termed *a mini-amputation of the pulp*. Using a sharp fissure bur in a low-torque ultraspeed handpiece, about 1.5 mm of the pulp tissue at the exposure sight is removed (**Fig. 5.12**). The bleeding is stopped by irrigation with sterile saline and slight compression with sterile cotton pellets. *A thin layer of calcium hydroxide paste is then applied to the pulp wound and the remainder of the cavity is filled with a paste of zinc oxide and eugenol which gives the necessary seal.* A temporary crown can then be cemented, and if leakage should occur between the tooth and the crown, the zinc oxide and eugenol matrial in the cavity will still provide a reliable pulpal seal. However, rather than restoring the tooth temporarily, a much more elegant method is to immediately restore the tooth with a semipermanent or permanent composite resin restoration using an acid-etch adhesive technique. The fractured dentin surface, including the zinc oxide and eugenol cement at the exposure site, is then covered with a hard-setting calcium hydroxide base material, the enamel is beveled, and after acid-etching, an adhesive is applied and the tooth is restored to its original shape (**Fig. 5.13**).

Follow-up Examination and Prognosis

Even when adhering to the narrow clinical indications outlined above, a failure rate of 10–20% will be observed after pulp capping, i.e., *the treatment will be unsuccessful in one to two of every 10 teeth treated.* The failures may not be clinically evident at once or even for a considerable time after the treatment, since, as is known, pulpal inflamma-

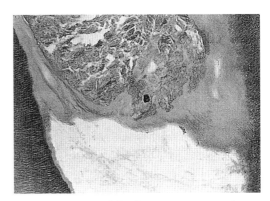

Fig. 5.11 Unsuccessful pulp capping in a monkey tooth. A dentin bridge has begun to form; however, the pulp has become necrotic (hematoxylin-eosin).

tion usually proceeds without symptoms. Thus, it is not unusual that failures after pulp capping are diagnosed after 2–3 or even more years. Follow-up examinations of pulp-capped teeth, therefore, are a must. They should be performed 3, 6, and 12 months after the treatment and later, once a year as deemed necessary.

The follow-up control should consist of a clinical examination with sensitivity tests and a radiographic examination. Although part of the incisal pulp is lost or has been removed, a meaningful sensitivity test can still be performed using the buccal surface of the tooth. Radiographically, the width of the root canal should be carefully examined and compared with the width of the canal of the contralateral or neighboring teeth. An increasing obliteration of the root canal may suggest a chronic inflammation in the pulp and failure of the treatment. A root canal that is wider than in the contralateral tooth usually means that the pulp has become necrotic, so that the formation of dentin on the root canal walls has stopped. Sometimes a failure becomes evident because of the presence of a periapical radiolucency.

During the follow-up controls it is important to check that the coronal restoration of the tooth is intact. The dentin bridge is important in that it renders a hard-tissue covering of the pulp. However, if bacteria are allowed to reach the bridge and colonize its surface, bacterial products will readily penetrate the bridge and cause pulpal inflammation. Obviously, this reaction is the same as may be observed under leaky restorations elsewhere in the mouth.

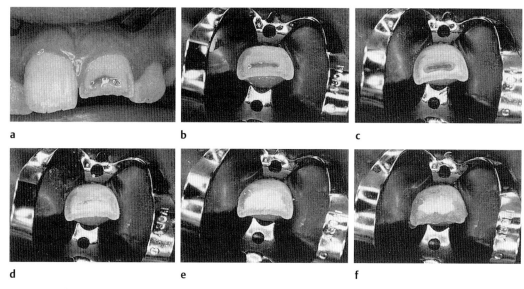

Fig. 5.12 Pulp capping: clinical procedures.

a Complicated crown fracture with pulp exposure of maxillary left central incisor. The patient is 12 years old and presents for treatment 2 hours following the accident.

b Rubber dam is applied and the field of operation is disinfected.

c Using a sharp sterile bur in a low-torque handpiece, about 1.5 mm of the pulp tissue at the exposure sight is removed. Bleeding is controlled.

d A thin layer of a paste of calcium hydroxide and saline is applied to the pulp wound.

e The remaining cavity is filled with zinc oxide–eugenol to establish a bacteria-tight seal.

f A temporary crown may then be applied or the tooth acid-etched and a composite resin restoration fabricated. (The eugenol-containing material is then covered with a cement compatible with the resin).

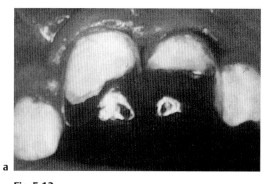

Fig. 5.13

a **Maxillary central incisors with complicated crown fractures.** After acid-etching, celluloid crown forms may be used with advantage to obtain the desired form of the teeth.

b Maxillary central incisors successfully restored with the acid-etch resin technique.

Certain additional factors have been considered to have an influence on the outcome of a pulp-capping procedure. The *size of the pulp exposure* is such a factor; in the literature it is often stated that the exposure should be less than 1 mm² in order for the treatment to be successful. However, there is no evidence to support this claim. On the contrary, it appears that the size of the pulp wound is without importance for the outcome of the treatment. An uninflamed pulp will form a large bridge just as readily as it forms a small bridge.

The *location of the exposure* has been another point of concern, and treatment of pulp wounds in the gingival third of the tooth has been considered by many to be contraindicated in that the local necrosis caused by calcium hydroxide in the cervical area might interrupt the blood supply to the coronal pulp. However, especially in young teeth, the area of necrosis will be small compared to the amount of pulp tissue, and the prognosis for pulp capping appears to be as good in the cervical region of the tooth as it is in a pulp horn.

The *age of the patient*, on the other hand, may affect the prognosis of pulp capping unfavorably. There is both clinical and experimental evidence to that effect, and in addition it is accepted today that age in general reduces the functional capacities of a tissue. However, advanced age is not a definite contraindication for pulp capping if other circumstances favor this treatment. On the other hand, *for fully formed teeth with exposed pulps, alternative treatment methods with exceptionally high success rates are available* (see p.97).

Capping of the Inflamed Pulp

Many attempts have been made to find pulp capping agents and develop methods that would give reliable results of pulp capping of teeth with carious exposures and inflamed pulps. The initial reaction to calcium hydroxide in these teeth is at least to some extent as described for teeth with healthy pulps. Thus, the local necrosis of the pulp tissue subjacent to the capping material is seen (**Fig. 5.14**). The inflammation in the tissue subjacent to the necrotic area, however, is much more pronounced, and it appears that the ability of calcium hydroxide to induce dentin bridge formation is impaired by the inflammation. On the whole, the reaction of the inflamed pulp to calcium hydroxide is erratic and unpredictable, and the percentage of unsuccessful cases will be intolerably high.

Promising clinical results have been obtained with *corticosteroid antibiotic preparations* as pulp-capping agents in teeth with inflamed pulps. These medicaments temporarily prevent or remove the symptoms of a pulpitis so that the treatment may appear successful in the short term. However, when such teeth are followed over time, the success rate steadily drops, and in one study it was down to 20% after 5 years. When the teeth of this study which were clinically successful after 5 years were extracted and examined under a microscope, the pulps in all teeth were necrotic. Antibiotics without corticosteroids have also been used, both systemically and locally on the pulp wound without success.

The best results in fact have been obtained in inflamed pulps with a paste of zinc oxide and eugenol as wound dressing, confirming old findings from the 1920s. However, dentin bridge formation will not occur under zinc oxide and eugenol materials, and consequently if the coronal restoration is lost, the pulp will again be exposed. On the whole it must be concluded that at present *the success rate of pulp capping of teeth with exposed, inflamed pulps is poor and that the treatment should not be carried out.* In mature teeth a pulpectomy should be performed, whereas in immature teeth where continued root formation is desirable, a pulpotomy is the treatment of choice.

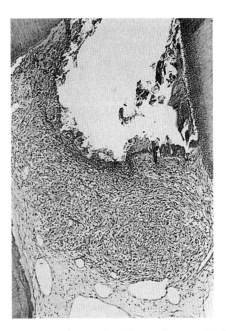

Fig. 5.14 Pulp capping of a monkey tooth with exposed, inflamed pulp. After 8 days, a necrotic area subjacent to the calcium hydroxide paste is recognized. In addition, a severe inflammatory reaction is seen in the vital pulp tissue (hematoxylin-eosin).

Pulpotomy

Pulpotomy, or pulp amputation, implies a *partial removal of the pulp.* Normally, the coronal pulp is removed to the level of the orifice of the root canal, but in certain instances if the pulp in the cervical region is visibly broken down, it is advantageous to amputate the pulp further apically in the root canal where the tissue clinically appears healthier. Such a procedure is referred to as *high amputation.*

Pulpotomy treatment developed as a logical consequence of the clinical experience that pulp capping of teeth with inflamed pulps is normally unsuccessful. Thus, the objective of a pulpotomy is the removal of the inflamed part of the pulp followed by application of a wound dressing (calcium hydroxide) to the remaining pulp tissue which then is allegedly free of inflammation (**Fig. 5.15**). If this is attained, the prognosis for a pulpotomy procedure is as good as for pulp capping of a tooth with an exposed pulp free of inflammation (**Fig. 5.16**).

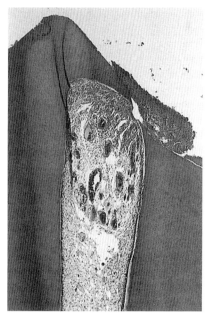

Fig. 5.15 Dog tooth with a complicated crown fracture. Two days following the exposure of the pulp, an inflammatory reaction is evident in the coronal pulp (hematoxylin-eosin).

Indications

The success rate of pulpotomy treatment depends to a great extent on the operator's ability to determine whether the pulpal inflammation is confined to the coronal pulp or has possibly progressed into the root pulp as well. Numerous studies have shown that this is not possible by clinical means, and that the diagnosis will be correct in only 50–60% of the teeth. *Consequently, the failure rate of pulpotomy treatment is high, and the treatment form is not considered acceptable as permanent therapy.*

None the less, pulpotomy has its definite place as a *temporary or semipermanent treatment method in teeth with incompletely formed roots where pulp capping is contraindicated because of diagnostic rea-*

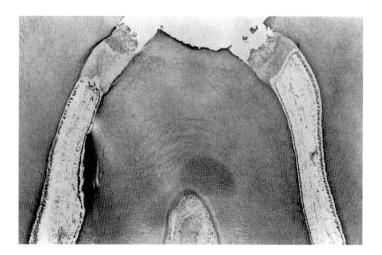

Fig. 5.16 Successful pulpotomy in a monkey tooth. Following calcium hydroxide treatment, dentin bridges have formed at the root canal orifices. The root pulps are healthy and free of inflammation (hematoxylin-eosin).

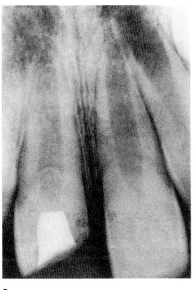
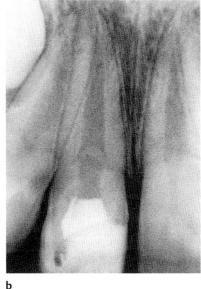

a

b

Fig. 5.17
a **Radiograph of the maxillary right central incisor of a 9-year-old.** Two months after pulpotomy treatment with calcium hydroxide, a dentin bridge is visible in the cervical area of the pulp.
b Follow-up radiograph after 6 months. The root development of the pulpotomized tooth appears to continue normally.

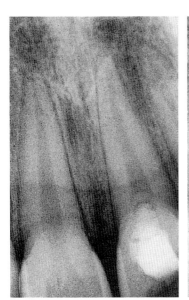
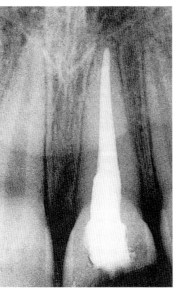

a

b

Fig. 5.18
a **This patient presented with severe symptomatic pulpitis in the maxillary left central incisor.** The radiographic examination revealed a previous, apparently successful, pulpotomy treatment of the tooth with dentin bridge formation in the cervical area of the pulp and normal root development when compared with the contralateral tooth. However, a late failure of the treatment is obvious at this time, underlining the fact that in good clinical practice a pulpotomy should be followed by a pulpectomy and root canal filling when symptoms are evident or when the root development is completed (**b**).

sons. The purpose of performing a pulpotomy in these teeth is to retain as much of the pulp tissue as possible, i.e., usually the root pulp, until the root development is completed (**Fig. 5.17**). What makes this a viable treatment form in spite of the diagnostic difficulties is the fact that the development of the root may continue even if the pulp is chronically inflamed. However, because of the risk of late failures, a pulpotomy should routinely be followed by pulpectomy and root canal filling as the final treatment when symptoms are evident or when the root development is completed (**Fig. 5.18**).

Wound Dressing and Tissue Reactions

Historically, as in pulp capping, phenol preparations and other strong antiseptics have been used routinely as wound dressing in pulpotomy treatment. However, since the late 1930s, *calcium hydroxide has been the dressing of choice.*

The tissue reactions to calcium hydroxide when used in pulpotomies are obviously the same as when the material is used as a pulp capping agent (**Fig. 5.16**). If applied to uninflamed tissue, there is local necrosis, formation of the dentin bridge, and healing of the underlying pulp. On the other hand, if applied to inflamed tissue, the reaction is unpredictable and anything from healing or a long-standing chronic inflammation to a rather immediate pulp necrosis may be seen.

Clinical Considerations

In teeth where a pulpotomy is performed, the pulp usually has severe local damage with inflamed areas and possibly areas with necrotic tissue which may be infected. After preparation of the access cavity, a rubber dam is applied and the field of operation, including the tooth and the exposed pulp, is thoroughly disinfected. The coronal pulp is then removed by means of a round bur in a low-torque ultraspeed handpiece or by means of a sharp excavator. The bleeding is controlled by irrigation with sterile saline and compression with sterile gauze or cotton pellets. Calcium hydroxide paste is applied. The pulp chamber is then filled with zinc oxide–eugenol cement, and in contrast to what is often the case after pulp capping, an adequate bacteria-tight seal is readily maintained in this situation since the temporary filling will be of adequate thickness and is easily retained in the pulp chamber and the access cavity of the tooth.

Follow-up Examinations and Prognosis

Pulpotomized teeth should be examined clinically and radiographically after 3, 6, and 12 months and then later once a year until symptoms or other signs of failure are evident or until a pulpectomy is performed. *As the pulp is usually amputated apically to the gingival margin, sensitivity tests cannot be carried out in these teeth.* The clinical examination, therefore, is limited to evaluating whether signs of inflammation are evident. The formation of the dentin bridge can be followed radiographically (**Fig. 5.17**). Still, the width of the root canal as it compares with the width of the canal of the contralateral tooth and other neighboring teeth is the most valuable indicator as to the state of the pulp. Sometimes internal resorption is seen in pulpotomized teeth. This is a definite sign of necrosis and infection of an area cervically in the residual pulp and a chronic inflammation in the canal at the resorption lacuna.

As discussed above, the prognosis of pulpotomized teeth is poor, probably in the area of 40%. It is important to understand and accept that even after the most thorough clinical and radiographic examination, it may not be possible to determine whether a pulpotomy is successful or not. It is good clinical practice, therefore, to always perform a pulpectomy in these teeth when necessary or when the root development is completed. The question then arises of whether it is really worthwhile going by way of a pulpotomy, or if these teeth should not be treated with a pulpectomy in the first place. There can be no doubt about the answer. The roots of the teeth of a 7–12-year-old child are so thin and weak that if the pulp is removed and the root canal is filled with gutta-percha and a sealer, the teeth will fracture either horizontally or vertically sooner or later. On the other hand, if the root pulp of these teeth is saved temporarily until the root development is completed, the roots of these teeth will be strong and, when root filled, may last a lifetime and serve effectively to retain any type of coronal restoration.

Pulpectomy

Pulpectomy implies *the removal of the vital pulp.* This form of therapy has developed as a logical consequence of the high failure rate of pulp capping and pulpotomy treatment of teeth with exposed, inflamed pulps. When a pulpectomy is performed, the pulp is severed near the apical foramen so that in all instances practically all inflamed tissue is removed. Consequently, the diagnostic problems that are unsolvable in conjunction with a pulpotomy procedure hardly exist with this method. Thus, in the treatment of teeth with exposed, inflamed pulps, pulpectomy is by far the treatment form with the widest indications, and until new diagnostic methods are available with which it will be possible to determine more accurately the preoperative condition of the inflamed pulp, pulpectomy will continue to be the treatment method of choice.

Indications

From a biological point of view, the treatment of a tooth by pulpectomy is simple. The pulp tissue is removed and the root canal is filled with a material or materials that are biocompatible and provide a long-lasting, bacteria-tight seal of the canal. If this is achieved, the tooth will remain healthy and functional. Thus, a pulpectomy may be carried out in all teeth with vital pulps, and the only limitations of the method would be possible practical ones like an unusually complicated morphology of a tooth. Considering the complexity of the root canal system, pulpectomy treatment is amazingly successful, and a success rate of 90–95% is within reach when optimal methods are used.

Treatment Principles

The vital pulp tissue, although it is usually inflamed, is potentially sterile. Even if the pulp is exposed to the oral environment, only the superficial area of the tissue may be infected. Thus, *when a pulpectomy is performed, it is normally not a question of combating an infection, but of preventing a contamination of the root canal during the treatment.*

Special conditions exist when the pulpitis has resulted in necrosis of the coronal part of the pulp. The necrotic tissue will be infected and is removed first. The pulp chamber is then thoroughly disinfected before the vital pulp tissue in the root canal is extirpated. Of course, teeth will be encountered in which the tissue necrosis is not confined to the coronal pulp, but has spread to the root pulp as well so that only the apical part of the pulp is vital. Similarly, in multirooted teeth, the pulp tissue in one of the roots may be necrotic whereas it is vital in another root. It should then be remembered that the front of infection is always at the transition zone between necrotic and vital tissue, and *the clinical rule is that, if in doubt about the presence of bacteria, a tooth should always be regarded as infected and be treated accordingly* (see Chapter 6).

Pulp extirpation and instrumentation.   When the pulp is extirpated it should be severed inside the root canal near the apical foramen. As a rule, the

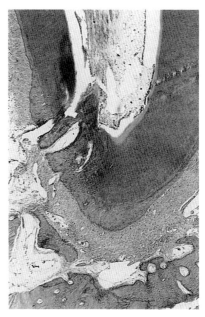

Fig. 5.19 Root end with apical periodontium. The apical foramen is situated laterally on the root at a distance from the apex of the tooth (hematoxylin-eosin).

foramen is not located at the radiographic apex of the tooth, and most often it is not possible to determine its exact position (**Fig. 5.19**). Consequently, in order to stay within the root canal, we have to be satisfied with the somewhat inexact rule that the pulp wound should be placed 1–3 mm short of the radiographic apex. With this rule in mind, and after careful study of the preoperative radiograph, the optimal apical level of instrumentation in each individual tooth is determined.

By severing the pulp inside the root canal, several advantages are achieved. It is technically possible to obtain a *clean wound* when the pulp is cut off against the hard root canal walls, thereby minimizing the apical tissue damage. Still, a wound is made, resulting in an inflammatory reaction in the apical tissue. The inflammation is usually combined with a transient root resorption and the severity of the reaction will depend on the gentleness with which the pulp wound is made. Normally, the inflammatory reaction is over in 2–3 weeks, and repair of the resorptive areas with apposition of a cementum-like tissue is seen at that time as well (**Fig. 5.20**).

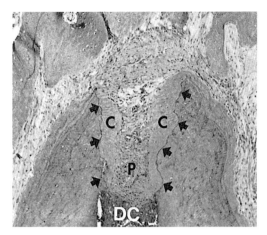

Fig. 5.20 Pulpectomy, monkey tooth. The pulp (P) was severed short of the apex and the resulting in-flammation caused transient root resorption (ar-rows). At 60 days, pulpal healing is completed with cemental repair (C) of the resorptive areas (DC = den-tin chips plug) (hematoxylin-eosin).

Another advantage of placing the pulp wound short of the apex is that *a possible apical delta of accessory root canals is left intact* (**Fig. 5.21**). Be-cause of the proximity of the root canal delta with the periodontal ligament and consequently a well-developed collateral circulation in the area, the tissue in the accessory canals will remain vital

if not encroached upon. This is undoubtedly a key to the high success rate of pulpectomy treatment.

A third advantage of an intracanal pulp wound is that *the periodontal ligament is not damaged.* However, in some instances the periodontal tis-sues will be impinged upon during the extirpation of the pulp, either because the working length has been incorrectly determined or, as is often the case, because the operator is unable to sever the pulp tissue within the root canal and conse-quently removes the entire pulp and maybe part of the periodontal ligament as well. In such in-stances the apical soft-tissue wound is much larger than a wound inside the canal, and since the tissue outside the root canal is not cut, but torn, the wound will be irregular and the tissue damage more severe. Consequently, the inflam-matory reaction that follows the extirpation will be more severe as well and, in addition to the re-sorption of the root, there may be a certain resorp-tion of the alveolar bone as well so that a slight periapical radiolucency becomes evident in a ra-diograph. This reaction is referred to as a *temporary failure,* since periapical repair usually occurs if the treatment is adequately completed.

The best approach to correcting the mistake of over-instrumentation is to ignore it. The root canal is prepared to the optimal level short of the radio-graphic apex and later obturated to this level (**Fig. 5.22**). The space in the canal apically to the

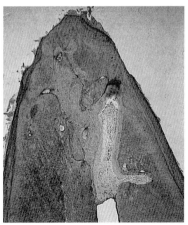

a

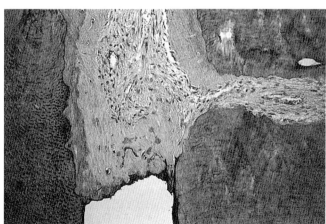

b

Fig. 5.21
a Pulpectomy of a maxillary central incisor with an extensive apical root canal delta. The pulp has been severed short of the area with the acces-sory root canals.

b Complete healing of the apical pulp tissue is evi-dent (hematoxylin-eosin).

root filling will be filled with tissue fluids and blood which, gradually, will be organized to new connective tissue. If there is no bacterial contamination of the root canal so that the blood clot becomes infected, the new tissue will form quickly and predictably. After 30 days or sooner, a well-vascularized and cell-rich connective tissue is seen (**Fig. 5.23**). Gradually the new tissue inside the root canal usually mineralizes and a cementum-like hard tissue will fill the root canal space apically to the root canal filling.

When the pulp has been extirpated and the instrumentation of the root canal is completed, *the canal should be obturated* (**Fig. 5.22**). In principle, the root canal can be filled with any biocompatible material that gives a bacteria-tight seal and neither shrinks, nor dissolves in tissue fluids, nor is resorbed, so that leakage and infection may cause problems at a later date. The healing after pulpectomy and root canal filling occurs in the same manner as after implantation of an inert material in connective tissue elsewhere in the body (**Fig. 5.24**). A fibrous capsule forms adjacent to the material and, as discussed above, the inflammation that always occurs when the pulp is removed, resolves, usually within weeks, provided that the root canal filling material is in fact tolerated by the tissues.

Apical dentin chips plug.   Unfortunately, the root filling materials we have today all cause at least a temporary tissue reaction when brought in contact with the apical tissue. Efforts have been made, therefore, to create a biocompatible interface between the pulp stump and the actual root canal filling. Materials like hydroxyapatite and ceramic powders have been used for this purpose with some success. However, the simplest and most elegant method is *to use dentin chips from the tooth itself and make an apical plug prior to obturating the root canal.*

The plug, which should be 0.5–1 mm thick, is made by filing dentin chips from the root canal wall, bringing them in an apical direction, and condensing them carefully against the apical tissue. Dentin chips have an ability to induce hard-tissue formation. As a result the chips in the plug are gradually "cemented" together and, in addition, a cementum-like tissue readily forms onto the plug against the vital tissue of the pulp stump or the periodontal ligament (**Fig. 5.25**). In this

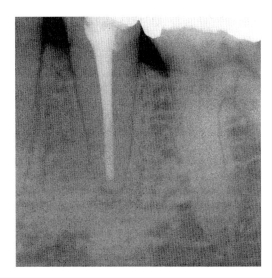

Fig. 5.22 Radiograph of a pulpectomized mandibular premolar. The root canal has been filled to an ideal level about 1 mm short of the radiographic apex.

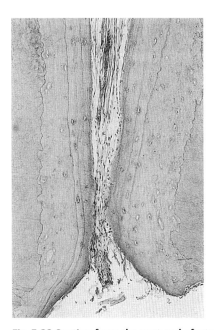

Fig. 5.23 Section from the root end of a tooth which was instrumented beyond the apex but filled short of the apex. Cell-rich connective (periodontal) tissue has grown into the root canal. Apposition of cementum-like tissue is seen on the root canal walls (hematoxylin-eosin).

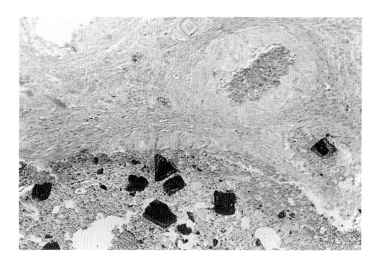

Fig. 5.24 Root filling materi-al–tissue interface. Repair with a fibrous capsule adjacent to the material is evident. A capsule also surrounds the small particles of material in the tissue (hematoxylin-eosin).

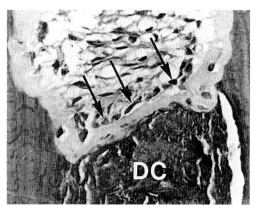

Fig. 5.25 Dentin chips plug (DC)–apical pulp stump interface in pulpectomized monkey tooth. Hard tissue-forming cells (arrows) have laid down a cementum-like tissue in areas with root resorption as well as on the dentin chips plug. This may result in a hard-tissue closure of the root canal (hematoxylin-eosin).

may play an important part in periradicular healing following pulpectomy, even if they are not used intentionally. Experimental findings have shown that, during instrumentation of the root canal, dentin chips are quite automatically pushed into pulpal ends of lateral and accessory canals (**Fig. 5.26**). Hard-tissue formation is induced and the pulpal openings of the canals are sealed off. Peripherally to the plug, the tissue in the lateral canals then remain vital and healthy.

Calcium hydroxide–induced apical bridge. An apical hard-tissue barrier may also be induced by means of calcium hydroxide (**Fig. 5.21**). However, it takes longer for the bridge to form apically in the root canal than in the coronal pulp, and a period of 3 – 6 months is not unusual. Still, in certain instances, especially in the treatment of teeth with incompletely formed roots, it is advantageous to delay the obturation of the canal until an apical hard-tissue barrier has formed.

Root canal obturation. Routinely the root canal is filled as soon as the instrumentation is completed, i.e., in the same visit as when the pulp is removed (**Fig. 5.22**). Since there is no infection to worry about in vital teeth, there is no reason not to complete the treatment in one visit. However, for practical clinical reasons, usually the lack of time, it may be necessary to postpone the obturation phase of the treatment to a second visit. It is then extremely important to protect the root canal from becoming infected during the period between the visits. An antiseptic medicament with

manner a hard-tissue closure of the root canal may be obtained, and the apical tissues are protected from possible adverse influences from the root filling materials. Moreover, the dentin chips plug effectively prevents overfilling of the root canal, even if obturation techniques with soft or softened materials are used. However, it should be emphasized that the dentin chips plug may not give a bacteria-tight seal of the canal and, even if a plug is made, it is the root canal filling materials that must provide the necessary seal.

It should also be mentioned that dentin chips

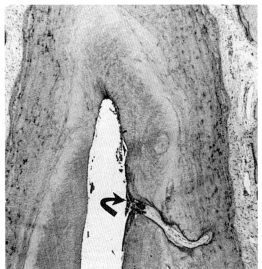
a

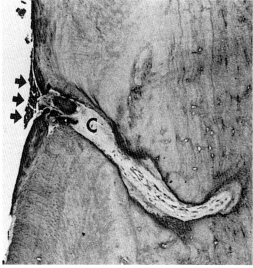
b

Fig. 5.26
a Pulpectomized monkey tooth with lateral root canal (arrow).
b Dentin chips have inadvertently been pushed into the orifice of the lateral canal (arrows) and a cementum-like tissue (C) has formed onto the chips. The tissue in the lateral canal is healthy and free of inflammation (hematoxylin-eosin).

long-lasting antibacterial effect which is well tolerated by human cells should be applied to the orifice of the root canal, or the root canal should be filled with a calcium hydroxide paste. The coronal access cavity is then sealed bacteria-tight (see p. 167).

Postoperative pain. If a pulpectomized tooth is asymptomatic when the treatment begins, it will usually be asymptomatic when the anesthesia wears off. However, the apical inflammation due to the extirpation of the pulp may cause a mild tenderness to percussion that normally will be gone in 1–2 days or even sooner. Obviously, if the tooth is tender to percussion at the beginning of the treatment, it will still be tender when the anesthesia loses its effect. However, also such a tooth will be asymptomatic within a short period of time. It should also be mentioned that pulpectomy with completion of the treatment in one visit does not cause additional postoperative symptoms, neither in frequency nor intensity.

Clinical Considerations (see Chapter 11)
When it has been ascertained that the pulp of the tooth is vital, anesthesia is given. Carious dentin and leaky fillings are removed and weak cusps are cut or reduced to prevent fractures. An access cavity to expose the pulp chamber is then prepared, followed by removal of the coronal pulp by means of large round burs or sharp excavators. The canal orifices are located and the access cavity completed. This part of the treatment is not performed aseptically, mainly for two reasons. First, it is difficult or even impossible to achieve asepsis as long as carious dentin and infected tissue are present. Second, in difficult teeth it is a lot easier to keep one's sense of direction and avoid perforations and other complications when locating the root canal orifices before the rubber dam is applied.

When the coronal pulp has been removed, further treatment should be performed under strictly aseptic conditions. A rubber dam is applied and the field of operation—the rubber dam, the rubber dam clamp, the tooth, and especially the pulp chamber with the exposed root pulps—is thoroughly and conscientiously disinfected. The used, nonsterile instruments are removed and a tray with sterile hand and root canal instruments is made available. A tooth-length radiograph is taken with a thin instrument in the canal or an apex locator is used. The pulp tissue is then removed with a reamer or file to the apical level judged to be optimal. The root canal is instrumented and prepared under irrigation with sodium hypochlorite. The cleansing and bleaching effect of sodium hypochlorite will effectively prevent discoloration of the tooth from the unavoidable bleeding during and after removal of the pulp tissue. A chelating agent, EDTA, is then used for a final rinse of the root canal to remove the smear layer from the canal walls (see Chapter 6). The canal is then dried with paper points and preferably permanently obturated. The obturation is checked radiographically. If an immediate obturation is not possible, the root canal is protected from infection until it can be filled. A simple and safe solution is to fill the canal with a calcium hydroxide paste and to seal the access cavity bacteria-tight with zinc oxide–eugenol cement. To be reasonably safe, the temporary filling in the access cavity should be at least 3 mm and preferably 4 – 5 mm thick. The rubber dam is then removed and, most importantly, the filling in the access cavity checked before the patient may close his mouth.

At the second visit, if necessary, the tooth is examined, a rubber dam is applied, and the field of operation is disinfected before the root canal is opened. The canal dressing is rinsed out, the instrumentation checked, and the root canal is dried and obturated.

Follow-up Examinations and Prognosis

A number of studies from many parts of the world comprising different techniques and root filling materials have shown that pulpectomy treatment has a very good prognosis. *The two factors which have the greatest impact on the outcome of the treatment are the adequacy of the obturation of the root canal, i.e., whether or not a bacteria-tight seal is accomplished, and the apical level of the root filling.* With regard to the latter factor, the best results are obtained when the root filling ends 1 – 2 mm, in some studies 1 – 3 mm, short of the radiographic apex. A success rate of 90 – 95 % can be obtained under optimal conditions.

However, failures do occur and clinical–radiographic follow-up examinations should take place 6 to 12 months after the completion of the treatment and then later as deemed necessary. As mentioned above, so-called "temporary failures" may occur after pulpectomy treatment. In such instances, a normal periodontal contour should be reestablished at the 1-year control.

Further Reading

Al-Dawood A, Wennberg A. Biocompatibility of dentin bonding agents. Endod Dent Traumatol 1993;9:1 – 7.

Cvek M. Partial pulpotomy in crown-fractured incisors—results 3 to 15 years after treatment. Acta Stomatol Croatica 1993;27:167 – 173.

Engström B, Spångberg L. Wound healing after partial pulpectomy. A histological study performed on contralateral tooth pairs. Odont Tidskr 1967;75:5 – 18.

Hasselgren G, Kerekes K, Nellestam P. pH changes in calcium hydroxide-covered dentin. J Endod 1987;8: 502 – 505.

Hasselgren G, Tronstad L. Enzyme activity in the pulp following preparation of cavities and insertion of medicaments in cavities in monkey teeth. Acta Odont Scand 1978;35:289 – 295.

Hilton TJ. Cavity sealers, liners and bases: current philosophies and indications for use. Oper Dent 1996; 21:134 – 146.

Kerekes K, Tronstad L. Long-term results of endodontic treatment performed with a standardized technique. J Endod 1979;5:83 – 90.

Ketterl W. Kriterien für den Erfolg der Vitalextirpation. Dtsch Zahnärztl Zeitschr 1965;20:407 – 416.

Mejare J, Mejare B, Edwardsson S. Effect of tight seal on survival of bacteria in saliva-contaminated cavities filled with composite resin. Endod Dent Traumatol 1987;3:6 – 9.

Murray PE, Garcia-Godoy F, Hargreaves KM. Regenerative endodontics: a review of current status and a call for action. J Endod 2007;33:377 – 390.

Nakashima M. Tissue engineering in endodontics. Aust Endod J 2005;31:111 – 113.

Nyborg H. Healing processes in the pulp on capping. Acta Odont Scand 1955;13:Suppl.16, 1 – 130.

Nygaard-Östby B, Hjortdal O. Tissue formation in the root canal following pulp removal. Scand J Dent Res 1971;79:333 – 49.

Pameijer CH, Wendt SL. Microleakage of "surface-sealing" materials. Am J Dent 1995;8:43 – 46.

Petersson K, Hasselgren G, Tronstad L. Clinical experience with the use of dentin chips in pulpectomies. Int Endod J 1982;15:161 – 167.

Petersson K, Söderström C, Kiani-Anaraki M, Levy G. Evaluation of the ability of thermal and electrical tests to register pulp vitality. Endod Dent Traumatol 1999;15:127 – 131.

Qvist V, Qvist J, Mjör IA. Placement and longevity of tooth-colored restorations in Denmark. Acta Odont Scand 1990;48:305 – 311.

Swift EJ, Perdiago J, Heyman HO. Bonding to enamel

and dentin: a brief history and state of the art. Quintessence Int 1995;26:95 – 110.

Tronstad L, Andreasen JO, Hasselgren G, Riis J. pH changes in dental tissues after root canal filling with calcium hydroxide. J Endod 1981;7:17 – 21.

Tronstad L, Mjör IA. Capping of the inflamed pulp. Oral Surg Oral Med Oral Pathol 1972;34:477 – 485.

Tronstad L. Reaction of the exposed pulp to Dycal treatment. Oral Surg Oral Med Oral Pathol 1974;38: 945 – 953.

Tronstad L. Tissue reactions following apical plugging of the root canal with dentin chips in pulpectomized teeth in monkeys. Oral Surg Oral Med Oral Pathol 1978;45:297 – 304.

Trope M, Rabie G, Tronstad L. Pulp capping of immature teeth with anatomic anomalies. Endod Dent Traumatol 1991;7:139 – 143.

Wennberg A, Hasselgren G, Tronstad L. A method for evaluation of initial tissue response to biomaterials. Acta Odont Scand 1978;36:67 – 73.

6

Treatment of Nonvital Teeth

By definition, *a nonvital tooth is a tooth with a necrotic pulp.* Pulp necrosis is suspected when a tooth does not react to thermal, electric, or mechanical stimulation, but the definite diagnosis is established only after inspection and probing of the pulp chamber and the root canal. As was discussed above, the necrotic pulp tissue and the root canal space are infected almost without exception, even in teeth which clinically appear intact (**Fig. 6.1**). Over time, bacteria in the root canal will induce inflammation outside the tooth, resulting in the formation of an apical granuloma or cyst (see p. 33). *Treatment of a nonvital tooth,* *therefore, invariably involves the treatment of an infectious disease process.*

The objective of treating a nonvital tooth is to remove the necrotic tissue and tissue breakdown products from the root canal, eliminate infection, seal the root canal bacteria-tight, and thereby establish a functioning tooth in a healthy periodontium. An apical periodontitis which is refractory to conservative endodontic treatment may be treated successfully by a surgical–endodontic approach in which the apical granulation tissue, which may be infected, is curetted out.

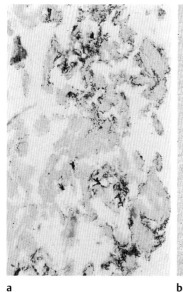 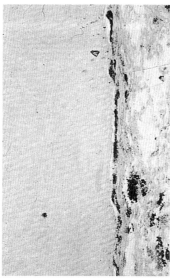 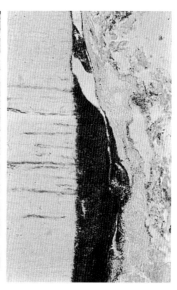

a b c

Fig. 6.1
a Colonies of microorganisms in necrotic tissue in a root canal.
b Bacterial colonies in tissue and on the root canal wall.

c Large bacterial colony in the cervical area of a root canal subjacent to dentin exposed to the oral cavity. The root canal of this tooth was sealed to the mouth, and the bacteria have gained access to the canal through the tubules of the exposed dentin (Brown–Brenn stain).

Conservative Endodontic Treatment

Indications

In principle, a conservative approach is indicated in the treatment of all nonvital teeth. Traditionally, there have been some doubts as to whether large periapical lesions would heal following treatment of the root canal, but with modern methods the size of the lesion is of no real concern when the treatment plan is made (**Fig. 6.2**). However, there is still no definite evidence that periapical cysts respond to nonsurgical treatment, although the circumstantial evidence to that effect is considerable (**Fig. 6.2**). *The main rule, therefore, is that all nonvital teeth with or without apical periodontitis should be treated conservatively.*

Treatment Principles

The treatment of the root canal of a nonvital tooth can be divided into three main phases:

1) Chemomechanical instrumentation of the canal with removal of necrotic pulp tissue and bacteria;
2) Final disinfection of the canal and creation of favorable conditions for periapical healing; and
3) Obturation of the canal with materials rendering a bacteria-tight seal.

Chemomechanical instrumentation. The mechanical instrumentation of the root canal is of the utmost importance in the treatment of nonvital teeth. During this phase the necrotic tissue with its colonies of bacteria is *physically removed* from the main root canal. By enlarging and preparing the canal and giving it its shape for obturation, most bacteria in the dentinal tubules are physically removed as well. However, *the mechanical instrumentation obviously has no effect in crevices and lateral or accessory root canals where the instruments do not reach.*

The effect of the mechanical instrumentation can be enhanced by the use of chemically active preparations during the instrumentation phase. These preparations are referred to as *root canal irrigants*, or irrigation solutions, and they are injected continuously or at intervals into the canal during the instrumentation. Different irrigants may be used in an alternate fashion to obtain a combined effect of the medicaments. Thus, medicaments are available which have a cleansing effect, an antibacterial effect, a detoxifying and denaturing effect, and a hard- and soft-tissue dis-

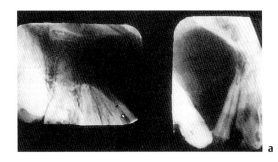

a

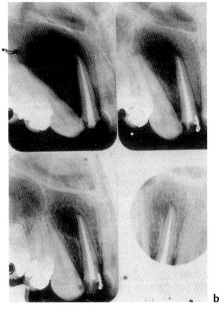

b

Fig. 6.2

a Radiographs showing a large radiolucent lesion extending from the maxillary right central incisor to the third molar. Note the deviation of the roots of the teeth. The right lateral incisor is nonvital.

b Radiographs showing resolution of the lesion over a 4-year period following endodontic treatment of the lateral incisor.

solving effect. Depending on the clinical situation, different medicaments may be selected. However, the main purpose of a root canal irrigant should be to aid in the removal of necrotic tissue and tissue components, bacteria, blood clots, exudate, and pus. Irrigants with a tissue-dissolving ability have a good cleansing effect, even in crevices and lateral canals where the mechanical instrumentation has no effect. The cleansing action and the tissue dissolution will further lead to an *exposure of bacteria* that are normally embedded in and protected by necrotic tissue and tissue components or by bacterial extracellular polymeric materials so that the antimicrobial action of the irrigant and other root canal antiseptics is maximized.

The classic root canal irrigant is *0.5% sodium hypochlorite at pH 9.* This solution was first used in medicine in the form of a drip in the treatment of soldiers with grenade wounds in World War I. By constantly dripping onto a wound surface, the sodium hypochlorite would cleanse the wound, dissolve necrotic tissue at the wound surface, and keep the wound clean and bacteria-free. The effect of the medicament is virtually the same in the root canal. It has an excellent cleansing ability, dissolves and detoxifies necrotic tissue, has a certain antibacterial effect, and is well tolerated by vital tissue. However, the effect of sodium hypochlorite is quickly neutralized by organic components like tissue remnants, blood, and exudate in the root canal, and consequently the irrigant has to be renewed continuously or at frequent intervals. An amount of at least 10 mL should be used during the instrumentation of a single-rooted tooth and comparably more in premolars and molars.

Sodium hypochlorite is used in concentrations between 0.5 and 10%. Since the medicament when used for irrigation is applied in excess, a low concentration will be about as effective as a solution with higher concentration, and it will be less toxic. Thus, a 5% solution is 10 times as toxic as a 0.5% solution, but has only about twice the antibacterial effect. However, in a 5% concentration, sodium hypochlorite has an improved tissue-dissolving effect. This may be beneficial when mechanical removal of tissue is difficult, as in side canals and in teeth with resorption defects.

Chlorhexidine gluconate is an antiseptic that is effective against oral bacteria and has been used in the treatment of periodontal disease for two generations. Lately, chlorhexidine has been used as a root canal irrigant to replace sodium hypochlorite, apparently since sodium hypochloride leaves an oxygen-rich surface in the root canal that might influence negatively the bonding action of resin-based root filling materials. Unlike sodium hypochlorite, chlorhexidine lacks bleaching and tissue dissolving properties. It is therefore not well suited for irrigation of the root canal during the instrumentation phase of the treatment.

Quaternary ammonium compounds are surface-active agents with a soap-like character, and because of these characteristics are widely used as root canal irrigants. They have a bacteriostatic effect and are well tolerated by the tissues. However, like sodium hypochlorite and chlorhexidine, their effect is quickly reduced by organic components, and renewed injection into the canal at frequent intervals is necessary for maximal effect. Like chlorhexidine, the quaternary ammonium compounds lack bleaching and tissue dissolving properties.

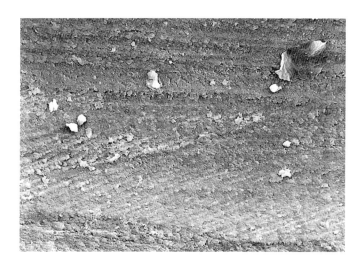

Fig. 6.3 Scanning electron micrograph of a root canal wall following instrumentation and irrigation with sodium hypochlorite. A smear layer is covering the wall so that the dentin surface cannot be seen (×470).

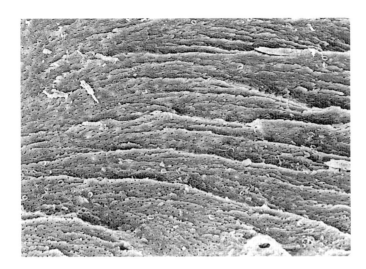

Fig. 6.4 Scanning electron micrograph of a root canal wall following instrumentation and irrigation with sodium hypochlorite as well as a final rinse with EDTA. The smear layer is removed and the dentin surface with its tubule orifices can be seen (×300).

Oxidizing agents like a 3% solution of *hydrogen peroxide* are used as root canal irrigants as well, usually in combination with sodium hypochlorite. However, sodium hypochlorite is as effective when used alone as when combined with hydrogen peroxide, and hydrogen peroxide, therefore, is presently not widely used.

None of the irrigants mentioned above has an effect on hard tissue or on the smear layer of the root canal walls (**Fig. 6.3**). However, irrigation of the root canal with a *chelating agent* like ethylenediamine tetraacetic acid (EDTA) which binds Ca^{++} ions, will effectively remove the smear layer and dentin chips remaining on the canal wall after the instrumentation (**Fig. 6.4**).

In the root canal ethylenediamine tetraacetic acid (EDTA) is used in a 15% solution at pH 7.4. A certain volume of the solution can only bind a limited number of Ca^{++} ions, and additional EDTA must be injected into the canal at frequent intervals in order for continued Ca^{++}-binding to take place. EDTA is well tolerated by soft tissues and, from a biological point of view, can be used safely. The most effective use of EDTA as an irrigant is in combination with sodium hypochlorite. These two irrigants supplement each other in that one has its effect on necrotic tissue, bacteria, and other organic components in the root canal system, whereas the other gives a clean root canal wall. Clinically, sodium hypochlorite and EDTA may be used alternately during the instrumentation phase. *Excellent results are also obtained when sodium hypochlorite is used during the instrumentation,* *and EDTA is used for a final irrigation of the canal after the instrumentation is completed.*

A new irrigating solution, MTAD, containing a mixture of a tetracycline isomer, an acid and a detergent has come on the market. It was initially meant to replace both sodium hypochlorite and EDTA, but is now recommended to be used together with sodium hypochlorite. The acid in MTAD may remove the smear layer of the canal walls, but the antibacterial effect of the combined use of sodium hypochlorite and EDTA is reported to be superior to the effect of the MTAD and sodium hypochlorite combination.

If at all possible, the chemomechanical instrumentation of the root canal should be completed in the first visit. If a partial instrumentation is done, the environment in the canal is changed and the balance that existed in the bacterial flora is altered as well. Chances are that certain pathogenic bacteria now may have an opportunity to dominate the infection and cause a flare-up or exacerbation of the periapical inflammation.

Iatrogenic flare-ups occur first and foremost during treatment of teeth with apical periodontitis, and with optimal treatment will be seen in about 5% of such teeth. The frequency with which flare-ups occur is an excellent indicator of a dentist's effectiveness and carefulness in endodontic treatment of nonvital teeth. If the overall frequency is much higher than 2–3% (5% in teeth with apical periodontitis), it is a clear message that something is wrong with the dentist's therapeutic approach, either conceptually, clinically, or both.

Disinfection of the root canal. A thorough and complete chemomechanical instrumentation in the first visit may render the root canal system bacteria-free. However, in most instances it results in only an effective reduction in the number of bacteria, and *an antiseptic medicament must be applied to the root canal for a period of time in order to assure that the last remnants of the root canal flora are eliminated.*

Presently, there is disagreement about how important this is. It is felt by many that it is of no clinical consequence that bacteria are left in the root canal system if only the root canal is obturated bacteria-tight. Remaining bacteria will then be sealed in the root and have no effect on the periapical tissues. However, from a medical point of view this concept may seem hard to defend. Firstly, pathogenic bacteria should not be left in a patient if they can be eradicated, and secondly, not all bacteria may be "blocked off," but be present in root canal deltas and lateral canals that are in continuity with the periodontium. With our present methods and techniques, therefore, endodontic treatment of a nonvital tooth should as a rule not be completed in the first visit, but in a second visit after a period of final disinfection of the root and root canal system.

In traditional endodontic treatment of nonvital teeth, little emphasis was put on instrumentation and tissue management, and much emphasis was put on disinfection. Sophisticated disinfection methods such as diathermy and iontophoresis were advocated, and a large number of imaginative concoctions of powerful antiseptics were used as well. Today, we know that *medicaments which are effective against microorganisms also, as a rule, kill human cells, and consequently may cause tissue damage.* The damage which is caused by uncritical use of medicaments in the root canal may, therefore, at times exceed the advantages of their use. Recognition of this fact led to attempts to find antiseptics which have the desired effect on the microorganisms of the root canal system without causing unacceptable injury to the periapical tissues (*selective toxicity*). Iodine and chlorine preparations as well as quaternary ammonium compounds and chlorhexidine have shown the best results in these studies, and from the point of view of selective toxicity, are suitable intracanal medicaments in the treatment of nonvital teeth.

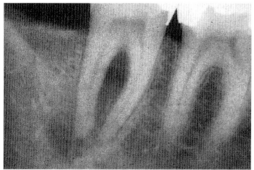

a

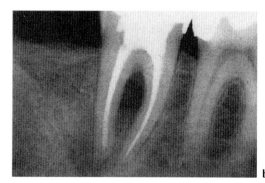

b

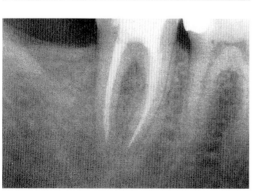

c

Fig. 6.5

a **Radiograph of a mandibular molar with apical and interradicular periodontitis.** The tooth was completely instrumented under irrigation with sodium hypochlorite and EDTA in the first visit and formocresol was placed in the pulp chamber by means of a cotton pellet.

b In the second visit after 1 week, the patient was asymptomatic and the root canals were dry. The canals were then obdurated.

c After 6 months, resolution of the lesion is observed.

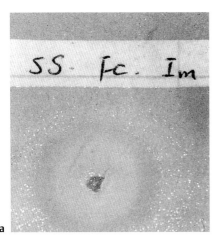

a

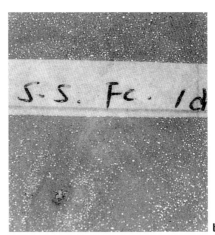

b

Fig. 6.6
a A cotton pellet with fresh formocresol is placed on a pour plate with *Streptococcus* species. After incubation for 24 h, a zone of inhibition of the growth of the bacteria is seen surrounding the cotton pellet with the medicament.

b Cotton pellet with formocresol which was sealed in the pulp chamber of an instrumented, nonvital dog tooth for 24 h is placed on a pour plate with *Streptococcus* species. After incubation for 24 h, the bacteria are seen growing in contact with the cotton pellet. The formocresol had lost its antibacterial effect.

Formocresol and monochlorphenol are other medicaments used widely for this purpose (**Fig. 6.5**).

Although the selective toxicity of the medicaments mentioned above varies, and thereby their suitability for use, they have one feature in common, namely the fact that *they are quickly rendered inactive by contact with the dental tissues and tissue fluids, usually within 24 hours* (**Fig. 6.6**). Thus, if any of these medicaments is used in the root canal, the canal will be unprotected 1 day after the placement of the medicament or even sooner. This means that if the bacteria in the root canal system are not killed during the first day, surviving organisms will begin to multiply again, since the canal will contain tissue fluids, exudate, and blood, which constitute an excellent substrate for bacterial growth. Also, when the root canal is no longer protected by the antiseptic, it may become reinfected by bacteria from outside the root canal system.

Ideally, a root canal antiseptic should have a long-lasting antimicrobial effect. In the future, intracanal medicaments in *controlled-release delivery systems* will undoubtedly be available (**Fig. 6.7**). At present, prolonged antibacterial action can be readily and effectively obtained by filling the root canal with a paste of calcium hydroxide and isotonic saline. The use of calcium hydroxide in the treatment of nonvital teeth developed empirically. It was noted that when placed in the root canal, calcium hydroxide has a striking effect on periapical exudation. This was taken as evidence that the material has *an anti-inflammatory effect*, i.e., it has the ability to bring a periapical inflammation from the exudative stage to a stage of repair. It was also noted that periapical lesions quickly show radiographic signs of healing in teeth with calcium hydroxide in the root canal, and that complete repair regularly occurs in 2–3 months (**Fig. 6.8**).

The *modes of action of calcium hydroxide* are only partially understood. When mixed with saline, the resulting paste has a pH of 12.5. Moreover, calcium hydroxide has a disassociation coefficient of 0.17, which means that if placed in the root canal, it will become ionized and dissolve slowly and steadily in the fluids of the dentinal tubules, the lateral and accessory canals, and the periapical tissue. In other words, there is a controlled, long-lasting release of Ca^{++} and OH^- ions from the paste in the root canal. *Consequently, calcium hydroxide will have a controlled, long-lasting therapeutic effect.*

The therapeutic effect of calcium hydroxide is clearly related to the hydroxyl ions, which will lead to a lowered oxygen tension and an increase in the pH in the inflamed periapical tissue. A low oxygen tension in the tissue favors bone forma-

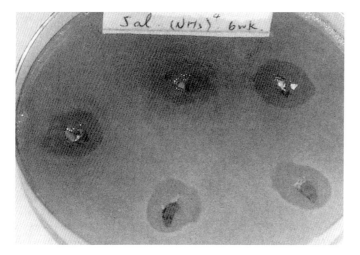

Fig. 6.7 Antiseptic in a controlled-release delivery system. The dispensers were sealed in the pulp chamber of instrumented, nonvital dog teeth for 6 weeks and were, after removal, placed on a pour plate with *Streptococcus* species. After incubation for 24 h, zones of inhibition of bacterial growth are seen surrounding the dispensers, indicating that the antiseptic is still being released after 6 weeks of contact with dentin and tissue fluids in the root canal.

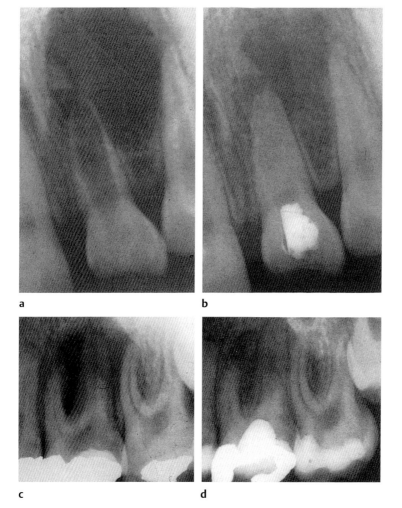

Fig. 6.8
a **Radiograph of a maxillary incisor with root fracture and a large radiolucency in conjunction with the fracture line.** Calcium hydroxide treatment of the coronal fragment (apexification) is initiated.
b After 2 months, near complete resolution of the radiolucent lesion is observed.
c Radiograph of a maxillary molar with interradicular periodontitis and suspected oral communication. Long-term calcium hydroxide treatment is initiated.
d After 10 weeks, resolution of the radiolucent lesion is evident.

a

b

c

d

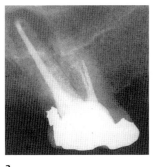 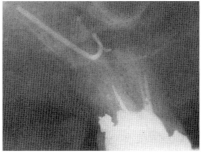 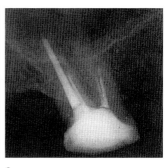

a   b   c

Fig. 6.9
a Radiograph of a maxillary molar with apical periodontitis and a palatal fistula from the palatal root. The tooth was completely instrumented in the first visit (buccal root canals calcified) and treated with calcium hydroxide for 3 weeks. At the second visit, the patient was asymptomatic, the fistula had closed, and the root canals were obturated.

b At 3-month control, the palatal fistula has recurred, the root filling is removed from the palatal canal and long-term calcium hydroxide treatment is initiated.
c The fistula closed immediately, and after 3 months the periapical lesion had resolved. Only then was the palatal root canal again permanently obturated.

tion and repair, and a favorable effect of an alkaline environment on mineralization is also evidenced by the high pH found in the growth plate at the mineralization front of bones. A possible therapeutic effect of the calcium ions is less well understood, but apparently they may have a stimulating effect on certain alkaline phosphatases, which are enzymes connected with hard-tissue formation. It is also possible that the calcium ions have a beneficial effect on the local immune response.

With a pH of 12.5, a calcium hydroxide paste has an excellent and exceptionally broad antibacterial effect. No known endodontopathogens can survive at this pH, and will be killed instantly when directly exposed to the paste. However, in crevices of the main canal and especially in lateral and accessory canals where the chemomechanical instrumentation has only a limited effect, the bacteria may be embedded in and protected by necrotic tissue components and bacterial extracellular material, and may survive the influence of an antiseptic for considerable time. Even in such inaccessible areas of the root canal system, the bacteria can be expected to eventually die out under the constant and long-lasting influence of calcium hydroxide, but a long-term exposure to the drug, i.e., weeks and even months may be necessary in some instances (**Fig. 6.9**).

The long-lasting antibacterial effect of the calcium hydroxide paste is highly dependent on a constant, high alkalinity of the paste. Thus, rather common root canal organisms like *Enterococcus faecalis* may survive in an environment with a pH up to 11. Blood, exudate, dental tissues, and tissue fluids will readily lower the pH of the calcium hydroxide paste, and in teeth with severe exudation from the periapical tissues, the paste in the apical part of the canal may have a pH of 8 within 2–3 weeks after placement. The paste will then have lost its antibacterial effect. However, due to its anti-inflammatory effect, even a severe periapical exudation may have stopped at this time. The "used" calcium hydroxide paste is, therefore, removed, the root canal is irrigated and dried, and new, clean calcium hydroxide paste with the right alkalinity is packed into the canal. Bacteria anywhere in the root canal system that might have survived the first application of calcium hydroxide should now effectively be killed. However, in most instances the root canal can be dried to such an extent at the first visit that a one-time application of calcium hydroxide for 2–3 weeks is sufficient to obtain a bacteria-free root canal system.

An additional aspect of the therapeutic effect of calcium hydroxide is its ability to denature proteins. *Necrotic tissue influenced by calcium hydroxide will swell to twice its size and be dissolved by sodium hypochlorite twice as fast as tissue untreated by calcium hydroxide.* Tissue remnants left behind in the root canal after the chemomechanical instrumentation can, therefore, readily be dissolved and rinsed out with sodium hypochlorite following a period of a week or longer with calcium hydroxide in the canal. Similarly, the content of lateral and accessory canals and other areas in the root canal system which cannot be reached by instruments will be influenced by the combined action of calcium hydroxide and sodium hypochlorite, resulting in an optimally cleaned root canal system.

It also appears that the *actual filling of the root canal* with a material with the properties of a calcium hydroxide–saline paste is beneficial for the periapical repair processes. When a traditional antiseptic is applied to an empty root canal by means of a cotton pellet, an exudate consisting of tissue fluids, cells, bacteria, and bacterial products and components will fill the canal. The exudate as such may maintain a periapical inflammation, but most importantly it is an excellent substrate for bacterial growth. The possibilities of reinfection of the root canal between visits under these circumstances are quite real. The use of calcium hydroxide, on the other hand, will effectively prevent exudate from filling the root canal, and by virtue of its presence and its long-lasting antibacterial effect will prevent reinfection of the canal.

Obturation of the root canal. The effectiveness of the chemomechanical instrumentation and disinfection of the root canal is normally evaluated clinically. *If the patient is asymptomatic and the root canal remains dry after the intracanal medicament has been removed and the canal has been irrigated and dried, it is assumed that the periapical inflammation is at a stage of repair.* This can be expected at the first visit following the visit with complete instrumentation of the canal, i.e., *usually in the second visit,* and the root canal can then be permanently obturated.

Sometimes the criteria for final obturation are not achieved in two visits. The reasons for the unfavorable tissue reactions should then be determined, if possible, before the treatment is continued. The primary concern is whether the chemomechanical instrumentation has been performed satisfactorily. The canal may not have been enlarged enough or a canal may have been missed. In any case, insufficient instrumentation with remaining infection is by far the dominating cause of persistent tissue reactions. Microbiological culturing of the root canal content may provide useful information in such instances (see p. 117).

If infection is suspected at the second visit, and the instrumentation of the root canal appears to have been carried out well, *the problem may be caused by reinfection because of a leaky temporary filling, inadequate old restorations, caries, cracks, fractures, or similar causes.* Therefore, after renewed chemomechanical instrumentation and application of the intracanal antiseptic, the coronal seal must be checked most carefully. Remember that a temporary filling should preferably be 4–5 mm thick in order to provide a safe bacteria-tight seal. If symptoms, exudation, or fistulae persist after repeated treatment of a tooth, it is useless to keep changing the intracanal dressing. An analysis of the probable causes of the problem must be carried out and effective therapeutic measures taken (see p. 116).

Clinical Considerations

The access cavity is prepared in the tooth and the root canal orifices are located *before a rubber dam is applied.* This is even more important in nonvital than in vital teeth in that, in these teeth, the root canals are often calcified because of a long-standing chronic inflammation before the pulp finally necrotizes. It may, therefore, be difficult to localize the root canal orifices, and calcified tissue may have to be removed with rotating instruments. In this situation it is helpful to see the entire tooth and the neighboring teeth with adjacent structures for orientation purposes so as to avoid root perforations and other mishaps (**Fig. 6.10**).

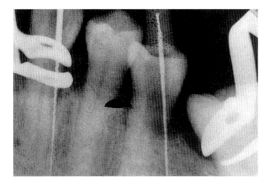

Fig. 6.10 Radiograph showing perforations of teeth in the cervical area during preparation of access cavities under a rubber dam. The operator has clearly misjudged the longitudinal direction of the teeth.

When the orifices are located, a rubber dam is applied and the field of operation is disinfected as described for vital teeth (see p.101). The treatment then continues with sterile instruments and under surgical–aseptic conditions. First, the length of the root canal is established by means of a tooth-length radiograph taken with an instrument in the root canal or with an apex locator. Theoretically, the root canal of a nonvital tooth should be instrumented to the apical foramen to ensure the removal of all necrotic tissue. However, as with vital teeth, it is usually not possible to determine the exact position of the foramen. Therefore, *the practical rule to follow in nonvital teeth is to end the mechanical instrumentation of the root canal 1 mm short of the radiographic apex.* In this way practically all necrotic tissue will be removed, and in most instances the instrumentation will be confined within the canal with the possibility of creating an apical stop to facilitate the obturation of the canal (**Fig.6.11**).

Remember that over-instrumentation of the root canal of nonvital teeth is an effective way to carry bacteria to the periapical tissues, often resulting in an exacerbation of an asymptomatic periapical inflammation.

As discussed above, the root canal will not routinely be bacteria-free after the chemomechanical instrumentation. Consequently, *the root canal in nonvital teeth should not be obturated in the first visit.* For further disinfection of the canal it is important to understand that *the antiseptic medicament used has to come in contact with the bacteria in order to kill them.* Thus, vaporizing medicaments like iodine- and formalin-containing drugs may be applied to the pulp chamber, whereas nonvaporizing medicaments will have to fill the root canal system to have an effect.

If calcium hydroxide is used, it is mixed with saline to a creamy mix. It is applied to the pulp chamber with a plastic instrument and introduced into the root canal by means of a lentulo. When the canal appears filled, excess water is removed with paper points and the paste is condensed with a plugger or similar instrument. Additional calcium hydroxide paste is then applied with the lentulo and condensed at the canal orifice with cotton pellets. When the canal is adequately filled, *excess paste on the walls of the access cavity is carefully removed* and a temporary filling which gives a bacteria-tight seal is finally placed in the access cavity.

The *time between the first and second visit* depends on the type of intracanal antiseptic used. With a traditional antiseptic the time should be short (days) since the medicament loses its effect within hours of placement in the canal. A third appointment may, therefore, become necessary before the criteria for obturating the root canal are fulfilled (asymptomatic patient, dry root canal). An antiseptic in a controlled-release delivery system offers greater convenience because the time interval between appointments may be considerably increased. Possible symptoms of an apical periodontitis may then have time to subside and periapical exudation may stop. At present a calcium hydroxide–saline paste appears to fulfill these requirements of an intracanal antiseptic the best. The paste in the canal will act as a depot and continuously release Ca^{++} and OH^- ions for weeks and months. A period of 2–3 weeks between appointments is as a rule enough in that the pH in the dentinal tubules reaches its peak during this

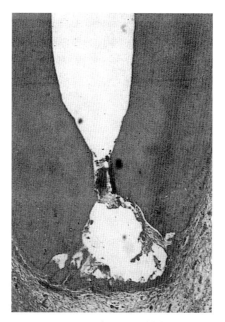

Fig.6.11 Section of a nonvital dog tooth. The instrumentation of the root canal has been carried out according to the apical box method and ends 1 mm short of the apex. In this way, a stop to facilitate the obturation of the canal has been created in spite of apical resorption. The root canal is clean and if the infection has been eliminated, periapical healing will be predictable and fast (hematoxylin-eosin).

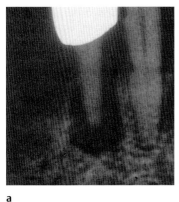 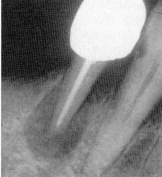 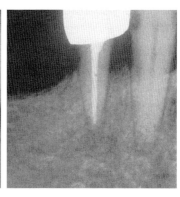

a   b   c

Fig. 6.12
a Radiograph of a mandibular premolar with asymptomatic apical periodontitis. The root canal is completely instrumented in the first visit and calcium hydroxide is packed into the canal to complete the disinfection of the root. (When an ill-fitting crown is not removed until after the endodon-

tic treatment, it is imperative to establish an intracoronal bacteria-tight seal.)
b In the second visit after 3 weeks, the patient remains asymptomatic and no periapical exudation is seen. The root canal is then obturated.
c At the 3-month control, resolution of the periradicular lesion is evident.

time. The bacteria in the root canal system and the root dentin should then be killed and the periapical inflammation will have subsided so that the root canal can be dried and filled under optimal conditions. This method, which is referred to *as short-term calcium hydroxide treatment*, makes for effective and problem-free endodontics (**Fig. 6.12**).

Long-term calcium hydroxide treatment may be the method of choice in special cases. It is used in the treatment of teeth with large periapical lesions, severe periapical exudation, incomplete root formation, progressive external inflammatory resorption, and in the retreatment of teeth where conventional treatment has failed. In other words, the long-term calcium hydroxide method is used in situations in which we want to maximize the effect of our treatment.

With this method the tooth is treated with calcium hydroxide until periapical healing is complete or is at least well under way, i.e., for 3–12 months or even longer (**Figs. 6.8, 6.9, 6.13, 6.14**). The medication is changed after 2–3 weeks and then if necessary after 3 months. The purpose of the treatment is to maximize the antibacterial treatment of the root canal system and to favorably influence hard- and soft-tissue repair processes in the tooth and periradicular tissues. An additional benefit of the method is that apical repair or, just as importantly, lack of repair can be

determined relatively quickly. This may be important for the overall treatment plan of the patient.

Antibiotics should be given prophylactically in conjunction with endodontic treatment of nonvital teeth to certain patients. They are patients with heart valve injury, acute glomerulonephritis, or diabetes that is difficult to control, patients on steroid therapy, and a steadily increasing number of patients who have undergone open heart surgery. Patients with implants and pacemakers should also be included in this group. Prophylactic antibiotic treatment should be performed with bactericidal medicaments, normally amoxicillin. The dose is given a half to 1 hour before the treatment begins, which means that the patient may receive the medicament in the waiting room. The regime for prophylactic use of antibiotics may differ somewhat from country to country. For legal reasons, therefore, one should use the regime exactly as recommended by local authorities, heart associations, or similar institutions.

Follow-up Examinations and Prognosis
Endodontic treatment of nonvital teeth has an excellent prognosis. For teeth with necrotic pulp without radiographically visible periapical inflammation, a success rate of 90–95% is within reach. This is the same success rate as for pulpectomy treatment of vital teeth. Temporary failures, which

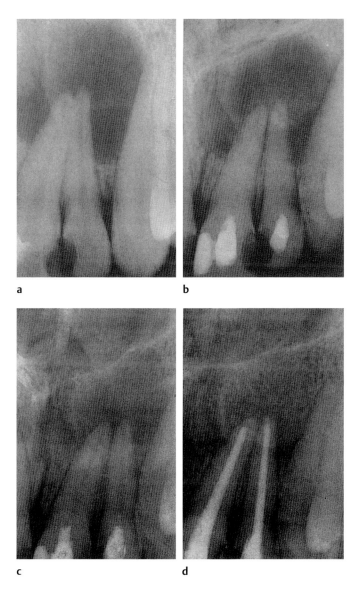

a

b

c

d

Fig. 6.13

a **Radiograph of the maxillary left central and lateral incisors with apical periodontitis and palatal abscess.** Both teeth are nonvital.

b To maximize the antimicrobial and anti-inflammatory treatment, long-term calcium hydroxide therapy is initiated. Calcium hydroxide-saline paste is packed into the canals and, to maintain the all-important high alkalinity, is changed after 3 weeks.

c When the periapical exudation has stopped, the paste is changed about every 3 months until periapical healing is complete or at least well in progress.

d The root canals are then obturated permanently.

are occasionally seen after pulpectomies, will not occur after correct treatment of nonvital teeth. However, severe over-instrumentation of the canal or excess root canal filling material in the periapical tissues, or both, may lead to periapical radiolucencies which may later disappear.

The prognosis of endodontic treatment of teeth with *radiographically visible apical periodontitis* may be 75–80%, which is 15–20% poorer than for vital teeth or nonvital teeth without periapical radiolucencies. Thus, good clinical and radiographic examination routines are important also

in this regard, since necessary endodontic treatment is best performed before an apical periodontitis has had a chance to develop.

Clinical and radiographic follow-up examinations of endodontically treated nonvital teeth must be performed. Intervals of 3–6 months initially, and, if necessary, once a year until healing has occurred are appropriate. When a periapical radiolucency has disappeared and a normal periodontal ligament space has been reestablished, the treatment can be considered successful and subsequent follow-up examinations are not necessary.

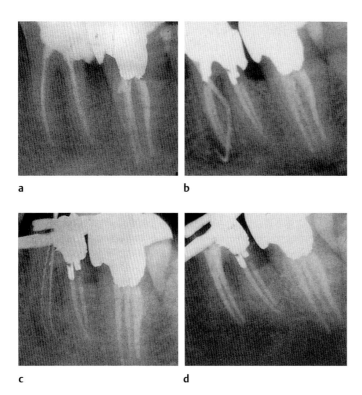

Fig. 6.14
a **Radiograph of mandibular molars with technically excellent root canal filings.**
b After 2 years, an intraoral fistula became evident. It was traced to the mesial root of the first molar where an apical radiolucency had developed.
c Retreatment of the mesial root is initiated and maximized by long-term calcium hydroxide therapy.
d When periapical healing is complete, the mesial root is again permanently obturated.

Periapical repair may occur relatively quickly and be completed within 3–6 months, but sometimes several years may pass before even small periapical radiolucencies disappear. If a radiolucency remains after 4 years in a symptom-free tooth with an adequately filled root canal, it will be necessary to make a decision whether the root filling should be revised, surgical treatment performed, or if the treatment should be considered successful. Periapical repair with the formation of fibrous connective tissue rather than bone does occur and makes this decision difficult in many instances (**Fig. 2.27**). However, the general rule should be that in healthy elderly patients, reserve should be exercised, and the follow-up examinations may be continued at 2–3 year intervals when small radiolucencies do not increase in size.

Apical Periodontitis Refractory to Endodontic Treatment

As discussed above, about 20% of nonvital teeth with apical periodontitis have been found to fail following conventional endodontic treatment. The reason for the failures are bacteria in the root, the root canal system, the periapical lesion, or in all of the above, which have survived the treatment and are able to maintain the inflammatory disease process in the periapical tissues after the treatment is completed. *Many of these teeth will heal following retreatment* (**Fig. 6.14**). However, a certain number of cases are refractory to conventional endodontic treatment, usually because of established extraradicular infections (**Fig. 6.15**) (see p. 37). These infections are usually polymicrobial and dominated by Gram-positive species known from studies of the microflora of the root canal and the periodontal pocket. However, in cases with long-standing fistulas or where root canals have been left open to the oral cavity for any length of time, superinfections with enteric and environmental microorganisms and yeast may occur. The refractory cases may heal following additional treatment, and treatment methods that have shown success singly or in combinations will be outlined.

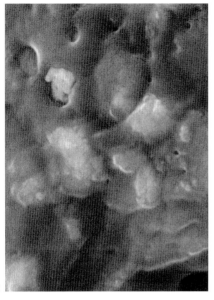
a

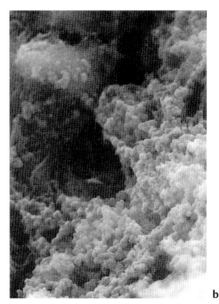
b

Fig. 6.15 Scanning electron micrographs of root surfaces of teeth with refractory apical periodontitis.
a Bacterial colonies in structureless material, prob-
ably extracellular polysaccharide, outside the apical foramen.
b Bacterial colonies in tissue on root surface within granuloma.

Systemic Antibiotic Treatment

The fact that bacteria in the periapical tissues may be the reason for the failure of the conventional methods immediately makes systemic antibiotic treatment a logical second alternative (**Fig. 6.16**). However, an increasing number of bacteria are resistant to one or more antibiotics so that the choice of drug often proves difficult. A microbiological sample, therefore, may be taken in these refractory cases to determine the type and sensitivity of the infecting bacteria. If the failure is apparent before the root canal is obturated, microbiological samples are taken from the canal. Otherwise samples may be taken through the opening of a fistula, or if need be, the periapical lesion may be exposed surgically so that microbiological samples can be taken directly from the lesion. *In all sampling procedures it must be remembered that the endodontic flora is, in principle, anaerobic; thus, an anaerobic culturing technique has to be applied.*

Bacteriological sampling from root canal. Before the sampling is performed, the root canal is left empty without an antiseptic for 1 week. During this period the access opening to the canal is sealed bacteria-tight, so that only bacteria in the dentinal tubules, lateral and accessory canals, periapical tissues, or in all of the above may enter the main root canal. Prior to the sampling, a rubber dam is applied to the tooth and the field of operation is cleaned and repeatedly washed with a surface antiseptic like chlorhexidine or povidone-iodine. The root canal is then exposed and sterile paper points are used to suck up exudate in the canal. If necessary, the canal is filled with sterile saline and further points are introduced into the canal, sometimes after a certain filing of the canal walls. The paper points are placed in vials with a transport medium for anaerobic bacteria, and the samples are sent to a microbiological laboratory for identification and testing of the bacteria's sensitivity to various antibiotics.

Bacteriological sampling from fistula. The area with the fistula is isolated as best as possible from the rest of the oral cavity with cotton rolls and gauze pads. The gingiva and mucosa, including the fistula, are then washed repeatedly with a surface antiseptic. If pus can be squeezed out of the fistula, this is collected on paper points. The mucosa is then stretched with two fingers so that the

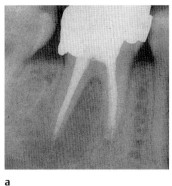
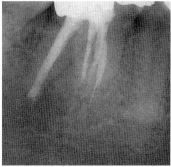
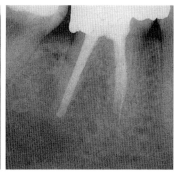

a   b   c

Fig. 6.16
a Radiograph of a mandibular molar with a non-responding periapical radiolucency on the distal root.
b Four weeks following apparently successful retreatment of the distal root, the patient returns with slight swelling and a fistula in the oral vestibule

from the distal root. A bacterial sample is obtained from the fistula and systemic penicillin treatment is initiated.
c The fistula closes and at the 1-year control, resolution of the periapical lesion is evident without further treatment.

fistula is maximally open and a paper point is introduced into the fistula to further suck up exudate. At least two paper points are used and the points are introduced into a vial with anaerobic transport medium.

Bacterial sampling from periapical lesion. The teeth, gingiva, and mucosa are washed repeatedly with a surface antiseptic. A full-thickness flap is raised and the periapical lesion is exposed and opened under aseptic conditions. Sterile paper points (at least three) are then introduced into the lesion toward the root end, and upon removal they are placed in a vial with anaerobic transport medium. When the granulation tissue has been curetted out, scrapings from the root tip or the root tip itself may be removed and introduced into the transport medium. In this way it should be fairly certain that the infecting bacteria are recovered for study.

Depending on the culturing results, an antibiotic is selected. Often a combination of drugs may offer therapeutic advantages over single preparations. *If culturing is not performed*, penicillin is the first drug of choice, both for medical and legal reasons. A combination of penicillin and metronidazole with its special effect on anaerobes may be an even better choice. Clindamycin is also an excellent alternative, and clindamycin is the drug of choice in patients allergic to penicillin.

Surgical Treatment (see p. 127)
Systemic antibiotic treatment of periapical lesions refractory to endodontic treatment may be very effective. Fistulae may disappear within days and regeneration of periapical bone may occur within months (**Fig. 6.16**). However, in some instances, this treatment has no appreciable effect and a surgical removal of the lesion may be required (**Fig. 6.17**). *The purpose of the surgical treatment is to remove the periapical lesion with possible surviving bacteria and preferably the apical 1–3 mm of the root tip which may have an apical delta of accessory canals which conceivably constitute a further habitat for endodontopathic bacteria.* In addition, the apical seal of the root canal may be checked and, if necessary, improved upon with a retrograde root filling.

The periapical surgical treatment is effective in that it is directed at the possible causes of failure, namely bacteria either in the apical part of the root, the periapical lesion, or both. Traditionally, therefore, surgical removal of a refractory lesion has not routinely been combined with systemic antibiotic treatment. However, failures after surgical treatment do occur, usually because of persistent infection, and *it is good clinical practice to cover the patient with an appropriate antibiotic beginning one day before the surgery and continuing after the surgery, normally for 4–5 days.* Many postsurgical failures will then be prevented.

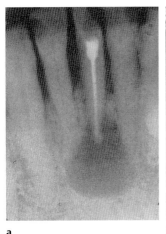

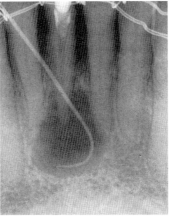

a

b

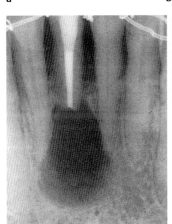

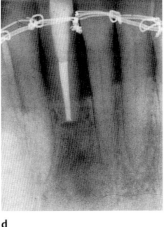

c

d

Fig. 6.17
a Radiograph of mandibular incisor 2 years following endodontic treatment. Periapical healing has not occurred.
b During retreatment, which was ineffective, a fistula to the oral vestibule opened up. Systemic antibiotic treatment following sampling and identification of infecting microorganisms was ineffective as well.
c The root canal was then obturated and an apicoectomy performed.
d At 6-month control, periapical healing is evident.

It should be noted that failures after surgical removal of refractory lesions occur either because bacteria which were present in the tooth, the lesion, or both, are not removed during the operation, or because the operator introduces new bacteria into the surgical wound. In this regard, irrigation of the wound with tap water should be particularly warned against, especially from the water syringe of the dental unit. The syringe, which is often heated, functions as an incubator for bacterial growth, and counts of 15 000 bacteria per mL have been observed in the water in the syringe. As an example, pathogenic organisms like *Pseudomonas aeruginosa* may survive in water for long periods of time, and if transferred to a surgical wound, may cause an infection that is extremely difficult to treat.

Prognosis

An innovative and aggressive systemic antibiotic therapy aimed at specific bacteria present in the individual case may save many teeth with apical periodontitis refractory to conventional treatment. When the systemic antibiotic therapy is combined with surgical removal of the periapical lesion, additional refractory cases can be successfully treated. This approach to the treatment of teeth which fail following conventional methods may conceivably bring the success rate of the treatment of nonvital teeth with apical periodontitis up to 90–95%.

Treatment of Immature Nonvital Teeth

From a biological point of view, the treatment of nonvital immature teeth does not differ from the treatment of nonvital fully formed teeth. The infected necrotic tissue in the root canal is removed by chemomechanical instrumentation, the root canal is disinfected, and when the canal is dry and the patient has no symptoms, the root canal is obturated. However, the obturation of the root canal in an immature tooth is extremely difficult because of the blunderbuss shape of the canal with its widest diameter at the apex of the tooth. *The treatment of choice in such teeth, therefore, is the induction of a hard-tissue barrier at the apical end of the root canal to facilitate the subsequent obturation of the canal without voids and excess material in the periapical tissues.* This treatment procedure is referred to as *apexification.*

Apexification

The *hard tissue-inducing effect of calcium hydroxide* known from, for instance, pulp capping, is utilized to attain apexification of nonvital immature teeth. The calcium hydroxide paste obviously has the same effect when used apically as when used in the coronal pulp, but the apical tissue is usually not pulp tissue, but periodontal tissue or even granulation tissue, and the apical hard-tissue response, therefore, is different from the pulpal response. Most often a cementum-like tissue is recognized in the apical hard-tissue barrier (**Fig. 6.18**). Other times the tissue is so irregular

that all that can be said about it is that it is a mineralized tissue. The hard-tissue barrier is usually also irregular in that it contains inclusions of soft tissue. The degree of irregularity apparently depends on the type of apical tissue. Thus, if vital pulp tissue is present at the apex, dentin is formed, and in such instances the Hertwig's root sheath may be fully or partially intact as well and the root development may continue (**Figs. 1.44, 6.19**). Otherwise, the apical hard-tissue barrier will always be a more or less complete bridge across the root canal at the level of the root where the development of the tooth had stopped when the pulp and the root sheath necrotized (**Figs. 6.18, 6.20**).

As appears from the above, *the apical hard-tissue bridge does not seal the root canal. It only renders a barrier against which a bacteria-tight seal of the canal may be achieved by means of the root filling materials.*

Technically, an apexification procedure follows the guidelines for long-term calcium hydroxide treatment of teeth with apical periodontitis. The calcium hydroxide paste is packed into the root canal with good contact to the periapical tissues. It is first changed 2–3 weeks later, at which time any periapical exudation will have stopped. Then, when new, clean calcium hydroxide paste has been introduced into the canal, it usually only needs to be changed every 3 months. However, in very young patients when the root canal is ex-

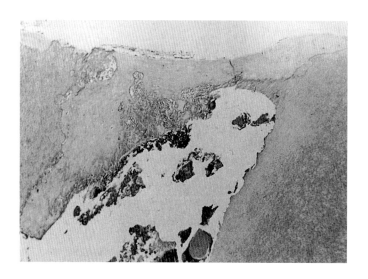

Fig. 6.18 Root end of an immature maxillary incisor. A cementum-like tissue is bridging the wide root canal at the apex of the root following calcium hydroxide treatment for 12 months (apexification; hematoxylin-eosin).

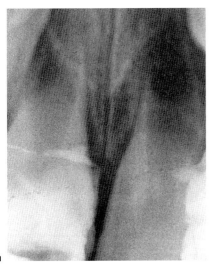

a

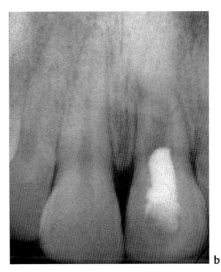

b

Fig. 6.19
a Radiograph of an avulsed and replanted maxillary right central incisor in a 7-year-old.

b Twenty-year follow up. Continuation of the root development following endodontic treatment is evident (apexigenesis).

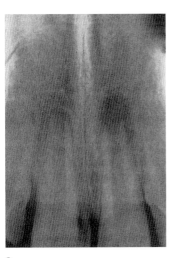

a

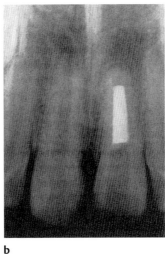

b

Fig. 6.20
a Radiograph of a nonvital, immature maxillary left central incisor with apical periodontitis. Long-term calcium hydroxide therapy is carried out to obtain resolution of the periapical lesion and apexification of the root.
b After 12 months, periapical healing is evident and an apical hard-tissue bridge has formed. The root canal is then obturated and the tooth is restored with the acid-etch resin technique. Note the difference in the root length of the central incisors.

tremely wide, the calcium hydroxide paste may dissolve and wash out from the root canal so quickly that, at least at the beginning of the treatment, it may have to be changed more often than every 3 months. Granulation tissue which often grows into the apical area of a wide open root canal is sometimes difficult to remove with instruments. However, it will necrotize when calcium hydroxide is packed into the canal, and at the second visit can be rinsed out of the canal with sodium hypochlorite (**Fig. 6.21**). *Usually it takes from 6–18 months for the apical barrier to form and be strong enough that the canal can be obturated.*

Follow-up Examinations and Prognosis

Due to the long-term nature of the apexification procedure, periapical healing is usually a fact long before the immature tooth is ready to be obturated (**Fig. 6.8**). It should be mentioned, however, that the formation of an apical hard-tissue barrier in itself is no criterion for periapical healing. Nonvital immature teeth are usually traumatized,

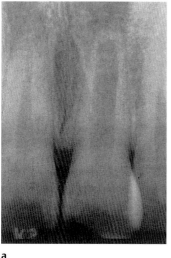
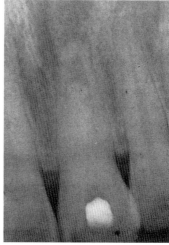
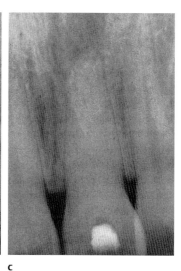

a   b   c

Fig. 6.21
a **Radiograph of a maxillary left central incisor with arrested root development and a wide root canal.**
b Apically in the canal, a tenacious granulation tissue is nearly impossible to remove with instruments.

Calcium hydroxide is then packed tightly against the tissue.
c At the next visit 1 week later, the apical tissue is necrotized due to the influence of calcium hydroxide. It is rinsed out and the entire root canal can be filled with the apexification paste.

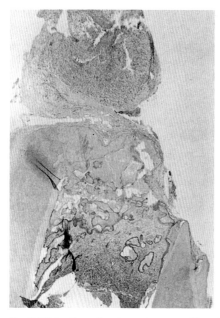

Fig. 6.22 Section of an immature maxillary incisor after 18 months of calcium hydroxide (apexification) treatment. Resolution of a periapical lesion did not occur. The tooth was extracted and a vertical root fracture became evident (hematoxylin-eosin).

and undiagnosed problems like vertical root fractures or marginal–apical periodontal communications may allow ingress of bacteria from the oral cavity to sustain a periapical inflammation. In such teeth an apical barrier may form without periapical healing (**Fig. 6.22**).

The frequency of periapical healing and apical hard-tissue closure of nonvital immature teeth after long-term calcium hydroxide treatment is in the range of 90– 95%, which shows that the treatment is predictable. For the sake of comparison it should be mentioned that if an apexification procedure is not performed prior to obturating the root canal of immature teeth, the success rate of the treatment is less than 50%.

However, the fact that an apical hard-tissue bridge takes months to form has led to attempts to use other methods to close off the open apex so that a blunderbuss root canal can be filled after a normal period of disinfection of 2–3 weeks. This has proved difficult in that any material that is condensed in an apical direction readily is pushed beyond the apex and into the periapical tissues, often without bridging the foramen sufficiently so that the canal can be filled bacteria-tight. Still, somewhat acceptable results have been obtained in parallel-walled root canals where the foramen is not too wide by scraping off dentin chips from the root canal walls and condensing them to a plug in the apical area. The dentin chips are exceptionally well tolerated by the periodontium since they are taken from the patient's own dentin. They are "cemented" together in the tissue fluids and root cementum forms onto and covers the periodontal surface of the plug (**Fig. 6.23**). Similar results have been reported by the use of a new cement, mineral trioxide aggregate (MTA), to form an apical plug after disinfection of the root canal. This material appears to be well tolerated by the periodontium and root cementum has been observed forming onto the periodontal surface of the MTA plug. Apparently this is due to the release of Ca^{++} and OH^- ions from the MTA material. Thus, the tissue reaction to MTA appears to be similar to or the same as the well known reaction to calcium hydroxide.

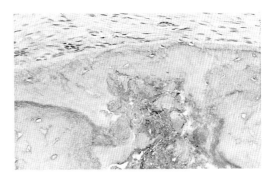

Fig. 6.23 Root tip of immature monkey tooth. Prior to root filling, dentin chips have been condensed to a plug in the apical area of the root canal. Root cementum has formed onto and covers the periodontal surface of the plug. The periodontal ligament is free of inflammation.

Endodontic Treatment of Root-Fractured Teeth

Only about 20% of root-fractured teeth will be in need of endodontic treatment, and by far the most endodontic problems are located to the coronal fragment of the teeth. The reason for this is that the coronal fragment may be displaced by the injury so that the pulpal blood vessels are severed at the fracture site. The pulp tissue of the coronal fragment will then become necrotic, whereas in the apical fragment, which was not displaced, the pulp tissue most often remains vital.

Thus, in general, endodontic treatment of a root-fractured tooth will entail treatment of a nonvital coronal fragment. The treatment follows the guidelines for the treatment of nonvital teeth and the root canal can be filled when it is dry and the patient is asymptomatic. However, root fractures often occur in young teeth with wide root canals. Long-term calcium hydroxide treatment of the coronal fragment with induction of a hard-tissue barrier toward the fracture line is then the treatment of choice (**Fig. 6.24**). The hard-tissue barrier then makes it possible to obturate the coronal root canal without impinging on the fracture line area. The treatment is performed as described for apexification of nonvital immature teeth (see p. 120). If the root canal is not too wide a "bridge" towards the fracture line may be made using a material like IRM, EBA cement, or MTA. However,

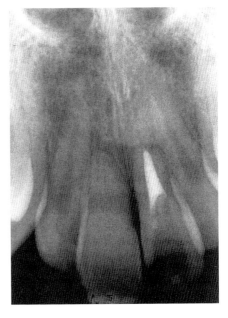

Fig. 6.24 Radiograph of maxillary central incisors with a fracture of their roots. In the right incisor the pulp remained vital in both fragments and obliteration of the root canal has occurred. In the left incisor the pulp of the coronal fragment became necrotic and infected, and endodontic treatment of this tooth to the fracture line has been performed.

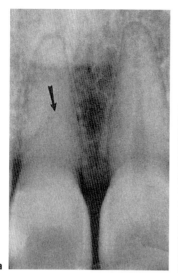

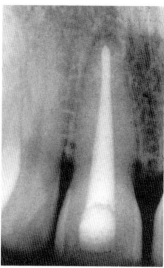

Fig. 6.25
a **Radiograph of a maxillary right central incisor with a root fracture** (arrow; root canal is obliterated because of previous trauma).
b The tooth was splinted for a period of 12 months and hard-tissue unification of the two fragments has taken place. When the tooth became symptomatic, endodontic treatment of both fragments through the fracture line was performed.

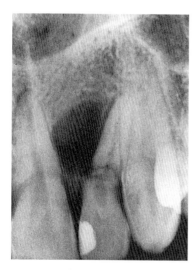

Fig. 6.26 Radigraph of a maxillary left lateral incisor. The pulp of the coronal fragment is nonvital and a lateral radiolucent lesion has developed adjacent to the fracture line.

this is a technique-sensitive approach in that the material inadvertently may be pushed into the fracture line area, which may prevent healing of the root fracture.

If the pulp of the apical fragment has become necrotic as well, endodontic treatment of *both fragments through the fracture line* is indicated. The treatment is performed as described for non-

vital teeth and calcium hydroxide should be used as the intracanal medicament in these teeth. The prognosis of the treatment will depend to a great extent on the efficacy of the emergency treatment when the fracture occurred. If the repositioning and splinting of the tooth is performed correctly so that an effective immobilization of the coronal fragment in juxtaposition to the apical fragment is attained for a sufficient period of time (6–12 months), a calcific bridging of the two fragments may occur.

Endodontic treatment through the fracture line will then have a near-normal success rate (**Fig. 6.25**). However, if the two fragments are apart, a lateral periodontitis often develops at the fracture site (**Fig. 6.26**). If the fracture is in the apical half of the root, surgical removal of the apical fragment may save the tooth. Similarly, if the root fracture is in the cervical area, surgical removal of the coronal fragment and orthodontic or surgical extrusion of the apical fragment may constitute an excellent therapeutic alternative (**Fig. 6.27**). Endodontic treatment of the apical fragment is then carried out as the clinical situation demands.

Endodontic treatment of root-fractured teeth is a rather delicate procedure and should be performed with optimal techniques and methods. The prognosis then is good, although no information on the actual frequencies of repair are available.

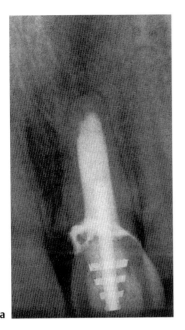
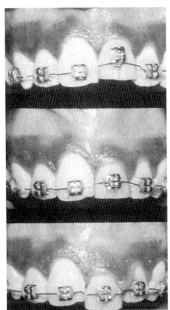
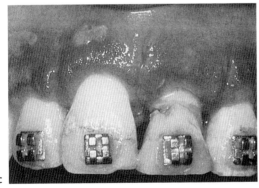
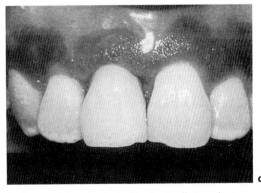

Fig. 6.27

a Radiograph of an immature maxillary left central incisor with a fracture of the root in the cervical area. The coronal fragment is temporarily retained by means of luting cement and a post.

b The tooth is extruded orthodontically in order to bring the apical fragment to a level where it can be used to hold a permanent coronal restoration.
c Surgical correction of the gingival margin level.
d Final restoration.

Endodontic Treatment of Endo–Perio Lesions

Endodontic treatment of teeth with endo–perio lesions follow the guidelines for treatment of teeth with apical periodontitis. As discussed above, diagnostic problems may exist in patients with possible endo–perio lesions, especially whether a periodontal probing depth is due to a periodontal pocket or an endodontic fistula alongside the root. Therefore, *an unbreakable rule is that, when in doubt, the* *endodontic treatment is initiated first* (**Fig. 2.16, 6.28**). Although it may take months before radiographic signs of periapical bone regeneration are evident, clinical signs will indicate within days or weeks whether the lesion responds to endodontic treatment or not. Such clinical signs are the closing of a fistula, a rapid reduction in probing depth, and a general firming up of the gingival tissues. If

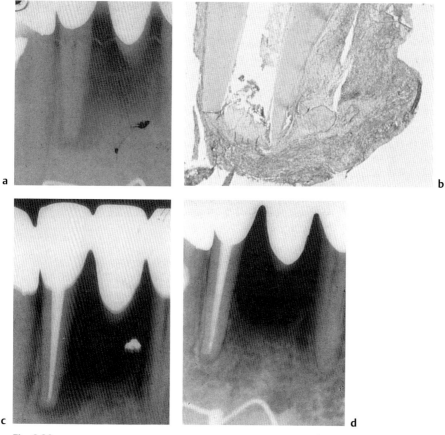

Fig. 6.28

a **Radiograph of a mandibular central incisor with an apical–lateral radiolucency of endodontic or periodontal origin.**

b Section from a tooth with an apical granuloma with an extension similar to the radiolucent lesion in **a** (hematoxylin-eosin).

c Since the tooth in **a** is nonvital, endodontic treatment is carried out first, and periodontal treatment is only initiated if and when it is clear that the endodontic treatment has had no effect.

d One-year control. Full resolution of the radiolucent lesion is evident following the endodontic treatment.

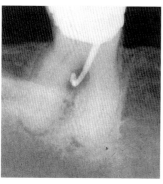
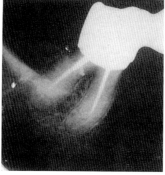

Fig. 6.29

a **Radiograph of mandibular molar with an intraoral fistula traced to a radiolucent lesion in the furcation.** The tooth is nonvital and no periodontal treatment is performed until the effect of the necessary endodontic treatment is known.

b One-year control. Full resolution of the furcation lesion is evident. Also, note that a lateral canal to the area of the furcation became visible after obturation of the root canals.

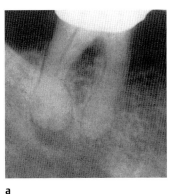 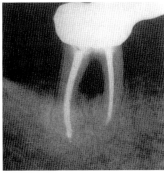

a   b

Fig. 6.30
a Radiograph of a mandibular molar with apical periodontitis and a radiolucent lesion in the furcation.
b Two-year control. Following endodontic treatment, periapical healing has occurred. However, the furcation lesion was of periodontal origin (see bone level in **a**) and did not respond to the endodontic therapy.

clear indications of healing are not seen 2–3 weeks after complete instrumentation of the root canal, periodontal treatment with scaling and root planing should follow, as the observed probing depth is then with great certainty due to a periodontal pocket.

On the other hand, if the treatment of a lesion of endodontic origin begins with scaling and root planing, the thin, delicate periodontal tissue which exists between the fistula and the root surface will be removed. Thus, the root is denuded and the fistula is in actual contact with the root surface. Epithelium then grows down and a periodontal pocket will form to the foraminal areas of the tooth. At this stage the lesion as a result of incorrect treatment has become a combined endo–perio lesion, which at best can only heal with a long junctional epithelial attachment.

The same considerations should be made regarding *furcation lesions*. If in doubt, and if endodontic treatment is indicated, this treatment should be initiated first (**Fig. 6.29**). Periodontal treatment then only follows if and when it is clear that the endodontic measures had no effect on the lesion (**Fig. 6.30**).

When decisions such as these are made about sequencing of therapy, it is important to understand that, if a periodontal pocket is deep enough to be mistaken for an endodontic fistula originating at or near the apex of the tooth, a postponement of the periodontal treatment for 2–3 weeks will have no negative effect on the outcome of such treatment that may subsequently prove necessary.

Surgical–Endodontic Treatment

Traditionally, the rationale for surgical–endodontic treatment of a tooth has been to attain a bacteria-tight seal of the root canal by means of a filling placed in a retrograde fashion in the root canal. This treatment is performed when an orthograde root filling is expected to be ineffective or to fail, usually because of complications during conventional treatment, or when conventional treatment has failed. A common practice before placing the retrograde root filling is to remove 1–3 mm of the root end, as this part of the root is most likely to contain accessory canals conceivably harboring the bacteria responsible for the failure of the conventional treatment. Today we also know that apical granulomas refractory to conservative treatment may contain bacteria capable of sustaining a

periapical disease process independent of the root canal (see p. 37). A meticulous removal of periapical granulation tissue is therefore an important aspect of surgical–endodontic treatment.

Indications

Primary surgical treatment. In principle, surgical treatment of apical periodontitis as the primary treatment form is performed only when a root is removed or a tooth is extracted. Primary surgical treatment may, however, be the last resort in certain teeth where an obliteration of the root canal makes it impossible to negotiate the canal. Such teeth may be tentatively treated with a retrograde root filling in an attempt to seal the ap-

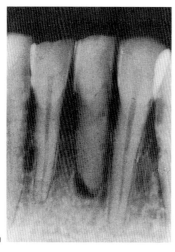

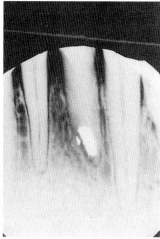

a

b

Fig. 6.31
a **Radiograph of a mandibular left central incisor with an obliterated root canal and apical periodontitis.** An attempt to locate and negotiate the root canal was not made and the tooth was treated with apicoectomy and retrograde root filling only.
b Two-year control. Periapical repair is evident.

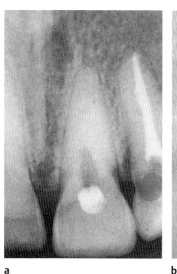

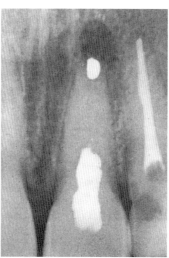

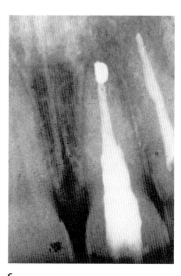

a   b   c

Fig. 6.32
a **Radiograph of a maxillary left central incisor with obliterated root canal.** The tooth is tender to biting. An attempt to locate and negotiate the root canal was abandoned.

b An apicoectomy with retrograde root filling was then carried out. Three months later the patient returned with symptoms.
c A renewed effort was made to find and instrument the root canal, this time successfully. At the 6-month control, periapical healing is evident.

ical end of the canal bacteria-tight (**Fig. 6.31**). However, even if a canal is clinically and radiographically obliterated, there will always be infected necrotic tissue in microscopic spaces in the root of such teeth. Leakage of bacterial products may, therefore, occur in spite of the retrograde filling and the treatment will fail (**Fig. 6.32**). *Surgical*

treatment of apical periodontitis should, therefore, if at all possible be performed in conjunction with orthograde treatment of the root canal.

Conventional treatment ineffective. Surgical therapy is indicated in the treatment of apical periodontitis when conventional treatment proves in-

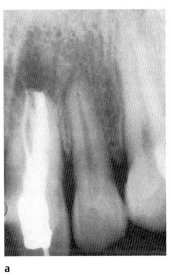 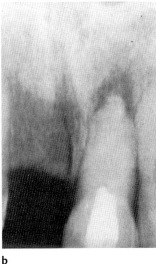

a   b

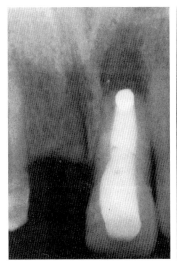 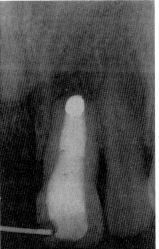

c   d

Fig. 6.33
a Radiograph of an immature maxillary left central incisor with inadequate root canal filling and a fistula to the vestibule.
b Retreatment with calcium hydroxide to obtain periapical healing and root apexification was initiated, but proved ineffective and the fistula did not close.
c The root canal was then filled and an apicoectomy was performed.
d Three-month control. The fistula is closed and complete periapical repair is evident.

effective. This is most often evidenced by a persisting fistula (**Figs. 6.17, 6.33**). In addition, a surgical–endodontic approach may be used for reasons of convenience. An optimal conservative approach may sometimes require several visits over several months and the patient may elect to have the periapical lesion surgically removed for more rapid periapical repair.

Retreatment. Most often a surgical–endodontic approach is indicated in the retreatment of failure cases after conservative treatment of teeth with apical periodontitis. As was discussed above, a

certain percentage of endodontic treatments will fail, and the failure rate will increase dramatically if the technical quality of the treatment is inadequate. In most instances this is evidenced radiographically by incompletely instrumented and sealed, or grossly overfilled root canals. If possible, i.e., if the root canal is not physically blocked by posts, instrument fragments, etc., failure cases should be retreated conventionally before surgical treatment is initiated (**Fig. 6.34**). *The objective of the conservative retreatment is the removal of possible causal factors for the failure in the tooth itself, such as missed canals, inadequate disinfec-*

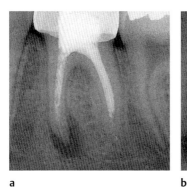
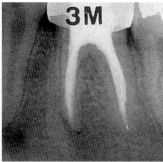

a   b

Fig. 6.34
a Radiograph of a mandibular molar with technically inadequate endodontic treatment and a periapical radiolucency on the mesial root.
b Following retreatment with thorough disinfection of the roots and proper root canal fillings, near full resolution of the periapical lesion is seen at the 3-month control.

tion, or incomplete seal of the root canal. However, only about 60% of unsuccessfully treated teeth will be successful after conservative retreatment, and in the remaining teeth a surgical approach will be the treatment of choice. The success rate of periapical surgical treatment is greatly enhanced by an adequately filled root canal. In addition, a retrograde filling may be placed for extra precaution and an optimal result of the treatment.

Post in the root canal. When an apical periodontitis has not healed and conventional retreatment is made difficult or impossible because the root canal is blocked coronally by a post, surgical treatment may be the method of choice. However, the possibilities of removing the post should be evaluated carefully, especially in teeth where the root filling is technically inadequate (**Fig. 6.35**). The quality of the root filling is then evaluated against the type and size of the post and the risk of root fracture and other complications if removal of the post is attempted. In this context it should be mentioned that the use of ultrasonically energized vibratory instruments to break the cement seal around a root canal post has greatly facilitated the ease and safety with which a post may be removed (**Fig. 6.35**).

In teeth with an inadequately filled but coronally blocked root canal, the canal should if at all possible be completely instrumented and filled bacteria-tight from the apical end to the root canal post during the surgical operation (**Fig. 6.36**). If the quality of the root filling appears satisfactory, a regular retrograde filling may be placed to secure the seal of the root canal (**Fig. 6.37**).

Instrument fragment in the root canal. Fracture of instruments inside the root canal occurs. Often

healing is observed in spite of this mishap, but failures must be expected. Instrument fragments, therefore, may have to be removed. New vibratory nickel-titanium tips are useful to loosen intracanal fragments (see Chapter 13), but often surgical–endodontic treatment is the only treatment alternative (**Fig. 13.11**). Ideally, the instrument fragment is removed apically, and an orthograde root filling is placed in the canal during the operation. If it proves impossible to remove the instrument fragment, the best possible retrograde root filling is placed.

Root perforations. A perforation of the root may occur *during root canal instrumentation.* Often, this may be managed with conventional endodontic methods by sealing the perforation opening through the root canal. However, in many instances a surgical approach may be the best or only alternative (**Fig. 13.11**). *Perforations in the furcation, on the other hand, should be treated conservatively.* If unsuccessful, a hemi-section of the tooth or removal of one root are usually the only alternatives.

Perforations are also seen in conjunction with root canal post preparations. A surgical exposure of the perforation and creation of a bacteria-tight seal of the perforation canal is often the treatment of choice in these teeth (**Fig. 13.13**). However, it should be noted that, depending on the location of the perforation, this is difficult treatment and the long-term success rate is far from good.

External root resorption. In most instances, progressive external inflammatory root resorption is treated conservatively through the root canal (see p. 146). However, in teeth with *cervical resorption,* surgical treatment is the only alternative (**Fig. 6.38**)

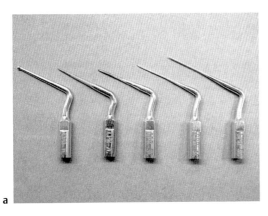

a

Fig. 6.35

a **Multipurpose vibratory instruments energized by an ultrasonic unit.** These instruments can be used to remove cement around a post, to loosen the post by breaking the cement seal, to instrument the root canal from the retrograde position, etc.

b Radiograph of a mandibular premolar with post-retained crown, inadequate root canal filling and apical periodontitis.

c The post and crown are removed and endodontic retreatment is carried out.

d The root canal is properly instrumented and obturated and a new post-retained crown is fabricated.

e Two-year control with repair.

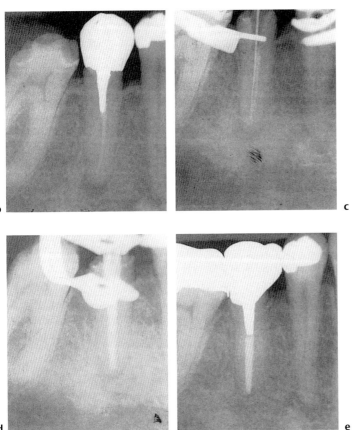

b

c

d

e

The resorptive cavity is then exposed surgically, the granulation tissue removed, and the cavity is filled with a restorative material. A very rapid apical resorption is occasionally seen in conjunction with large excesses of root filling material. In these instances, surgical removal of the excess material is effective treatment and should be considered together with a bevelling of the root end (**Fig. 13.22**).

Root fracture. In teeth with horizontal root fractures, the pulp of the apical fragment of the frac-

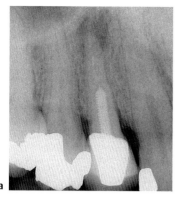
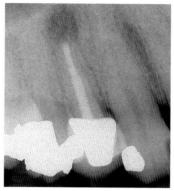

a

b

Fig. 6.36

a Radiograph of maxillary premolar with symptomatic apical periodontitis. The root of the tooth is narrow with long and thick post. No root filling is visible. Because of the radiographic findings, a decision was made not to remove the post, but to treat the tooth from the retrograde position.

b Radiograph of tooth following treatment. The root tip has been cut off and the root canal has been instrumented and filled with IRM-cement to the level of the root canal post. An ultrasonic tip (see **Fig. 6.35a**) was used for the instrumentation.

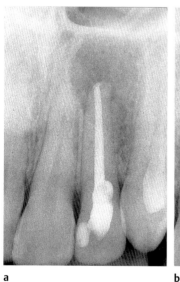
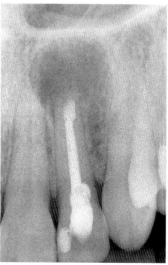
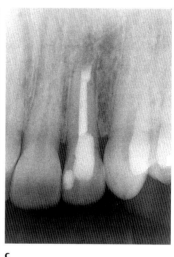

a

b

c

Fig. 6.37

a Radiograph of root-filled tooth with persisting apical periodontitis.

b The root filling is considered technically adequate and an apicoectomy with retrograde filling of IRM-cement is carried out.

c Six-month control with repair.

tured tooth occasionally becomes necrotic and may cause an apical periodontitis. Endodontic treatment through the fracture line is often unsuccessful and surgical removal of the apical fragment may save the tooth if the fracture is in the apical half of the tooth.

Asepsis

In endodontic surgery as with all surgical procedures, the bacteria count of the field of operation should be as low as at all possible. This means that the patient's oral hygiene must be evaluated, and if necessary, professional tooth cleaning

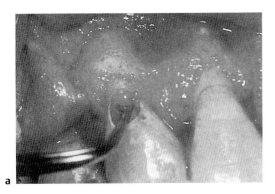

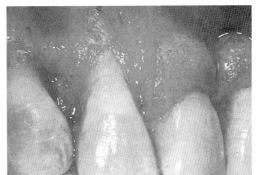

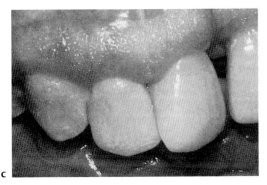

Fig. 6.38
a **Maxillary canine with a cervical resorption lacuna on the buccal surface after reflection of a sulcular flap.**
b The resorption lacuna is cleaned and restored with the acid-etch resin technique.
c Three-month control with good clinical conditions.

should be carried out prior to the surgical intervention. Placing the patient on a program of chemical plaque control for some days prior to the operation may also be advantageous. At the time of surgery, the area to be operated on is washed repeatedly with a surface antiseptic like chlorhexidine and is isolated as much as possible from the rest of the mouth with cotton rolls and gauze pads.

Flap Design and Surgical Access
In the design of the flap it must be remembered that the pathological lesion as a rule is larger than what appears radiographically. Thus, the incision must be extended well beyond the apparent area of pathosis and include at least one tooth on each side of the one to be operated on. Frequently, a larger area is included in the flap to improve either the visibility, the surgical access, or both. Both marginal and submarginal incisions are used in endodontic surgery and with one or two releasing incisions as found necessary (**Fig. 6.39**). In most situations, a marginal full-thickness flap with one vertical incision is the flap of choice. This design gives good surgical access and visibility, maintains

an intact mucosal vasculature, causes minimal postoperative swelling and discomfort, and heals by primary intention. A conceivable disadvantage of the marginal incision is that the sulcular area of the teeth with subgingival plaque and an abundance of bacteria is infringed upon. As a result, a direct or circulatory translocation of periodontal bacteria to the surgical site will occur. *This is avoided with a submarginal incision.* Still, this type of incision should not be used indiscriminately in that it may come in conflict with the area of pathosis. It also disrupts the vascular supply of the gingiva to some extent and scarring may occur (**Fig. 6.40**). However, in patients with a wide, attached gingiva, the submarginal incision may be preferable and give the required surgical access. A submarginal incision is also used in patients with crowns on their maxillary incisors, allegedly to prevent recession of the gingiva and to obtain the best possible aesthetic results. However, if the gingiva is not perfectly healthy, a submarginal incision will cause a recession. On the other hand, if the gingiva is healthy, a well-executed marginal incision will cause a recession of only about 0.5 mm, which clinically may not be noticeable.

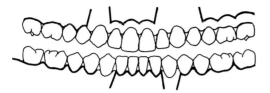

Fig. 6.39 Diagram illustrating commonly used flap designs in endodontic surgery. Both marginal and submarginal incisions are used with one or two releasing incisions as deemed necessary for access and visibility.

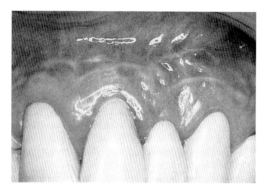

Fig. 6.40 Gingiva in the maxillary anterior region. Multiple scars following submarginal incisions can be seen.

A nontoxic surgical pencil is used to mark the gingiva and mucosa where the incisions are planned (**Fig. 6.41**). For an inexperienced surgeon this is quite helpful in that the markings help visualize the flap before the actual incisions are made. A sharp scalpel, usually no. 15, cuts through the periosteum to the bone, following the markings of the pencil. A no. 12 scalpel is used to loosen the delicate gingival tissues around the teeth. The flap is elevated by means of a sharp periosteal elevator with great care taken not to damage gingival papillae or otherwise tear the tissues.

When the flap is reflected, a periapical lesion may have broken through the buccal cortical bone so that the location of the root tip is readily recognized (**Fig. 6.41**). In other instances when the cortical plate is intact, it may be difficult to locate the root tip, or even more so, a root perforation site or a lateral or cervical resorption lacuna. A small piece of radiopaque material, for instance, gutta-percha, may then be placed on the buccal bone, and a radiograph is taken. This procedure may, if necessary, be repeated until the location of the lesion is determined as exactly as possible. Round burs no. 6 – 12 are then used in an ultraspeed, low-torque handpiece under continuous and copious irrigation with sterile isotonic saline to expose the apical granuloma, perforation site, etc.

Microbiological and Microscopic Examination

In cases with indications that the "normal" antibiotic regime may be ineffective, a microbiological sample may be taken from the lesion in order to identify infecting bacteria. This may make it possible to select a "correct" antibiotic to support the postoperative healing (see p. 118). The periradicular lesion is then removed as much as possible in one piece by means of endodontic spoons and curettes and placed in formalin for subsequent microscopic examination. Remember that the reason for the surgical operation may well be extraradicular infection and consequently all granulation tissue should be removed.

Resorption Lacunae and Perforation Defects

When surgical access has been obtained, a resorption lacuna, or perforation defect, is given undercuts for retention and is then restored. The restorative material used will become an implant and as such should tolerate the influence of tissue fluids and cells without being resorbed, washed out, or otherwise broken down. Over the years, various amalgams have been used for this purpose, and at present the modern copper-containing spherical amalgams might still be a good alternative. When used together with a copal varnish to coat the cavity walls, they give good immediate and long-lasting seal of the cavity (**Fig. 6.41**). However, the use of dental amalgam is frowned upon in many circles, and in some countries its use is simply prohibited. We therefore have a definite need for an alternative retrograde obturation material. Resin-reinforced zinc oxide–eugenol cements and EBA-cements give an adequate seal and have so far been shown to hold up well in the tissue for 12 – 15 years and more. If esthetic factors are of importance, a defect, for example, a cervical resorption lacuna, is acid-etched and restored with a bonded composite resin restoration (**Fig. 8.13**).

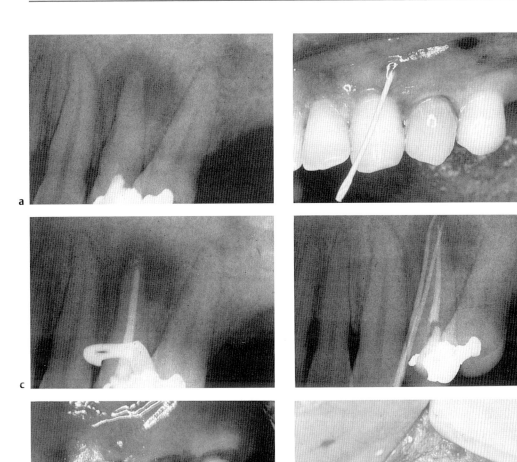

Fig. 6.41

a, b Maxillary premolar with apical periodontitis with fistula.

c Following instrumentation and disinfection of the root, the fistula closed and the root canal was obturated.

d At the 3-month control, the fistula had recurred and the decision to carry out a surgical retreatment was made.

e The radiolucent lesion is large with an extension toward the cervical area of the tooth. Thus, a marginal (sulcular) flap is designed and the incision is outlined with a nontoxic pencil.

f The flap is reflected and, typically, the lesion is bigger than indicated radiographically.

g The root tip is cut off.

h The granulation tissue is curetted out.

i A retrograde cavity is prepared.

j A copal varnish is applied to the retrograde cavity by means of a paper point.

k A retrograde amalgam filling is inserted.

l Radiographic control of the surgical site and the retrograde filling.

m The flap is sutured in place with interrupted sutures.

n The gingiva on the day of suture removal.

o Three-month control with repair.

[(**Fig. 6.41g–o**, see pp. 136, 137)]

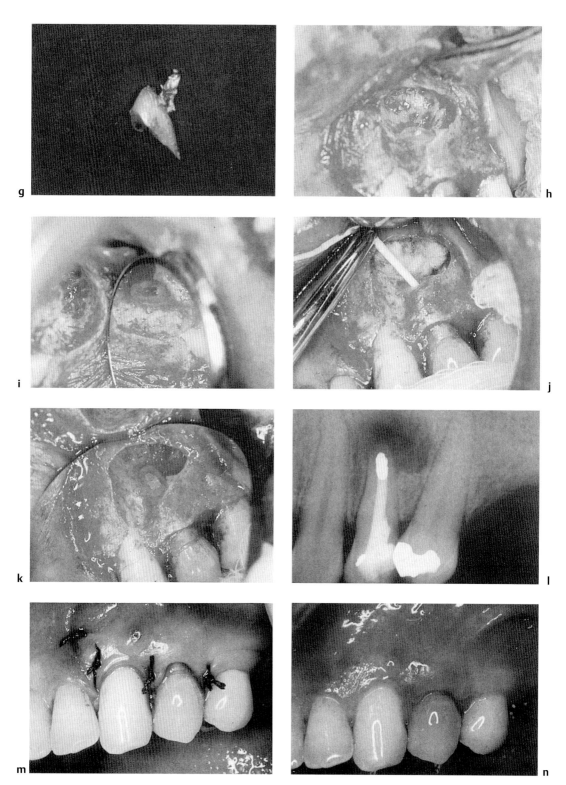

Fig. 6.41 cont.

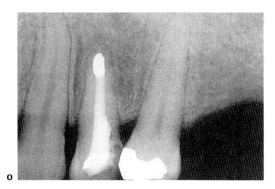

o

Apicoectomy

In teeth with apical periodontitis, the root tip may be of etiological importance in that an apical root canal delta may harbor bacteria. The root tip should, therefore, routinely be reduced 1–3 mm during surgical–endodontic treatment of apical periodontitis, and in addition, the root should be bevelled as needed in a buccal (or palatal) direction to facilitate access to the root canals.

Retrograde instrumentation of the root canal will be necessary if the root filling is not considered to give an adequate seal of the root canal. It can be carried out by means of a microhandpiece and a round or inverted cone microbur, usually no.3 (**Figs. 6.41**, **9.14**). A retrograde cavity should at least encompass the outline of the root canal and be 2–3 mm deep. Even with the smallness of a microhandpiece this may be difficult to achieve. It is recommended, therefore, that *ultrasonically energized microsurgical tips or retrotips* be used to prepare retrograde cavities (**Fig. 9.15**). The retrotips are made of steel and may be coated with diamond or zirconium particles to improve their effectiveness. Because of their small size and special design, access to the root end is readily obtained with these instruments, and retrograde cavities that follow the long axis of the root canal to the desired depth may be prepared.

In teeth with an unfilled or inadequately filled but coronally blocked root canal, the canal has to be instrumented and obturated in its entirety from the apical end during the surgical operation (**Fig. 6.36**). Traditionally, such canals were instrumented by the use of blades of K-files or Hedstrom files held in a hemostat. Today root canal instruments that can be screwed into an ultrasonic handpiece are available. These instruments may be bent once according to the needs of the clinical situation. They are then introduced into the root canal and energized and the entire canal can be cleaned and enlarged to the coronal blocking with relative ease. Copious irrigation with sterile saline is carried out in conjunction with the use of all ultrasonically energized instruments.

As mentioned above, a retrograde cavity may be filled with a copper-containing spherical amalgam after that a copal varnish is applied to the cavity (**Fig. 6.41**). If amalgam is not used, either for biological or legal reasons, reinforced zinc oxide–eugenol cements (IRM or EBA cements) give reliable bacteria-tight seals and appear to be the materials of choice. If larger parts of the root canal have been instrumented from the retrograde position, it may be convenient to use the materials normally used for orthograde obturation, such as gutta-percha cone(s) and a sealer, or a retrograde material may be used to fill the entire canal.

The surgical site is then thoroughly irrigated with sterile physiological saline, the flap is repositioned, and gentle pressure is applied to the flap by means of moist gauze for 1–2 minutes to ensure good adaptation to the underlying tissues. The flap is then secured, preferably by means of interrupted sutures, beginning at the angle between the horizontal and vertical incisions (**Fig. 6.41**). The sutures are removed after 4–7 days to avoid unnecessary tissue irritation.

Intentional Replantation

Sometimes desired surgical–endodontic treatment of a tooth may not be feasible for anatomical or other reasons. *A planned extraction with repair of the tooth outside the mouth and subsequent replantation* may then be the treatment of choice. This treatment method is usually referred to as *intentional replantation* (**Fig. 6.42**).

The success of this method depends on whether the tooth can be extracted with minimal damage to the periodontal ligament, especially to the cementoblast layer on the root surface. Moreover, it is important that the extraoral time is as short as possible (5–10 minutes), and that the periodontal tissues on the root are not touched and are kept wet at all times. This is best achieved by performing all aspects of the treatment that do not require a dry cavity with the tooth submerged in sterile isotonic saline. The tooth is taken out of the saline for only the very short time it takes to seal a retrograde cavity, a root perforation, or similar, and even during this time the soft tissue on the root surface is kept wet.

As soon as the repair is completed, the tooth is replanted with great care to avoid further injuries to the delicate tissue on the root surface. It will usually be necessary to splint the tooth to a neighboring tooth for about 5–7 days. Most conveniently, an acid-etch resin splint is used.

The primary periodontal healing is usually uneventful. Ankylosis and replacement resorption will occur if extensive areas of the root surface are denuded during extraction and replantation. However, if the technical aspects of the treatment are well controlled, reestablishment of a normal periodontal ligament can be expected to occur (**Fig. 6.42**).

Aftercare

Little postoperative care is needed following surgical–endodontic treatment. The patient should be advised not to manipulate the tissues, but protect the flap for quickest possible healing without bleeding or other complications. An ice pack may be held to the face for 15–20 minutes of every hour for the first few hours after the surgery to prevent swelling. Also, a regime with chemical

plaque control is advisable during the first week when tooth-brushing is difficult. With the new knowledge that bacteria may be present extraradicularly, antibiotic therapy is indicated. Mild to moderate postoperative pain will occur when the anesthesia wears off. Nonnarcotic analgesics like acetaminophen, aspirin, and especially ibuprofen give excellent relief.

Follow-up Examination and Prognosis

The patient should be examined 2 days after surgery, on the day of suture removal, after 1, 6, and 12 months, and later as needed (**Fig. 6.41**). Bone regenerates gradually and a period of 3–12 months may be needed for complete repair. It should be noted that new cementum forms on the bevelled root surface. A periodontal ligament with fibers between the cementum and the new alveolar bone forms as well. However, sometimes a fibrous rather than a bony repair occurs (**Figs. 2.27, 6.43**). This is especially the case when the periapical lesion has destroyed the buccal or lingual periosteum of the alveolar process, or both. It also occurs quite commonly in older patients and make the evaluation of periapical repair in these patients somewhat difficult.

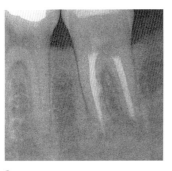
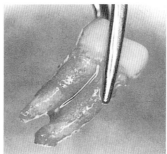

a

b

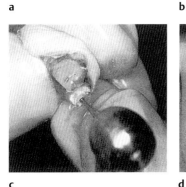
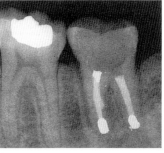

c

d

Fig. 6.42 Intentional replantation.
a Radiograph of a mandibular molar with strip perforation to the furcation and apical perforation of the mesial root. The tooth is tender to biting 6 months following endodontic treatment.
b The tooth was extracted with great care and immediately submerged in sterile isotonic saline.
c The cement in the furcation was removed and apicoectomies with retrograde fillings were performed extraorally. After 8 minutes extraoral time (about 5 of the 8 minutes in saline), the tooth was carefully replanted and splinted.
d One-year control. The mobility of the tooth is normal, periapical healing is evident, and the tooth is functioning normally. The patient is asymptomatic.

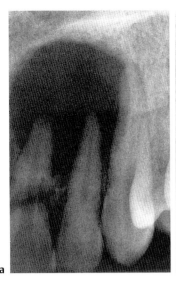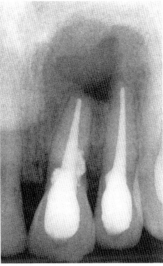

a

b

Fig. 6.43
a Radiograph of nonvital maxillary central and lateral incisors with a large radiolucent periapical lesion 18 years following a traumatic injury (a blow) to the area. The teeth are treated endodontically and the lesion is curetted out surgically.
b At the 1-year control, repair of the radiolucent area with a central fibrous scar can be seen.

On the whole, surgical–endodontic treatment is an invaluable complement to conservative endodontic treatment. It is especially valuable in problem cases as discussed above, and clearly contributes to the reliable and consistently good results of endodontic treatment.

Further Reading

Ari H, Yasar E, Belli S. Effects of NaOCl on bond strengths of resin cements to root canal dentin. J Endod 2003;29:248–251.

Banchs F, Trope M. Revascularization of immature permanent teeth with apical periodontitis: new treatment protocol? J Endod 2004;30:196–200.

Barnett F, Axelrod P, Tronstad L et al. Ciprofloxacin treatment of periapical *Pseudomonas aeruginosa* infection. Endod Dent Traumatol 1988;4:132–137.

Barnett F, Trope M, Khoja M, Tronstad L. Bacteriologic status of the root canal after sonic, ultrasonic and hand instrumentation. Endod Dent Traumatol 1985; 1:228–231.

Barnett F, Trope M, Kreshtool D, Tronstad L. Suitability of controlled release delivery system in root canal disinfection. Endod Dent Traumatol 1986;2:71–74.

Basrani BR, Manek S, Sodhi RNS, Fillery E, Manzur A. Interaction between sodium hypochlorite and chlorhexidine gluconate. J Endod 2007;33:966–969.

Baumgartner JC, Jobal S, Marshall JG. Comparison of the antimicrobial efficacy of 1.3% NaOCl/BioPure MTAD to 5.25% NaOCl/15% EDTA for root canal irrigation. J Endod 2007;33:48–51.

Baumgartner JC, Mader CL. A scanning electron microscopic evaluation of four root canal irrigation regiments. J Endod 1987;13:147–157.

Byström A, Claeson R, Sundqvist G. The antibacterial effect of camphorated paramonochlorphenol, camphorated phenol and calcium hydroxide in the treatment of infected root canals. Endod Dent Traumatol 1985;1:170–175.

Byström A, Sundqvist G. Bacteriologic evaluation of the efficacy of mechanical instrumentation in endodontic therapy. Scand J Dent Res 1981;89:321–328.

Byström A, Sundqvist G. The antibacterial effect of sodium hypochlorite and EDTA in 60 cases of endodontic therapy. Int Endod J 1985;18:35–40.

Cvek M. Endodontic management of traumatized teeth. In Andreassen JO, Andreassen FM, eds. Textbook and color atlas of traumatic injuries to the teeth. 3rd ed. Copenhagen: Munksgaard 1994, 517–586.

Dahlén G. Microbiology and treatment of dental abscesses and periodontal-endodontic lesions. Periodontology 2000 2002;28:206–39.

Dorn SO, Gartner AH. Retrograde filling materials: a retrospective success-failure study of amalgam, EBA and IRM. J Endod 1990;16:391–393.

Friedman S. Retrograde approaches in endodontic therapy. Endod Dent Traumatol 1991;7:97–107.

Gutman JL, Saunders WP, Nguyen L, Guo IY, Saunders EM. Ultrasonic root end preparation: part 1. SEM analysis. Int Endod J 1994;27:318–24.

Hasselgren G, Olsson B, Cvek M. Effects of calcium hydroxide and sodium hypochlorite on the dissolution of necrotic porcine muscle tissue. J Endod 1988; 14:125–127.

Kaufman B, Spangberg L, Barry J, Fouad AF. Enterococcus spp. in endodontically treated teeth with and without periapical lesions. J Endod 2005;31:851–856.

Kerekes K, Tronstad L. Long-term results of endodontic treatment performed with a standardized technique. J Endod 1979;5:83–90.

Koh ET, McDonald F, Pitt Ford TR, Torabinejad M. Cellular responses to mineral trioxide aggregate. J Endod 1998;24:543–547.

McComb D, Smith DC. A preliminary scanning electron microscopic study of root canals after endodontic procedures. J Endod 1975;1:238–242.

Messer HH, Chen RS. The duration of effectiveness of root canal medicaments. J Endod 1984;10:240–45.

Molander A, Reit C, Dahlén G, Kvist T. Microbiological status of root filled teeth with apical periodontitis. Int Endod J 1998;31:1–7.

Molander A, Warfinge J, Reit C, Kvist T. Clinical and radiographic evaluation of one- and two-visit endodontic treatment of asymptomatic necrotic teeth with apical periodontitis: a randomized clinical trial. J Endod 2007;33:1145–1148.

Nygaard-Östby B. Chelation in root canal therapy. Odont Tidskr 1957;65:3–11.

Safavi KE, Nickols FL. Alteration of biological properties of bacterial lipopolysaccharide by calcium hydroxide treatment. J Endod 1994;20:127–129.

Sato I, Ando-Kurihara N, Kota K, Iwaku M, Hoshino E. Sterilization of the infected root canal dentine by topical application of a mixture of ciprofloxacine, metronidazole and minicycline in situ. Int Endod J 1996;29:118–124.

Siqueira JF, Magalbaes R, Roças IN. Bacterial reduction in infected root canals treated with 2.5% NaOCl as an irrigant and calcium hydroxide/camphorated parachlorphenol paste as an intracanal dressing. J Endod 2007;33:667–672.

Siqueira JF, Paiva SSM, Roças IN. Reduction in the cultivable bacterial populations in infected root canals by a chlorhexidine-based antimicrobial protocol. J Endod 2007;33:541–547.

Socransky SS, Haffajee AD. Dental biofilms: difficult therapeutic targets. Periodontology 2000 2002;28:12–55.

Sultan M, Pitt Ford TR, Ultrasonic preparation and obturation of root end cavities. Int Endod J 1995;28:231–8.

Sunde PT, Olsen I, Debelian GJ, Tronstad L. Microbiota of periapical lesions refractory to endodontic therapy. J Endod 2002; 28:304–310.

Thibodeau B, Teixeira F, Yamauchi M, Caplan DJ, Trope M. Pulp revascularization of immature dog teeth with apical periodontitis. J Endod 2007;33:680–689.

Torabinejad M, Cho Y, Khademi AA, Bakland LK, Shabahang S. The effect of various concentrations of sodium hypochlorite on the ability of MTAD to remove the smear layer. J Endod 2003;29:233–239.

Torabinejad M, Pitt Ford TR, McKendry P et al. Histologic assessment of Mineral Trioxide Aggregate as root-end filling in monkeys. J Endod 1997;23:225–228.

Tronstad L, Andreasen JO, Hasselgren G, Riis I. pH changes in dental tissues after root canal filling with calcium hydroxide. J Endod 1981;7:17–21.

Tronstad L, Cervone F, Barnett F. Periapical bacterial plaque in teeth refractory to endodontic treatment. Endod Dent Traumatol 1990;6:73–77.

Tronstad L, Kreshtool D, Barnett F. Microbiological monitoring and results of treatment of extraradicular endodontic infection. Endod dent Traumatol 1990;6:129–135.

Tronstad L, Trope M, Doering A, Hasselgren G. Sealing abilities of dental amalgams as retrograde fillings in endodontic therapy. J Endod 1983;8:551–553.

Tronstad L, Yang Z-P, Trope M, Barnett F. Controlled release of medicaments in endodontic therapy. Endod Dent Traumatol 1985;1:130–134.

Trope M, Bank M, Barnett F, Tronstad L. Surgical access for endodontic treatment of intruded teeth. Endod Dent Traumatol 1986;2:75–78.

Trope M, Delano EO, Ørstavik D. Endodontic treatment of teeth with apical periodontitis: single vs. multivisit treatment. J Endod 1999;25:345–350.

Wallace JA. Transantral endodontic surgery. Oral Surg Oral Med Oral Pathol 1996;82:80–84.

Waltimo TMT, Sirén EK, Torkko HLK et al. Fungi in therapy-resistant apical periodontitis. Int Endod J 1997;32:94–98.

Wang JD, Hume WR. Diffusion of hydrogen ion and hydroxyl ion from various sources through dentin. Int Endod J 1988;21:17–21.

Weiger R, Manucke B, Werner H, Löst C. Microflora of sinus tracts and root canals of non-vital teeth. Endod Dent Traumatol 1995;11:15–19.

Weldon JK, Pashley DH, Lonshine RJ, Weller RN, Kuisbourg WF. Sealing ability of mineral trioxide aggregate and Super EBA when used as furcation repair materials: a longitudinal study. J Endod 2002;26:467–470.

7

Endodontic Emergency Treatment

Approximately 60% of patients with oral or maxillofacial pain are in need of endodontic emergency treatment. *The immediate goal of the emergency treatment is to mitigate the patient's symptoms and, if possible, it should also constitute the first phase in the permanent treatment of the condition.*

Since emergency treatment usually takes place between regular patients in a busy schedule, the therapeutic procedures should be as simple as possible and in keeping with the objective of relieving the patient's pain.

Emergency Treatment of Vital Teeth

About 90% of vital teeth that need endodontic emergency treatment are carious teeth or teeth previously restored because of caries (**Table 7.1**). Approximately 2% of the teeth will have symptoms because of traumatic occlusion. Exposed dentin and tooth fractures are other conditions causing pain in vital teeth.

Teeth with Symptomatic Pulpitis

In teeth with symptomatic pulpitis, either carious dentin must be excavated or existing restorations removed, or both. *The subsequent treatment will then depend on the clinical findings, mainly on whether the pulp is exposed or not.*

Symptomatic teeth without pulp exposure. When carious dentin and possible restorations have been removed, the cavity is cleansed with a spray of water and air, and while still wet is filled with zinc oxide–eugenol cement (see p.86). This is a simple, rapid, and effective method which, over a 5-year period, has been found to give relief from pain in 97% of the teeth (**Table 7.2**). Remember, however, that when the final treatment is planned,

absence of symptoms does not in any way guarantee a healthy pulp.

Symptomatic teeth with pulp exposure. If the pulp is found to be exposed after excavation of carious dentin or removal of a restoration (or both), there are three possible methods for emergency treatment. While the three procedures are not equally effective, they are all acceptable and provide a reasonable choice according to the time available for the emergency treatment.

Anodyne medicament. The simplest treatment method is to apply a cotton pellet with a medicament with an anodyne effect, preferably eugenol, directly on the exposed pulp. The cavity is subsequently filled temporarily with a material which gives a bacteria-tight seal, usually a zinc oxide–eugenol cement. This treatment is simple, rapid, and amazingly effective, and gives temporary relief from pain in about 90% of these cases until a pulpectomy can be performed (**Table 7.2**).

Emergency pulpotomy. The second method is to amputate and remove the coronal pulp of the symptomatic tooth. The bleeding is controlled and

Table 7.1 Reasons for pain in vital teeth in an emergency clinic over a 5-year period

Clinical findings, vital teeth	Patients (n = 3723)	
	Number	Percent
Caries, unrestored or restored	3300	88.6
Cusp fractures, complete or incomplete	214	5.8
Hypersensitive teeth	136	3.6
Traumatic occlusion	73	2.0

Table 7.2 Efficacy of emergency teatment methods in teeth with symptomatic pulpitis

Symptomatic pulpitis, emergency treatment	No. of patients	Relief of symptoms
No pulp exposure		
Excavation of caries or removal of a restoration; zinc oxide–eugenol cement	868	842 (97%)
Pulp exposure		
Anodyne medicament on the pulp wound; bacteria-tight seal	234	215 (92%)
Emergency pulpotomy; anodyne medicament in the pulp chamber; bacteria-tight seal	1884	1848 (98%)
Pulp extirpation; anodyne medicament in the root canal; bacteria-tight seal	57	52 (91%)
Pulpectomy with complete debridement; calcium hydroxide in the root canal; bacteria-tight seal	257	256 (99%)

a cotton pellet with an anodyne medicament (eugenol) is applied on the remaining pulp stump. The cavity is then sealed bacteria-tight as described above. This method is most effective and will give relief from pain in more than 95% of these cases (**Table 7.2**). It is somewhat more time-consuming than the first method, but it is still a simple procedure in that no root canal instrumentation is performed. The emergency pulpotomy *should be regarded as the routine method in emergency treatment of vital teeth with exposed pulp.*

Pulpectomy. The third possibility is to carry out the permanent treatment directly in the emergency situation. A pulpectomy *with complete instrumentation* and permanent root filling with gutta-percha or temporary root filling with calcium hydroxide paste is then performed. This is the most reliable method and will give relief from pain in more than 99% of these cases (**Table 7.2**). However, it is time-consuming compared to the two methods described above, and for that reason cannot be considered a routine method in an emergency situation.

In this context it is important to be aware of the fact that if a simple pulp extirpation is carried out without proper root canal instrumentation, the effectiveness of the treatment to relieve pain is reduced to 90%, possibly because tissue remnants are left behind in the root canal. Thus, the efficacy of a pulp extirpation with the placement of an anodyne medicament in the root canal is no greater than when the medicament is placed directly on the pulp exposure in the cavity of the tooth (**Table 7.2**).

Crown Fractures

Crown fractures may lead to symptoms because of exposure of dentin. The symptoms are controlled by restoring the tooth or simply covering the exposed dentin surface with a zinc oxide–eugenol cement, usually by means of a temporary crown. If the fracture is incomplete, one fragment should be removed if at all possible and the tooth treated as described above. However, an incomplete fracture may be present in the form of a crack and be directed in such a way that a fragment cannot be removed without sacrificing the tooth. Such teeth may be saved for considerable periods of time by restoring them with a crown to "hold the tooth together" and thereby to prevent further progression of the fracture. Reduction of the occlusal height of an incompletely fractured tooth and instruction to the patient to avoid biting on the tooth may give adequate relief from pain until a crown can be made.

Dental Hypersensitivity

Dental hypersensitivity is most often due to the fact that dentin has become exposed, usually in the cervical area of the tooth. Immediate relief from the pain can be achieved by *blocking the exposed dentinal tubules, for example, with a cavity varnish* (**Fig. 7.1**). Obviously, as soon as the varnish has dissolved, usually after a few days, the sensitivity may be back, but often to a lesser degree than before.

A wide variety of agents have been used to reduce or eliminate dental hypersensitivity on a more permanent basis, and many agents are commercially available, usually in toothpastes. The effect of most of these agents is at best uncertain. Toothpastes with potassium nitrate as the active ingredient have shown some promise. The most reliable long-term results have been obtained with good oral hygiene and meticulous local plaque control in combination with the use of fluoride preparations. Occasionally, and especially after periodontal treatment, the symptoms from a hypersensitive tooth may be so severe that a pulpectomy has to be performed to bring the patient the necessary relief.

Traumatic Occlusion

Traumatic occlusion may cause symptoms similar to a symptomatic pulpitis. The condition is suspected when a traumatic situation exists or is suggested by bite facets on tooth surfaces or restorations. Emergency treatment, which may also be the permanent treatment, is to relieve the occlusion by selective grinding of the symptomatic tooth, its antagonist, and possibly neighboring teeth. This treatment will be effective in about 85% of these cases. The rest of the patients with this diagnosis will return with persisting symptoms, and incomplete fractures, symptomatic pulpitis, and even necrotic pulps are usually found after renewed examinations.

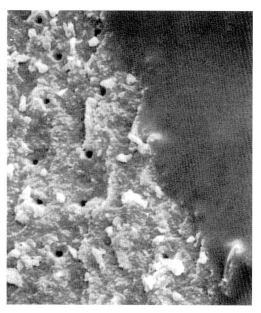

Fig. 7.1 Scanning electron micrograph of dentin surface with transversely exposed dentinal tubules. To the right, a film of copal varnish is covering the dentin and blocking the tubules (×900).

Emergency Treatment of Nonvital Teeth

Symptomatic Apical Periodontitis

In nonvital teeth, pain is associated with symptomatic apical, lateral, or interradicular periodontitis. The following factors are of special importance in obtaining relief from pain in these conditions.

Drainage. The most important cause of the symptoms is elevated pressure in the tissues. Accordingly, the emergency treatment should be aimed at a normalization of the tissue pressure which, as soon as it is achieved, results in relief from pain for the patient. If the patient's condition allows access to the symptomatic tooth, the pulp chamber is opened. Direct drainage of pus through the root canal may then take place. However, sometimes the purulent breakdown occurs in an area which does not have contact with the tooth in such a way that drainage may take place. *It is then important to remember that it is the infection of the root canal that has caused the*

painful periodontitis and even in the absence of drainage the emergency treatment should be complete chemomechanical instrumentation of the root canal.

If drainage from the root canal occurs, it is good clinical practice to have the patient sit in a dental chair for a short period of time until the exudation has stopped or has been reduced significantly. Chemomechanical instrumentation of the root canal is then performed, a suitable antiseptic dressing is applied, and the access cavity is sealed with a bacteria-tight temporary filling. More than 90% of patients will soon have relief from pain following this treatment, regardless of the severity of the clinical situation (**Table 7.3**). If instrumentation of the root canal is not possible, usually because of trismus or extreme tenderness of the tooth, the placement of a medicament (eugenol) in the pulp chamber before sealing the access cavity will bring relief in about 70% of these patients.

Table 7.3 Efficacy of emergency treatment methods in teeth with symptomatic apical periodontitis

Symptomatic teeth Emergency treatment	No. of patients	Persistening symptoms	Pain	Swelling
Pulpitis	463	1 (0.2%)	1	
Apical periodontitis	253	6 (2.4%)	2	4
Apical periodontitis with abscess	73	2 (2.7%)	2	
Total	789	9 (1.1%)		

It has been believed that teeth with symptomatic apical periodontitis should not be sealed in an acute situation, but should remain open to the mouth for rapid and reliable relief of pain. However, controlled clinical studies indicate that this is a misconception, and that leaving teeth open when the exudation has stopped only postpones, at best, the problems at hand. Open root canals will be filled with saliva and be colonized by bacteria from the oral cavity, and new, more severe exacerbations often occur when teeth that have been left open finally are instrumented and closed. *Only on rare occasions when the periapical exudation is so severe and persistent that it is virtually impossible to close a tooth, should it be left open.* Thus, in one 5-year retrospective study comprising 2184 patients with symptomatic apical periodontitis, only 11 teeth were left open because of persistent exudation. In these instances it is good practice to have the patient come back and to perform the chemomechanical instrumentation and begin the antimicrobial treatment of the root canal as soon as possible, preferably within 24 hours. In this way, the formation of biofilm in the open canal is limited to a minimum. It is relatively easily removed and since the new infection is not yet well established, the bacteria are readily killed.

Effective drainage may further be obtained by the incision of a fluctuant abscess (**Fig. 7.2**). In most instances this will lead to a dramatic relief from pain for the patient. If possible, the incision should be performed in addition to and not as a substitute for, the chemomechanical instrumentation of the root canal of the symptomatic tooth. In the 2184 patients referred to above, incision alone or incision combined with systemic antibiotic therapy was the sole emergency treatment in only 81 instances.

Antibiotics (see p. 114). Symptomatic apical periodontitis can usually be treated without antibi-

otics. If good drainage has been established, the symptoms will disappear relatively quickly and the situation can be corrected with routine endodontic treatment. However, there are situations in which the use of antibiotics is indicated. If a patient's general health is influenced by the periapical inflammation, or if a patient's medical status is poor, antibiotics should be given. Furthermore, antibiotics should be used for abscesses in the floor of the mouth, for perimandibular abscesses, or for any other dramatic inflammatory condition with severe swelling, especially when the symptomatic tooth cannot be reached for instrumentation or surgical drainage is not achieved otherwise. Remember that the inflammatory process involved in these situations occurs in the face–throat region with anatomically determined routes of spread to the brain as well as the mediastinum. In the actual situation it does not help much to think about statistics or to worry about general abuse of antibiotics. On the contrary, the clinician is responsible for the health of each individual patient and must provide the best treatment that is available at any time.

Occlusion. A tooth with symptomatic apical periodontitis will be pushed slightly out of its socket by the exudate in the periapical tissues. Consequently, each time the patient closes on the tooth, the periodontal tissues, which are already hypersensitive due to the exacerbation, are traumatized. Careful reduction of either the crown of the tooth, its antagonist, or both to avoid the traumatic occlusion normally has a distinct palliative effect. What also results from the occlusal adjustment is that the tooth is, in a way, *immobilized*. This is both correct and effective therapy in such a situation.

Pain and anxiety control. In addition to local treatment and necessary systemic antibiotic therapy, most patients with symptomatic apical perio-

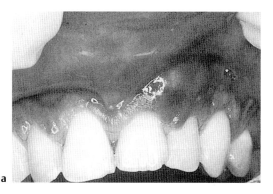

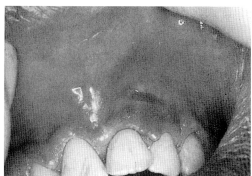

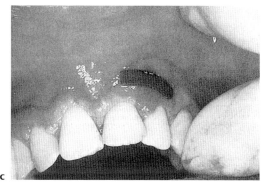

Fig. 7.2
a Fluctuant abscess in the oral vestibule.
b To obtain optimal drainage, the incision is made at the low point of the swelling.
c An H-shaped drain made of a rubber dam is used to keep the incision open.

dontitis should be on a mild analgesic regime. *Nonnarcotic drugs are preferable and in most instances more than adequate.* Analgesics with an anti-inflammatory effect, like ibuprofen, have proven to be especially effective and for pain control are the drugs of choice. If patient fear or anxiety presents a problem, a tranquilizer like diazepam should be used and not a narcotic analgesic. In some instances sleeping pills may be helpful as well.

In this context it must also be remembered that *a most important factor in pain and anxiety control is a dentist who exhibits security and authority as well as warmth and understanding for the situation at hand.* The dentist's behavior can make an uneasy patient calm and confident. If this is achieved, the patient will be better prepared to tolerate the potentially painful treatment and the postoperative period of discomfort that are often unavoidable.

Further Reading

Abbott PV, Hume WR, Pearman JW. Antibiotics and endodontics. Austr Dent J 1990;35:50–60.
Bjerkén E, Wennberg A, Tronstad L. Endodontisk akutbehandling. Tandläkartidn 1980;72:314–319.

Torabinejad M, Kettering JD, McGraw JC et al. Factors associated with endodontic interappointment emergencies of teeth with necrotic pulps. J Endod 1988; 14:261–266.

8

Endodontic Aspects of Root Resorption

The mineralized tissues of the permanent teeth are not normally resorbed. They are protected in the root canal by the predentin and the odontoblasts and on the root surface by the precementum and the cementoblasts. If the predentin or the precementum becomes mineralized or, in the case of precementum, is mechanically damaged or scraped off, osteoclast-like cells will colonize the mineralized or denuded surfaces and resorption will ensue. However, resorbing cells require continuous stimulation during phagocytosis, and stimulation by a denuded dentin or cementum surface is not sufficient to sustain the resorptive process for long. A phagocytic colonization of denuded areas of the root, therefore, will be transient without additional stimulation of the cells, and repair with formation of a cementum-like tissue will occur both in the root canal and on the root surface (**Fig. 8.1**). This type of resorption is referred to as transient root resorption.

Transient root resorption occurs quite frequently in traumatized teeth and in teeth which have undergone orthodontic and periodontal treatment, but is also seen in other teeth apparently as a result of wear and tear. Transient root resorption is without clinical importance and the resorption defects are usually too small to be detected, even radiographically.

Root resorption which is initiated by a denuded area of the root surface may be sustained by mechanical irritation, increased pressure in the tissue, or infection of the root canal and tubules of the crown and root dentin.

Mechanical stimulation of osteoclasts to sustain a progressive resorption is seen, for example, in root-fractured teeth where the sharp edges of the root fragments are selectively resorbed. Only when the fragments are well rounded and cause no further tissue irritation will the resorption stop (**Fig. 8.2**).

Pressure resorption in the permanent dentition may be seen during tooth eruption, especially of maxillary canines and mandibular third molars, and in patients with certain tumors impinging on

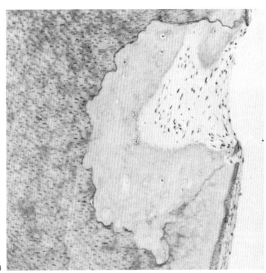 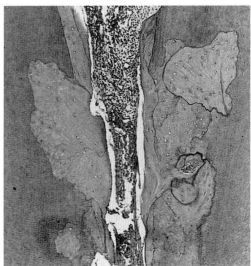

a   b

Fig. 8.1 Transient root resorption (a) on the root surface and (b) in the root canal. A cementum-like tissue is laid down in the resorption lacunae at both locations.

the roots of the teeth. Pressure resorption is also commonly seen during orthodontic movement of teeth, usually in the form of apical resorption and a shortening of the roots (**Fig. 8.3**). Pressure resorption may be quite destructive if diagnosed late on. However, the resorptive process will be arrested when the stimulation of the resorbing cells stops.

Root resorption sustained by infection is by far the most important clinical condition from an endodontic point of view. It can occur in the root canal (called internal resorption; **Fig. 8.4**), or on the root surface (referred to as cervical resorption; **Fig. 8.5** or *external inflammatory resorption*; **Fig. 8.6**), depending on whether the microbial stimuli come from the gingival sulcus or from the root canal. An infectious inflammation is accompanied by the production and release of cytokines

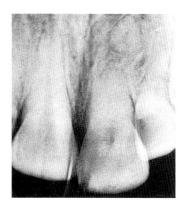

Fig. 8.2 Radiograph of a maxillary left central incisor 24 years following a traumatic injury resulting in a fracture of the root of the tooth. Note selective resorption of the sharp edges of both root fragments and repair.

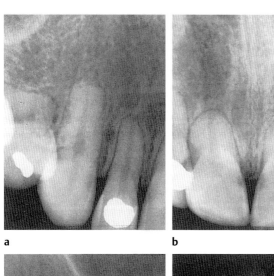

Fig. 8.3 a–d Radiographs of maxillary and mandibular teeth with apical root resorption following orthodontic tooth movement. The root resorption in this case is severe and the etiology may not be fully understood.

a

b

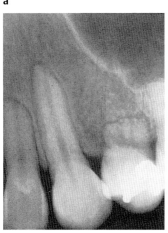

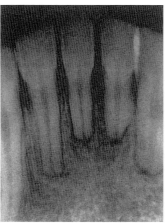

c

d

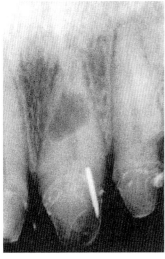
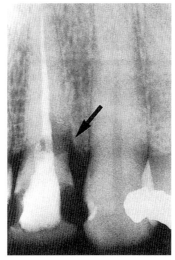
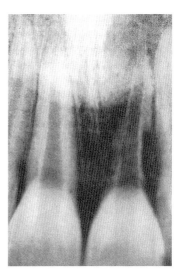

Fig. 8.4   Fig. 8.5   Fig. 8.6

Fig. 8.4 Radiograph of a maxillary central incisor with a midroot radiolucent area indicating internal root resorption.

Fig. 8.5 Radiograph of an endodontically treated maxillary incisor with a cervical radiolucent lesion in the tooth and adjacent bone (arrow) indicating cervical root resorption. Note the difference in the location of the resorption cavity and the proximal restorations of carious lesions.

Fig. 8.6 Radiograph of a maxillary left central incisor with external inflammatory resorption. Four months following a luxation injury, most of the root is resorbed. Note that the outline of the entire root canal can be recognized.

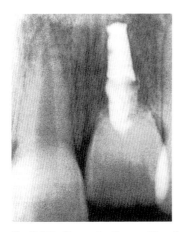

Fig. 8.7 Radiograph of a maxillary left central incisor with replacement resorption. The tooth is ankylosed and in infraocclusion, and the root has been replaced by bone. Note that endodontic treatment has had no effect on this type of resorption.

such as interleukin-1, tumor necrosis factor, and lymphotoxin, which are mediators of hard-tissue resorption. In addition, prostaglandin E_2, bacterial products, and components such as endotoxins will be present. A resorptive process sustained by infection can therefore progress quite rapidly, and in a short time may lead to complete destruction of the root (**Fig. 8.6**).

Replacement or endosteal root resorption is seen in teeth which have suffered dentoalveolar ankylosis because of necrosis of the periodontal ligament. With time, the roots of these teeth will be replaced by bone (**Fig. 8.7**).

Internal Root Resorption

Traditionally, internal resorption has been associated with a long-standing, chronic inflammation in the pulp (**Fig. 8.8**). This may hold true in the sense that the *transient type* of internal resorption discussed above may occur if the odontoblasts in an area of the root canal are destroyed so that the predentin becomes mineralized. However, in teeth with *progressive* internal resorption where the resorption lacunae are large enough to be diagnosed radiographically, the resorptive activity is sustained by infection of necrotic tissue coronally in the root canal. Bacterial products may then reach areas of the canal with vital pulp tissue through the dentinal tubules (**Fig. 8.9**). Thus, in order for progressive internal resorption to occur, the dentinal tubules have to have a special and fortuitous course. They have to be open to an area of the root canal where the tissue is necrotic and infected so that microorganisms may enter the tubules, and then lead to an area of the canal with vital pulp tissue. This is a rather unlikely occurrence and probably explains why progressive internal resorption is a rarity in permanent teeth.

An internal resorption lacuna when seen radiographically is a definite sign that endodontic treatment is indicated. Clinically in such teeth, one will find pulp necrosis in the pulp chamber and usually in the root canal to a level somewhere coronally to the resorption lacuna. The resorptive area and the root canal apical to this area will con-

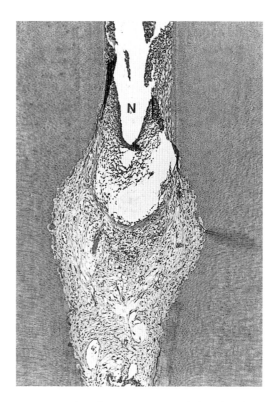

Fig. 8.8 Interface between necrotic (N) and vital inflamed tissue in a root canal. Resorption of the root canal walls (internal resorption) near the inflamed area of the pulp can be seen (hematoxylin-eosin).

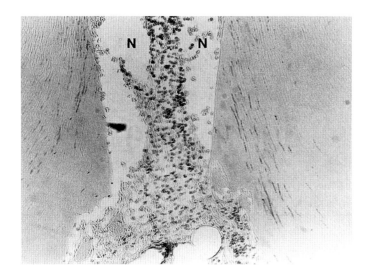

Fig. 8.9 Interface between necrotic (N) and vital tissue with an internal resorption lacuna in a root canal. Bacteria are present in the dentinal tubules leading from the area of the root canal with necrotic (infected) tissue to an area with vital tissue and internal resorption (Brown–Brenn stain).

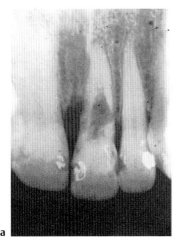
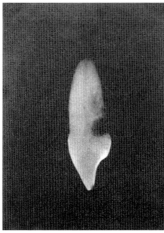

a   b

Fig. 8.10
a **Radiograph of a maxillary incisor with a radiolucent lesion due to cervical resorption.** Cervical resorption lacunae located on the buccal or lingual root surfaces are often mistakenly diagnosed as internal resorption.
b Radiograph of the extracted tooth shows the external nature of the resorption defect.

tain vital tissue. In some instances, the entire pulp will be necrotic. The resorptive process will then have stopped since obviously vital cells are needed for the resorption to continue. In root canals with vital tissue it may prove difficult to remove the tissue in the resorption lacuna since this cannot be reached by instruments. Irrigation with copious amounts of 5% sodium hypochlorite may have some effect, but the treatment of choice is to pack the canal and the resorption lacuna with calcium hydroxide paste. By the next visit, the calcium hydroxide will have necrotized any remaining tissue in the lacuna, and the necrotic remnants are readily removed by irrigation with sodium hypochlorite.

A rather common finding at the second visit is vital granulation tissue and bleeding in the resorptive area of the root canal. This can only mean that there is a *communication between the root canal and the periodontal ligament*. The communication may be due to a perforation of the root by progressive internal resorption. However, in most instances it will be due to an external resorptive process having perforated to the root canal. Cervical root resorption is the type of external resorption most often misdiagnosed as internal resorption (**Fig. 8.10**).

Cervical Root Resorption

Cervical root resorption is a rather commonly occurring, not well-recognized, late complication after traumatic injuries to the teeth (**Fig. 8.5**). It may also occur after orthodontic tooth movement, orthognathic and other dentoalveolar surgery, bleaching of teeth, and a wide variety of other "traumatic" conditions. In many instances the history is obscure. Cervical resorption appears to follow injury to the cervical attachment apparatus of the tooth, most importantly to an area of the cervical root surface below the epithelial attachment. It is most often an inflammatory type of resorption with clast-like cells colonizing the damaged area of the root. The necessary stimulation of the resorbing cells to maintain the resorptive process is seemingly provided by bacterial products via

the tubules of the cervical dentin from the gingival sulcus and the surface of the tooth.

If the local injuries lead to local necrosis of the periodontal ligament, cervical resorption may take the form of *ankylosis and replacement resorption*. This has reportedly been seen following the use of 30% hydrogen peroxide in conjunction with bleaching of teeth.

As the name implies, *cervical resorption begins in the cervical area of the tooth below the epithelial attachment* (**Fig. 8.11**). The damaged area of the root surface where the resorption starts may be very small. The resorbing cells will penetrate the tooth through the small denuded area and cause a spreading of the resorption inside the dentin of the root. At first the resorptive process will not penetrate to the pulp because of the protective qualities of the predentin, but rather spread around the root canal in an irregular fashion. Because of this pattern of spreading inside the root, cervical resorption is also referred to as *external–internal*, or *invasive resorption*.

With time, the resorptive process will usually penetrate to the root canal. In addition, cervical resorption will include the alveolar bone adjacent to the resorption lacuna in the tooth. Radiographically, therefore, the condition may have the appearance of periodontal disease with an infrabony periodontal pocket (**Fig. 8.5**).

Cervical resorption is not a pulpal reaction nor is it maintained by pulp necrosis or root canal infection. However, the condition is of considerable endodontic importance because by penetrating to the root canal it becomes an endodontic problem that requires endodontic treatment. Cervical resorption is usually asymptomatic and as a rule will be diagnosed in a routine radiographic examination. However, *the patient may present with pain of pulpal origin if the resorption has perforated to the root canal and exposed the pulp.* If the resorptive process reaches a supragingival area of the crown, the well-vascularized granulation tissue of the resorption lacuna may be visible through the enamel and the patient will present with a so-called *pink spot* or *pink tooth* (**Fig. 8.12**). Traditionally, this condition has been thought to be caused by internal resorption. However, in most instances it is due to cervical resorption.

With regard to *therapy*, the most effective approach is to expose the resorption lacuna surgically and remove the granulation tissue (**Figs. 8.12, 8.13**). The resorptive defect is then shaped as a cavity with necessary retentive areas and restored, preferably with a bonded restoration.

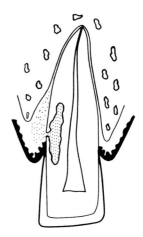

Fig. 8.11 Diagram of a tooth with cervical resorption defect. The resorption begins in a denuded area of the root below the gingival attachment and is apparently sustained by bacterial products from the sulcus. Cervical root resorption is always accompanied by resorption of the adjacent marginal bone, giving the radiographic appearance of an infrabony pocket.

Teeth in which a perforation to the root canal has occurred obviously need endodontic treatment. If a perforation to the root canal is ascertained or strongly suspected during the examination of the patient, the root canal treatment should be performed prior to a surgical exposure of the resorption lacuna (**Fig. 8.13**). This has the advantage that resorption lacunae with minute external openings may be cleaned out and obturated from the root canal (**Fig. 8.14**). However, if this method is used, follow-up examinations are especially important to make sure that the resorptive process really has been arrested.

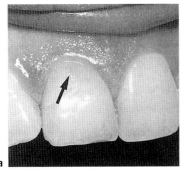

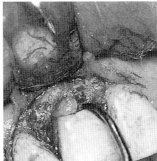

Fig. 8.12
a Maxillary right central incisor with a pink spot in the cervical area of the buccal surface (arrow).
b Envelope flap is raised, exposing resorption cavity with granulation tissue.

a   b

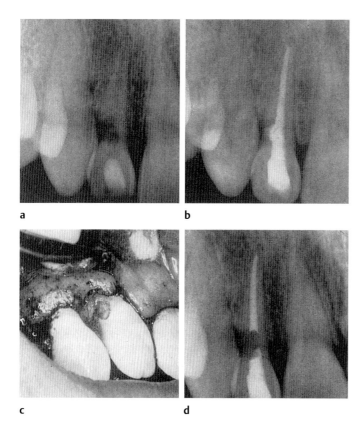

Fig. 8.13
a **Radiograph of a maxillary lateral incisor with cervical root resorption.** The patient presented with severe symptomatic pulpitis because of exposure and infection of the pulp through the undiagnosed resorption cavity.
b Pulpectomy with root canal filling is performed.
c The cervical resorption lacuna is exposed, cleaned, and restored with the acid-etch resin technique.
d Postoperative radiograph (radiolucent resin was used for cervical restoration).

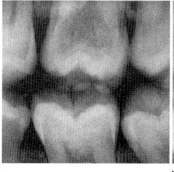

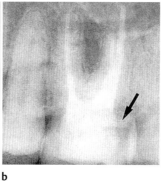

Fig. 8.14
a **Radiograph of a maxillary first molar with a cervical resorption lacuna encompassing the greater part of the coronal dentin.**
b Following pulpectomy and root canal filling, the pulp chamber, including a minute distolingual opening to the periodontium (arrow), was restored with the acid-etch resin technique

External Inflammatory Root Resorption

The condition referred to as external inflammatory root resorption is a commonly occurring complication following displacement of the teeth, i.e., after luxation and avulsion injuries. The extrusion or intrusion of the tooth as well as subsequent repositioning or replantation procedures will inevitably cause damage to the root, resulting in denuded areas on the root surface which will be chemotactic to phagocytes. Transient root resorption will then ensue.

In addition, displacement of the teeth leads to a disruption of the pulpal blood vessels at the apical foramina and to ischemic pulp necrosis (see p. 25). Microorganisms may then reach the root canal through enamel–dentin cracks and exposed dentinal tubules, and establish an infection, usually after a few days. The transient root resorption induced by the denuded areas of the root surface may now have exposed the tubular root dentin. Bacterial products from the infected root canal can then reach the resorptive areas on the root surface through the dentinal tubules and sustain the resorption of the root (**Fig. 8.15**).

Thus, external inflammatory root resorption is initiated by mechanical trauma, resulting in the removal of cementoblasts, precementum, and sometimes cementum in areas of the root surface. The resorptive process is then maintained by bacterial products from the infected root canal which provide the necessary continuous stimulation of the resorbing cells. *The condition can be recognized radiographically after a few weeks as periradicular radiolucent areas encompassing areas of the root and the adjacent alveolar bone* (**Fig. 8.16**). If allowed to progress, the resorptive process may destroy the tooth completely in a few months. However, by means of endodontic treatment, i.e., removal of the irritants from the root canal, the external inflammatory resorption can be arrested.

Any adequate endodontic treatment method will have an effect on the resorptive process. However, there is considerable clinical evidence that long-term treatment with calcium hydroxide provides the most predictable results. When calcium hydroxide is placed in the root canal, it will effectively kill the bacteria and, in addition, it will influence the local environment at the resorption sites on the root surface through the dentinal tubules (**Fig. 8.17**). Because of its high pH, calcium hydroxide will neutralize the lactic acid from the osteoclasts, thus preventing a dissolution of the mineral component of the root. Moreover, an alkaline pH at the resorption site will be unfavorable for the collagenase and acid hydrolase activity of the resorbing cells, and may also stimulate alka-

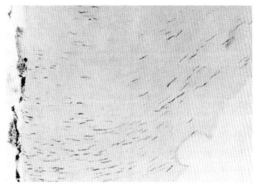

Fig. 8.15 Section of the root end of a nonvital tooth. Microorganisms are seen in necrotic tissue in the root canal (to the left) and in the dentinal tubules leading to external resorption lacunae (Brown–Brenn stain).

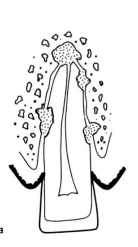

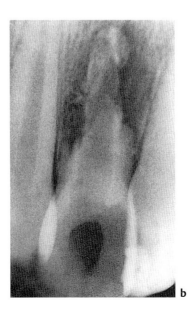

Fig. 8.16
a Diagram of a tooth with external inflammatory resorption. The resorption of the root is associated with resorption of the adjacent bone.
b Radiographically, radiolucent lesions are seen in the periodontium adjacent to external resorption lacunae.

a

b

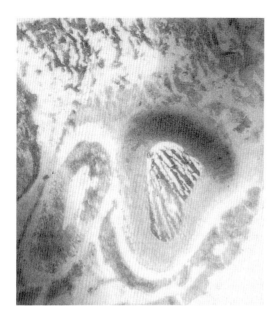

Fig. 8.17 Transverse section of a monkey tooth with calcium hydroxide in the root canal for 30 days. A pH indicator brought in contact with the root dentin reveals high alkalinity (pH > 11) of the content of the dentinal tubules.

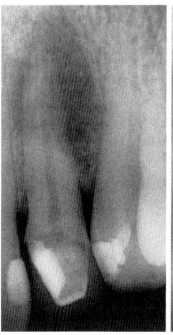 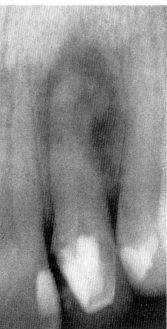 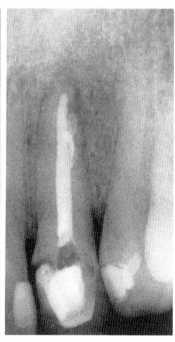

a   b   c

Fig. 8.18

a **Radiograph of a nonvital maxillary lateral incisor with a periradicular radiolucency and external inflammatory resorption.**

b Long-term calcium hydroxide treatment is initiated. Extrusion of calcium hydroxide paste to the external resorption lacuna has occurred, indicating that the resorptive process has led to a perforation of the root.

c After 6 months, resolution of the periradicular radiolucent lesion and reestablishment of the periodontal ligament space are evident and the root canal is permanently obturated.

line phosphatases, which play an important part in hard-tissue formation and repair. It appears, therefore, that calcium hydroxide would prevent a continuation of the resorptive process and, in addition, might stimulate repair. The calcium hydroxide treatment is discontinued when a contin-

uous periodontal ligament space is observed along the root, usually within 6–12 months. The root canal is then permanently obturated (**Fig. 8.18**). A success rate of 96% has been reported for the treatment of external inflammatory root resorption with this method.

Replacement Resorption

Dentoalveolar ankylosis occurs after extensive necrosis of the periodontal ligament with formation of bone on the root surface. Clinically, the condition is most often seen as a complication of luxation and avulsion injuries, especially in avulsed teeth which have been out of the mouth long enough for the cells of the periodontal ligament attached to the root to die (**Fig. 8.19**).

If less than 20% of the root surface is involved, reversal of the ankylosis may occur (**Fig. 8.20**). If not, ankylosed teeth are incorporated into the alveolar bone and will become part of the normal remodeling process of the bone. Consequently,

they will gradually resorb and be replaced by bone, hence the term replacement resorption (**Fig. 8.7**). The resorbing cells in replacement resorption are the osteoclasts normally involved in bone remodeling.

Clinically, dentoalveolar ankylosis will be recognized because of the lack of mobility of ankylosed teeth. These teeth will also have a special, metallic percussion sound, and after some time they will be in infraocclusion (**Fig. 8.21**). Radiographically, dentoalveolar ankylosis may be recognized by the absence of a periodontal ligament space (**Fig. 8.19**). Also, replacement resorption with ingrowth of

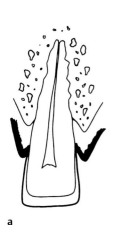

a

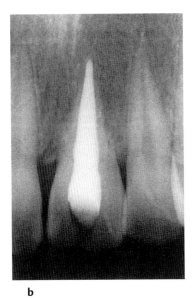

b

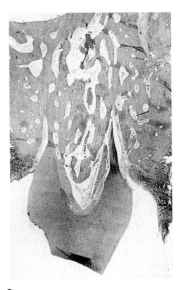

c

Fig. 8.19

a Diagram of an ankylosed tooth with replacement resorption. During remodeling of the alveolar bone, the dental tissues in contact with the bone by mistake are resorbed as well and are replaced by bone.

b Radiograph of an ankylosed maxillary central inci-

sor undergoing replacement resorption. Note the moth-eaten appearance of the root and the absence of a periodontal ligament space.

c Section of an ankylosed dog tooth with advanced replacement resorption. Note that not only the hard tissues of the root, but also the pulp is being replaced by bone (van Gieson stain).

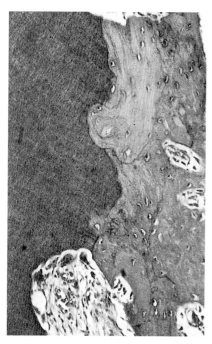

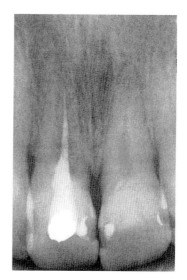

Fig. 8.21 Radiograph of an ankylosed maxillary right central incisor in infraocclusion undergoing replacement resorption. The tooth was avulsed and replanted 28 years earlier.

Fig. 8.20 Section of a tooth with ankylosis in a small area of the root surface ("spot ankylosis"). Because of stimulation from the use of the tooth, osteoclasts will sometimes resorb small ankylosed areas so that the ankylosis "breaks up." Cemental repair of the root surface with a normal periodontal ligament may then develop (hematoxylin-eosin).

bone into the dental tissues will give the tooth a characteristic moth-eaten appearance. There is presently no treatment for this condition and ultimately the crown of the tooth will break at the gingival crest and fall out. It should be known, however, that the speed with which the tooth is replaced by bone may vary and is usually quite slow. In most instances it takes years, sometimes decades, before the root is fully resorbed (**Fig. 8.21**). One should therefore never exaggerate or dramatize this situation for a patient or a parent of a patient when replacement resorption is diagnosed. Rather, one should stress the fact that the process progresses slowly and that by the time the tooth might fall out it can usually be adequately replaced.

Further Reading

Andreasen JO, Hjörting-Hansen E. Replantation of teeth. II. Histological study of 22 replanted anterior teeth in humans. Acta Odont Scand 1966;24:287–306.

Cvek M. Treatment of non-vital permanent incisors. II. Effect of calcium hydroxide on external root resorption in luxated teeth compared with the effect of rootfilling with gutta-percha. Odontol Revy 1973; 24:143–154.

Fuss Z, Tsesis I, Lin S. Root resorption: diagnosis, classification and treatment choices based on stimulation factors. Dent Traumatol 2003;19:175–182.

Hammarström L, Blomlöf L, Lindskog S. Dynamics of dentoalveolar ankylosis and the associated root resorption. 1989;4:163–175.

Hammarström L, Blomlöf LB, Feiglin B, Andersson L, Lindskog S. Replantation of teeth and antibiotic treatment. Endod Dent Traumatol 1986;2:51–57.

Heithersay GS. Invasive cervical resorption. Endod Topics 2004;7:73–92.

Lindskog S, Pierce AM, Blomlöf L, Hammarström L. The role of the necrotic periodontal membrane in cementum resorption and ankylosis. Endod Dent Traumatol 1985;1:96–101.

Makkes PG, Thoden van Velzen SK. Cervical external root resorption. J Dent Res 1975;3:217–222.

Pierce A, Lindskog S. The effect of an antibiotic cortico-steroid combination on inflammatory root resorption in vivo. Oral Surg Oral Med Oral Pathol 1987; 64:216–220.

Tronstad L. Pulp reactions in traumatized teeth. In: Gutmann JL, Harrison JW, eds. Proceedings of the International Conference on Oral Trauma. Chicago: American Association of Endodontists. 1984, pp 55–78.

Tronstad L. Root resorption – etiology, terminology and clinical manifestations. Endod Dent Traumatol 1988;4:241–252.

Trope M. Root resorption due to dental trauma. Endod Topics 2002;1:79–100.

Wedenberg C, Lindskog S. Evidence for resorption inhibitor in dentin. Scand J Dent Res 1987;95:205–211.

9

Endodontic Instruments

A variety of instruments are available for the extirpation of the pulp and the instrumentation, preparation, and obturation of the root canal. Although almost all these instruments were designed between 50 and 100 years ago, important changes have occurred in recent years with regard to their quality, efficacy, and standardization. Root canal instruments are available as hand instruments and many of them as engine-driven instruments.

Root Canal Instrumentation

Hand Instruments

Broaches and rasps. These instruments represent the oldest forms of root canal instruments (**Fig. 9.1**). They are made from round steel wire blanks and working edges are created by cutting into the wire at an angle to its long axis and then elevating the edges of the cuts. The depth, angle, and number of cuts (barbs) will determine how the instrument is used.

The *broach* is used to extirpate the vital pulp. It is introduced into the pulp and rotated so that the barbs engage the tissue. The pulp can then be removed, often in one piece. In modern endodontics this method is not recommended, as the pulp tissue is torn somewhere near the apical foramen, often impinging on the periodontal ligament as

well. Rather, an instrument is used that cuts the pulp tissue at the desired apical level before it is removed.

The rasps, or "rat tail files," are used to instrument and enlarge the root canal. Cutting occurs by longitudinal movement of the rasp toward the canal wall. The instrument is effective, but is not widely used today, since the barbs readily fall off during instrumentation and end up in the root canal.

Recently, two instruments with a cutting surface somewhat similar to that of the rasp have been brought onto the market, namely the Rispi file and the Sonic Shaper (**Fig. 9.2**). These instruments have circumferential grooves rather than single barbs and they hold up in use considerably better than the rasps. At present these instruments are available only with automated devices.

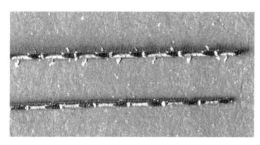

Fig. 9.1 Root canal broaches. A new broach with barbs is visible (top). The barbs have fallen off during use of the broach in the root canal (bottom).

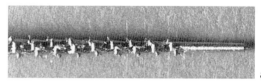
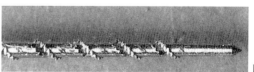

Fig. 9.2
a Rispi file.
b Sonic Shaper file. These instruments have "barb-like" cutting surfaces and smooth ends to avoid ledging of the root canal wall.

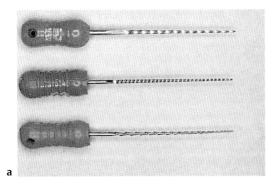

a

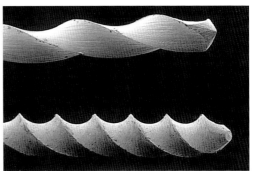

c

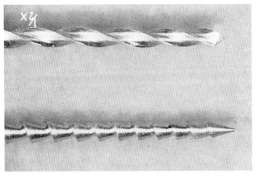

b

Fig. 9.3
a **K-reamer, K-file, and Hedstrom file (from top).**
b The K-type instruments (top) are twisted to give the working end a spiral form. They are used with longitudinal filing and rotary cutting actions. The flutes of the Hedstrom file (bottom) constitute a continuous, screw-like spiral. The file is used with longitudinal filing actions and is *not* a rotary cutting instrument.
c Scanning electron micrograph of K-type instruments with sharp, cutting tip (top) and rounded, noncutting tip (bottom).

Reamers and files.   Reamers and files are by far the most widely used root canal instruments. Traditionally, this group of instruments has been made from stainless steel and comprises two basic designs, the K-type instruments (K-files and K-reamers) and the Hedstrom file (**Fig. 9.3**).

The *K-type instruments* are made from rectangular or triangular blanks. They are twisted to give the working end of the instruments a spiral form. The number of spirals or cutting flutes may differ, but is higher in the file than in the reamer. Another difference is that the file is usually made from a rectangular blank, whereas the reamer has a triangular cross section. Because of its fewer flutes and triangular cross section, the K-reamer is a much more flexible instrument than the K-file. However, triangular K-files with increased flexibility are now available, as are files with a rhomboid-shaped cross section.

The *K-file* is used to enlarge the canal with a longitudinal filing and a rotational cutting action, or rather by a combination of the two. The *reamer* may be used in an identical fashion, but is most effective as *a rotary cutting instrument*. Recently new technology has been developed whereby K-type reamers and files are machined from round wires rather than twisted from square or triangular blanks. This has opened up interesting perspectives in terms of properties like stiffness, sharpness, and flexibility of the instruments. Another modification that has proven to be clinically useful is the rounding off of the original sharp, cutting tip of the K-type instruments (**Fig. 9.3**). Instruments with an inactive *noncutting tip* follow the root canal better than instruments with active tips. Still, stainless steel instruments are rigid enough that they should be *precurved* to match the curvature of the root during instrumentation of curved canals.

The versatility of the K-type instruments was further greatly improved by the introduction of instruments made of nickel-titanium. This material is superelastic and *instruments made of nickel-titanium are extremely flexible* (**Fig. 9.4**). With a noncutting tip they will follow curved canals well. The instrumented canals will be well centered and inner-curve strip perforations and apical outercurve "elbows" or perforations that might occur with the more rigid steel instruments are basically not seen. Thus, in curved canals the nickel-titanium instruments offer real advantages because of their flexibility.

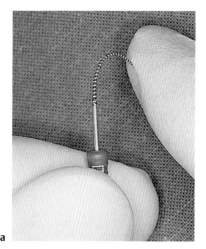

a

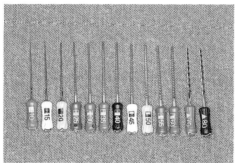

b

Fig. 9.4

a A nickel-titanium instrument is bent to show its flexibility.

b Practical sequence of K-type instruments. The size 10, 15, and 20 instruments are in stainless steel. The instruments size 25 – 60 are in nickel-titanium, and from 70 and up again in steel.

The nickel-titanium files are machined from round wires since, because of the flexibility of the material, they cannot be twisted. K-files are made in sizes 10–60. They are not nearly as sharp and effective as matching instruments made of stainless steel. Still, because of their extreme flexibility they will often be the instruments of choice. However, the smallest nickel-titanium instruments (sizes 10–20) are so flexible that they become ineffective and very difficult to use. *It is therefore good clinical practice to use steel files in the smallest sizes since they are flexible enough and then to begin the nickel-titanium instruments with size 25* (**Fig. 9.4**).

The *Hedstrom file* is made from a round blank. The flutes of the file are machined into the blank

and constitute a continuous spiral like in a screw (**Fig. 9.3**). The angle of the flutes to the long axis of the instrument is close to 90°. Thus, *the Hedstrom file is designed to be used with longitudinal filing motions and is not a rotary cutting instrument*. The Hedstrom file is by far the most effective hand instrument for root canal instrumentation. However, to reach its full potential it should be used in combination with rotary cutting instruments.

Attempts have been made to improve the rotary cutting ability of Hedstrom-type files by decreasing the flute angle of the instruments. However, this leads to a decreased efficacy of the instruments when used with longitudinal filing motions, and at present these instruments do not enjoy a wide acceptance.

Standardization of instruments. K-type instruments and Hedstrom files are today standardized (**Fig. 9.4**). This means that all manufacturers make their brand of instruments according to a standard or specification for root canal instruments as determined by standardization organizations. The numbering of the instruments is identical with the diameter of the instruments at their tip (D1) expressed in hundredths of a millimeter (**Fig. 9.5**). Thus, no. 40 instrument has a diameter at the tip (D1) of 40/100 mm, which is 0.4 mm. The standardized instruments are manufactured in numbers or sizes from 10–150. In the sizes 10–60 there is an instrument for each 5/100 mm increment at Dl, whereas from size 60 and above the increment is 10/ 100 mm. K-type instruments are available in a size 8 as well.

The standardized instruments are made in lengths of 21, 25, and 31 (30) mm. However, the length of the part of the blade with cutting flutes is always the same, namely 16 mm. Also, the flare of the blade is always the same regardless of the size of the instrument. Thus, the diameter of the blade where the cutting flutes end (D2) is the diameter at the tip (D1) plus 0.32 mm. This means that the taper of the instruments is 0.02 mm per mm. The manufacturing tolerance is 0.02 mm. Accordingly, the diameter of two instruments with the same number may vary as much as 0.04 mm. The colors white, yellow, red, blue, green, and black are used on the handles of the instruments to indicate their size. Since originally instrument no. 15 was the smallest instrument, the standardized color coding begins at this size. Thus, no. 15 instruments are white, no. 20 yellow, no. 25 red,

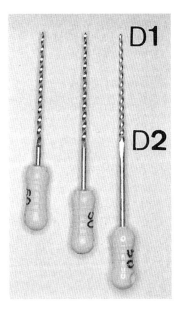

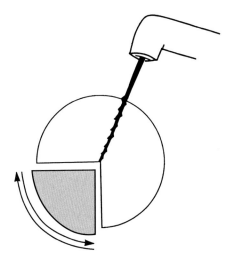

Fig. 9.6 Diagram of an endodontic handpiece giving root canal instrument rotary reciprocal action through a 90° arc.

Fig. 9.5 Standardized root canal instrument no. 50 of 21, 25, and 30 mm length. The numbering of the instruments is identical with the diameter at their tips (D1) expressed in hundredths of a millimeter. Note that the length of the cutting end of the instruments (D1–D2) is always 16 mm regardless of the total length of the instrument.

no. 30 blue, no. 35 green, and no. 40 are black. No. 45 instruments have white handles again, and the color coding is repeated. In addition, no. 10 instruments have purple-colored handles and no. 8 instruments have silver-colored ones.

Engine-Driven Instruments

Instruments with reciprocal rotary action. Most of the traditional stainless steel hand instruments are available with latch key grips and may be used with a rotary action in a regular slow-speed handpiece. However, with this technique instrument fractures will readily occur and perforations of the root will be a routine observation. Steel instruments should therefore not be used with engine-driven, continuous rotary action.

Better results have been obtained with handpieces especially made for root canal instrumentation. These devices are designed to give the root canal instruments a movement that will facilitate the instrumentation of the canal with a minimum of instrument fractures and other mishaps. A well-known design used by several manufacturers is a handpiece that operates *by a rotary reciprocal action through a 90° arc* (**Fig. 9.6**). Combined with suitable root canal instruments, these devices work well, although the rotary action will invariably lead to some instrument fractures.

An interesting concept is available in contra-angles used with a slow-speed handpiece where the basic pattern of movement is a lengthwise, vibratory motion of the root canal instrument at a variable range between 0.3 mm and 1.0 mm. The vibration amplitude is inversely related to the resistance during instrumentation. Thus, if the resistance is nil, the root canal instrument will have a linear motion. If a forward motion is not possible (stop in the canal), the linear movement is replaced by a 90° rotary reciprocal action. With moderate resistance the instrument in the canal will have a forward motion plus a certain rotary reciprocal movement. This automated system has been found to be as efficient as systems with a pure reciprocal action in all canal configurations. However, fewer mishaps are seen when the instruments are allowed freer, more complex movements in the canal.

Nickel-titanium rotary instruments. The introduction of the superelastic and flexible nickel-titanium alloy in endodontics created a wave of innovation. It soon became clear that *continuous*

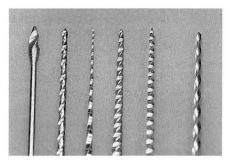

Fig. 9.7 A selection of engine-driven nickel-tita-nium root canal instruments showing innovation in design.

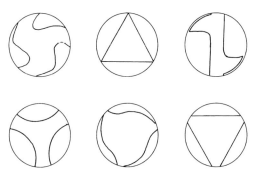

Fig. 9.8 Diagram indicating cross sections of six engine-driven nickel-titanium root canal instruments. In spite of the variations in appearance, two basic design ideas may be recognized: instruments that are sharp and instruments where the cutting edges have been "flattened" to reduce their aggressiveness.

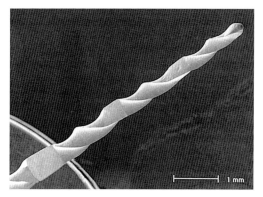

Fig. 9.9 Nickel-titanium rotary instrument (RaCe) which combines spiraled and nonspiraled sections along its working length. This design minimizes frictional resistance inside the canal. Also, the instrument has a triangular cross section guaranteeing cutting efficiency. Note the rounded tip of the instrument.

rotary instrumentation of the root canal might be attainable with flexible nickel-titanium instruments, and several companies set out to design instruments, handpieces, and motors, and to devise techniques that would be effective and safe. Presently more than 10 different systems of nickel-titanium instruments designed for engine-driven continuous rotary instrumentation of the root canal are available (**Fig. 9.7**).

Basically all endodontic instruments are designed like *screws* with one or more cutting helixes. When used with motorized rotation they therefore have a tendency to screw into the root canal until they become stuck or break. In order to avoid this phenomenon, several designs have been proposed and various measures have been taken. Thus, several manufacturers have chosen to

flatten the cutting edges of the instruments in order to reduce their agressiveness (**Fig. 9.8**). However, this leads to a reduction in cutting efficiency which almost unavoidably leads to an increased use of force and a higher working torque. The result then will be an increased rather than a reduced fracture risk. Thus, *instruments meant for motorized rotation also should be sharp. Also, a rotary instrument should have variable helical flute angles.* This will reduce the screwing-in effect, and debris will be removed from the canal in an efficient manner. One instrument is unique in this regard in that it combines spiraled and nonspiraled (straight) sections along its working length (**Fig. 9.9**). This design feature practically eliminates the screwing-in effect. Also, this instrument has the triangular cross section of a K-file with sharp edges, guaranteeing cutting efficiency. The instrument has been succcessfully designed to minimize frictional resistance inside the canal and thereby reduce torque demands.

A reduction in working torque has moreover been achieved by designing instruments with *different tapers* so that only a part of the root canal can be instrumented at a time. Most engine-driven systems offer instruments with tapers from the standard 0.02 mm to 0.10 mm. Three instruments with taper 0.10, 0.08, and 0.06 mm are usually short (16 – 19 mm) and used to open up and enlarge the coronal half of the canal. Instruments with taper 0.06 – 0.02 mm of normal length and sizes are then available to instrument the apical half of the canal. Thus, a sequence of instruments might be 40/0.10, 35/0.08, 30/0.06, 30/0.04, and 25/0.02 (see p.187). Such a sequence of instruments would follow the golden rule of engine-driven instrumentation: *maximize efficiency, minimize engagement, and maintain safety*. In narrow canals the instrument 40/0.10 or even 35/0.08 might not be used. In many canals, the instrument 30/0.06 might go to working length. Thus, not all instruments are used in all canals, but it is practical and safe to have the entire sequence available. Instruments with 0.02 mm taper are preferable for the instrumentation of severely curved canals since the working torque is the lowest in these instruments. This minimizes *cyclic fatigue* from compression and tension in the instruments as they are rotated around a curve. Cyclic fatigue is insidious and not readily noticeable, but must not be forgotten when the decision is made whether an instrument should be discarded or used again.

A final important design feature to permit safe use of engine-driven nickel-titanium instruments is the *safety tip*. The tip should be rounded and be noncutting or near noncutting (**Fig. 9.9**). This will allow the flexible instrument to follow the root canal so that stripping, transportation, or even perforation of the canal is avoided. A well-centered canal with smooth canal walls can be expected following instrumentation with these instruments and this technique.

The fracture risk of the instruments is further influenced by the *working speed*. Thus, instruments run at 1000 rpm will break twice as fast as instruments run at 500 rpm. The design of the instruments as far as it influences its working torque is important in this regard. Instruments with flattened cutting edges and high torque demands should be operated at 150–300 rpm, whereas sharp, low-torque, nonscrewing instruments may be run at 500–600 rpm with the same degree of safety. Also, the *type of motor* used is of importance for the risk of fracture. The handpiece of a standard dental unit has a working torque of about 2.5 Ncm, whereas nickel-titanium rotary instruments may break at torque levels below 1 Ncm. Low-torque and torque-limiting motors have, therefore, been designed specifically to be used with the rotary instruments. One motor can even be set to operate below the maximum permissible torque limit of each rotary instrument, regardless of taper and size. Theoretically, an instrument fracture should then not occur. In any case, controlled experiments show a significant reduction in instrument fractures when low-torque motors are used.

Root Canal Obturation

Hand Instruments

Root canal spreaders and pluggers. *Root canal spreaders* are tapered, pointed metal instruments with a smooth surface (**Fig. 9.10**). They are used for lateral condensation of filling materials in the root canal. Root canal spreaders are available in different sizes with different tapers and different flexibilities. They can have long handles like an explorer or they can be equipped with the short handle of a root canal instrument. In the latter instance they are called *finger spreaders*.

Root canal pluggers are slightly tapered and flat-ended metal instruments with a smooth surface (**Fig. 9.10**). They are used for vertical condensation of filling materials in the root canal. Like the spreaders, they are available with long or short handles. In the latter instance they are called finger pluggers (**Fig. 9.10**).

Lentulo spirals. The lentulo is a wire spiral attached to a latch key grip so that it can be mounted in a slow-speed handpiece (**Fig. 9.11**). The lentulo is also called a spiral filler or a paste carrier and is used to introduce paste-like materials into the root canal. Today it is widely used for the application of calcium hydroxide paste into the canal. It can also be used with permanent root canal sealers, but should then be hand-held rather than engine-driven in order to avoid overfilling the canal.

Gutta-Percha Guns

Devices are now available whereby thermoplasticized gutta-percha may be injected into the root canal. Fairly large needles are necessary for the gutta-percha to flow so that a rather wide enlargement of the root canal is necessary to bring the needle close enough to the apical part of the root canal.

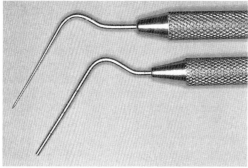
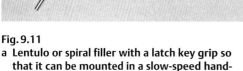

a

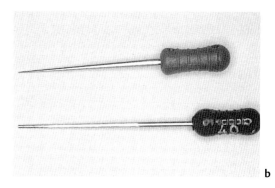

b

Fig. 9.11
a Lentulo or spiral filler with a latch key grip so that it can be mounted in a slow-speed hand-piece.

b The lentulo is used to introduce paste-like materials into the root canal

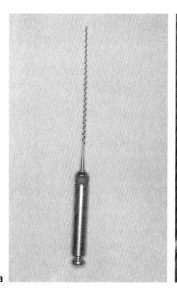
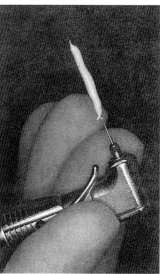

a

b

Fig. 9.10
a Examples of a root canal spreader (top) and root canal plugger (bottom). The spreader is tapered and pointed. The plugger is less tapered and has a flat end.
b Finger plugger (left) and finger spreader (right).

Surgical Instruments

Preferably, a no. 12 *scalpel blade* is used to free gingival tissues with the dental papillae from the teeth (**Fig. 9.12**). Otherwise a no. 15 scalpel is a good all-round instrument. A good *elevator* to reflect the flap in endodontic surgery should be sharp (**Fig. 9.13**). *Tissue retractors* vary from blunt blades to sharp-toothed claws. A blade-type retractor should preferably be used, so that it can rest on bone during the operation. *Round burs* no. 6–12 in a low-torque high-speed handpiece are used to remove necessary bone. *A long-shank*

fissure bur no. 557 or similar instrument is used to bevel the apex of the tooth or to remove the root tip. A *microhandpiece* and round or inverted cone *microburs* may be used for the preparation of retrograde cavities (**Fig. 9.14**). In difficult-to-reach areas, *ultrasonically energized multiangle tips* are used (**Fig. 9.15**). These so-called *retrotips* can be diamond-coated for improved effectiveness. Ultrasonically energized instruments are also available for retrograde instrumentation of unfilled root canals (**Fig. 6.35**). Mirrors of shapes and sizes so that they can be used in the surgical cavities are useful (**Fig. 9.16**), and pluggers in a variety of sizes and angulations that have been designed specifically for the filling of retrograde cavities are available (**Fig. 9.17**).

A *serrated needle holder*, thin-tipped scissors, and atraumatic needles with attached 4 – 0 or 3 – 0 sutures are needed for closure of the wound.

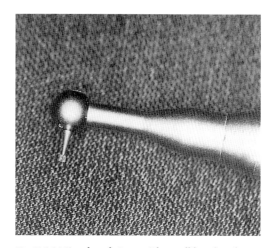

Fig. 9.14 Microhandpiece with small head and short (micro)bur is used to prepare retrograde cavities if access to the root end is sufficient.

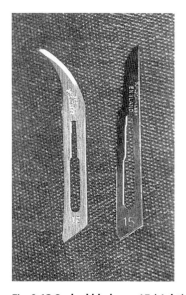

Fig. 9.12 Scalpel blade no. 15 (right) is a good all-round blade in endodontic surgery. Blade no. 12 (left) is best used to free gingival tissues.

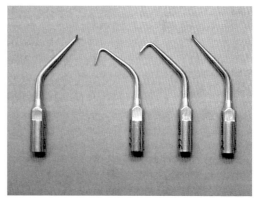

Fig. 9.15 Multiangle vibratory tips (retrotips) for the preparation of retrograde cavities. The retrotips are energized by an ultrasonic unit. Because of their size and shape they can be used to prepare ideal root end cavities at most locations in the mouth.

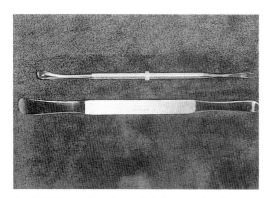

Fig. 9.13 Examples of a useful elevator (top) and tissue retractor (bottom).

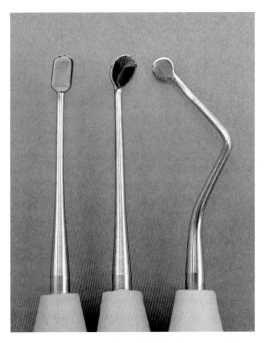

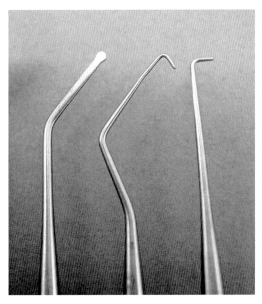

Fig. 9.17 Plastic instrument and pluggers designed specifically for the filling of retrograde cavities.

Fig. 9.16 Mirrors used in endodontic surgery. The mirrors have shapes and sizes so that they may be used in surgical cavities.

Further Reading

Deplazes P, Peters O, Barbakow F. Comparing apical preparations of root canals shaped by nickel-titanium rotary instruments and nickel-titanium hand instruments. J Endod 2001;27:196 – 202.

Gambarini G. Rationale for the use of low-torque endodontic motors in root canal instrumentation. Endod Dent Traumatol 2000;16:95 – 100.

Gutmann JL, Harrison JW. Posterior endodontic surgery: anatomical considerations and clinical techniques. Int Endod J 1985;18:8 – 34.

Kazemi RB, Stenman E, Spångberg LSW. Machining efficiency and wear resistance of nickel-titanium endodontic files. Oral Surg Oral Med Oral Pathol 1996; 81:596 – 602.

Pettiette MT, Metzger Z, Phillip SC, Trope M. Endodontic complications of root canal therapy performed by dental students with stainless steel K-files and nickel-titanium hand files. J Endod 1999;25:230 – 234.

Shäfer E. Root canal instruments for manual use: a review. Endod Dent Traumatol 1997;13:51 – 64.

Schäfer E, Hoppe W. Wurzalkanalinstrumente aus Titan-Aluminium, Nickel-Titan oder Edelstahl. Zahnärztl Welt 1995;104:612 – 616.

Schäfer E, Lan R. Comparison of cutting efficiency and instrumentation of curved canals with nickel-titanium and stainless steel instruments. J Endod 1999; 25:427 – 30.

Stenman E, Spångberg LSW. Root canal instruments are poorly standardized. J Endod 1993;19:327 – 334.

Sultan M, Pitt Ford TR. Ultrasonic preparation and obturation of root-end cavities. Int Endod J 1995;28: 231 – 238.

Tronstad L, Niemczyk SP. Efficacy and safety tests of six automated devices for root canal instrumentation. Endod Dent Traumatol 1996;2:270 – 276.

Tronstad L, Barnett F, Schwartzben L, Frasca P. Effectiveness and safety of a sonic vibratory endodontic instrument. Endod Dent Traumatol 1985;1:69 – 76.

Walia HM, Brantley WA, Gerstein H. An initial investigation of the bending and torsional poperties of Nitinol root canal files. J Endod 1988;14:340 – 351.

Wuchenich G, Meadows D, Torabinejad M. A comparison between two root end preparation techniques in human cadavers. J Endod 1994;20:279 – 282.

Yared GM, Bon Dagher FE, Machtou P. Influences of rotational speed, torque and operator's proficiency on ProFile failures. Int Endod J 2001;34:47 – 53.

10
Endodontic Materials

Endodontic materials in the widest sense are:
1) Cavity base materials with a therapeutic effect,
2) Pulp capping agents,
3) Materials used for temporary closure of access cavities in teeth during endodontic treatment,
4) Root canal filling materials, and
5) Materials used for retrograde filling of the root canal, repair of root perforations, etc.

Of these, base materials and pulp capping agents have been discussed above (see p. 86 and p. 88).

Temporary Filling Materials

An absolute requirement of a material for temporary closure of an access cavity is that it provide a *bacteria-tight seal*. In other words, the material must prevent oral bacteria from reaching the unfilled root canal. Most widely used for this purpose is a *paste of zinc oxide and eugenol*. Such a paste gives a good seal and has an antibacterial effect which adds to its protective properties. The thickness of the temporary filling is another factor which contributes to its sealing ability, and a zinc oxide–eugenol-type filling should be at least 3–4 mm and if at all possible 5 mm thick (**Fig. 10.1**). The root canal will then be well protected for several weeks. If longer periods of protection are required, a *resin-reinforced zinc oxide–eugenol material like IRM cement* may be used.

Eugenol is a substance that inhibits the polymerization reaction of resins, and can therefore interfere with the bonding of a final composite resin restoration in the access cavity. However, if the right precautions are taken, the influence of eugenol on the cavity walls can effectively be eliminated. The dentin should be cleaned mechanically with small burs and then washed with alcohol. A normal acid-etch and rinse technique may then be used, resulting in a resin–dentin bond as strong and reliable as if a eugenol temporary cement had not been used.

A temporary filling material, *Cavit*, which is based on zinc oxide and calcium sulfate, is another alternative. Cavit is available in tubes and jars ready-mixed to be inserted into the access cavity. The material will set under the influence of moisture (saliva) and it gives a reliable bacteria-tight seal when used in the necessary thickness (3–5 mm).

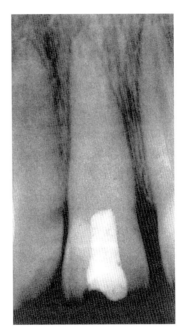

Fig. 10.1 Radiograph of a maxillary incisor with a zinc oxide–eugenol temporary filling. The filling seals the access cavity as well as the pulpal ends of possibly exposed dentinal tubules in the cervical area of the tooth.

Filling materials like amalgams, resins, and most cements will not give an adequate bacteria-tight seal of an access cavity. If it is desirable that such materials be used between endodontic visits for strength or esthetic reasons, the orifice of the root canal has to be sealed bacteria-tight first before the restorative material is inserted.

Root Canal Filling Materials

Root canal filling materials are protected by the dentin wall of the root canal and by occlusal or incisal restorations. However, the materials are in close contact with soft connective tissue apically in the root canal so that tissue–material interactions occur. *The root canal filling, therefore, is comparable to an implant elsewhere in the body.*

Ideally, a root canal filling material should permanently seal the root canal bacteria-tight. It should not irritate the apical tissues and it should not dissolve or disintegrate as a result of influences from tissues or tissue fluids. Also, a material used in the root canal should be radiopaque so that it can be determined radiographically whether a tooth has been treated endodontically or not. Moreover, radiographic examination is the only method by which the apical extent of a root canal filling and, very importantly, its technical quality can be determined. A root canal filling material should also be easily removed from the canal, as retreatment of teeth often becomes necessary because of treatment failure and because root canals are frequently used for retention of posts in the restoration of endodontically treated teeth.

A great number of materials and material modifications have been used as root canal filling materials, *but there is still no material available today which fulfills all of the above-mentioned criteria. As a consequence, a combination of materials is most often used to fill the root canal.* A tissue-compatible core material which can readily be removed from the canal but which does not give the necessary seal is used to fill the bulk of the root canal space. In addition, small quantities of a paste-like material that provides a bacteria-tight seal is used to fill minor spaces between the core material and the root canal wall. Thus, root canal filling materials may be divided into two distinct groups: core materials and sealing materials, or root canal sealers.

Core Materials

There are two types of core materials in common use, gutta-percha and a resin-based material (Resilon). In addition, points of metallic silver were widely used to fill root canals and may still be used in some areas.

Gutta-percha. Gutta-percha is a polymer, mainly polyisoprene, which is extracted from a tropical tree in Malaysia. At room temperature it is 60% crystalline, while the rest of the mass has an amorphous structure. As is normal for polymers, the material is viscoelastic, which means that it has a certain elasticity, but at the same time it has the characteristics of a viscous fluid. When heated, gutta-percha is softened and deformed and it becomes liquid when the temperature exceeds 65 °C. The material can also be dissolved in organic solvents such as chloroform, xylene, and eucalyptol. If gutta-percha is exposed for some time to light and air, it oxidizes and becomes hard and brittle. It can be reconditioned by means of warm water (40 °C).

Already at the beginning of the 19th century, attempts were made to use gutta-percha in dentistry, but without success. Not until it was learned how to alter its physical characteristics by adding zinc oxide and other substances did it receive real attention. It has been in continuous use as a root canal filling material since the 1860s and is still by far the most widely used material for obturation of the root canal space. Today, gutta-percha is available in two types of point, standardized points and accessory points (**Fig. 10.2**). The composition of the points may vary from one manufacturer to the other, but generally they contain 60–70% zinc oxide, up to 17% heavy metal salts, and 1–4% waxes, resins, antioxidizing agents, etc.

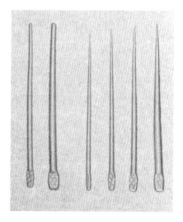

Fig. 10.2 Gutta-percha points for root canal filling. Standardized points nos. 50 and 80 (left); accessory points of the sizes A, B, C, and D (right).

The actual amount of gutta-percha in the points, therefore, is only about 20% of the total content.

The *standardized gutta-percha points* are manufactured to correspond in size and shape to the standardized root canal instruments (**Fig.10.3**). However, due to the nature of the material, the manufacturing process of standardized sizes is difficult, and diameter tolerances of ±0.05 mm have to be accepted at the present time. This is unfortunate, as two points of allegedly the same size may vary in diameter as much as 0.10 mm, which in points smaller than no.60 may represent 3 instrument sizes. Still, even with its present weaknesses, the standardization of the gutta-percha points is extremely helpful when selecting a master point to fit as well as possible in the apical part of the root canal. In addition to the standardized master points with taper 0.02 mm, standardized points with tapers 0.04 mm and 0.06 mm are also available.

The *accessory gutta-percha points* have a pointed shape (**Fig.10.2**). They are available in assorted sizes and are used to supplement the standardized master point to fill the coronal flared part of the root canal.

Gutta-percha points fulfill most of the requirements of a root canal filling material. An important characteristic of the material is its favorable biological properties in that it is virtually nonirritating to contacting connective tissue. Moreover, with a sensible technique, it is relatively easily inserted into the root canal. It does not discolor the tooth, it provides good radiographic contrast, and it is readily removed from the canal. However, *gutta-percha does not provide a bacteria-tight seal of the root canal*. Attempts have been made to overcome this weakness by softening the points in an organic solvent, usually chloroform. In this manner, the material can be molded according to the shape of the canal to fill it completely in three dimensions. However, the material loses its dimensional stability when exposed to a solvent, and when the solvent has evaporated, shrinkage will occur. Gutta-percha will shrink if softened by heat as well and regardless of method, the more it is softened, the larger is its shrinking potential. *Thus, gutta-percha points should preferably not be softened at all, but even if they are, they should always be used in combination with a second material, a root canal sealer, to obtain the necessary bacteria-tight seal of the root canal.*

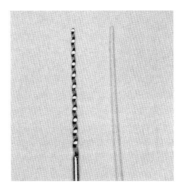

Fig. 10.3 Standardized root canal instrument (K-reamer) and standardized gutta-percha point. The standardized points correspond in size and shape to the standardized instruments.

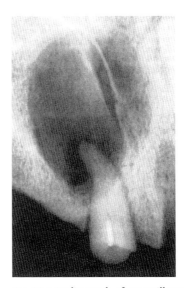

Fig. 10.4 Radiograph of a maxillary incisor with a metallic root canal filling in an ancient man (approximately 200 B.C.). Note that a large radiolucent periapical lesion has developed.

Silver points.   Metals have been used as root canal filling materials for thousands of years (**Fig.10.4**). Gold, silver, and lead were especially popular due to the relative softness and ductility of these metals. Historically, the largest area of use was the filling of extracted teeth which were to be transplanted from one individual to another.

Since the 1920s, metallic silver points have been used as root canal filling material (**Fig.10.5**). One reason silver was preferred to other metals

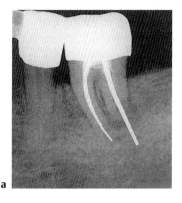

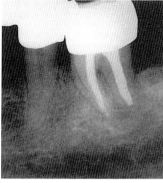

Fig. 10.5
a **Radiograph of a mandibular molar with silver point root canal fillings.** The case is failing and apical radiolucencies and root resorption are evident.
b Periapical repair after the removal of silver points, retreatment of the tooth and obturation of the root canals with gutta-percha.

a

b

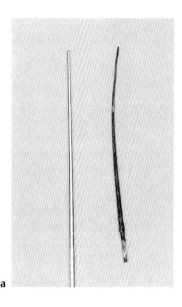

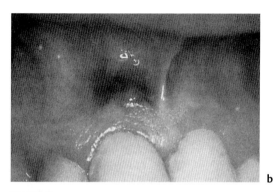

b

a

Fig. 10.6
a **Endodontic silver points.** A new, unused point (left); a point retrieved from the root canal during retreatment of a tooth (rigt). This silver point is corroded (black) in its entire length because of contact with tissue fluids.
b Tattoo in the oral vestibule due to corrosion products from silver point root filling of a maxillary right central incisor.

was its alleged oligodynamic effect, i.e., the silver points were believed to release silver ions with a bactericidal effect due to their affinity for certain bacterial enzymes. Moreover, silver is relatively soft, which permits adaptation of a straight point in curved canals.

Today, we know that silver ions in fact do have an antibacterial effect, but also that they are not released spontaneously from metallic silver. On the contrary, pure metallic silver is nontoxic and nonirritating to human cells as well as to bacteria. However, when silver has been in contact with tissue and tissue fluids for some time, as, for example, in the root canal, it corrodes (**Fig. 10.6**). Among the corrosion products are silver–sulfur compounds and others which are extremely toxic and

may cause inflammation in adjacent tissues. *For this reason silver points are used less and less in endodontic therapy and should preferably not be used at all.*

Thus, biological considerations have in fact made silver unsuitable as a root canal filling material in modern endodontics (**Fig. 10.5**). With regard to its physical properties, it should only be mentioned briefly that silver points are relatively easy to insert into the canal, provide an excellent radiographic contrast, and obviously do not seal the canal on their own and have to be used in combination with a root canal sealer. In instances of retreatment, which will be a rather frequent occurrence with this technique, the silver points may be easily removed if the correct obturation technique has been used. However, it may also be extremely difficult or sometimes impossible to remove them from the root canal.

Resin-Based Material (Resilon).   The Resilon material consists of a vinyl polyester with methacrylate polymer, glass filler particles and opacifiers added. Its appearance and handling properties are similar to gutta-percha. Master points with taper 0.02 mm and 0.04 mm are available as are pointed accessory points of normal ISO recommended sizes. Resilon fulfills most of the requirements of a root canal filling material. With a sensible technique it is easily inserted into the root canal, and it is nonirritating to contacting connective tissue. It does not discolor the tooth, it provides good radiographic contrast, and it is readily removed from the root canal with various techniques (e.g., dissolves in chloroform). However, like gutta-percha, Resilon does not provide a bacteria-tight seal of the root canal, and has to be used together with a second material, a root canal sealer. It may seem that Resilon could be used in combination with any type of sealer. However, the manufacturer requests that the material be used only with an obturating sealer, Epiphany, which utilizes a dentin adhesive technology.

Root Canal Sealers

As discussed above, core materials must be used together with another material, a sealing material, or root canal sealer. The materials in this group are generally unacceptable as root canal filling materials without core material, either because of shrinkage, difficulties in removing the material, or other reasons. The most important requirement of a sealer is that the material provide a bacteria-tight seal of the canal that sufficiently prevents ingress and growth of bacteria. Moreover, it should not shrink, be resorbable, or dissolve in tissue fluids, and it should be tissue-compatible. Several types of root canal sealers are available. For practical reasons they may be divided into sealers based on zinc oxide and eugenol, synthetic resins, gutta-percha and/or natural resin(s), and sealers with an alleged therapeutic effect.

Sealers based on zinc oxide and eugenol.   The sealers most widely used throughout the world are found in this group. Common to all the products is the fact that the powder consists to a great extent of zinc oxide (about 50%) and the liquid of

Table 10.1 Recipe of commonly used zinc oxide–eugenol root canal sealer (Grossman's sealer)

Powder		Liquid
Zinc oxide	42 parts	Eugenol
Staybelite resin	27 parts	
Bismuth subcarbonate	15 parts	
Barium sulfate	15 parts	
Sodium borate	1 part	

eugenol. A natural resin is usually added to the powder in order to give the paste a smoother texture. The resin is also said to favor-ably influence the long-term stability and sealing ability of the material. In some of the cements, finely distributed silver is added to provide radiographic contrast. These materials have a dark color, may cause discoloration of the teeth, and should not be used in modern endodontics. Normally barium or bismuth salts, or both, are used to give radiographic contrast (e.g., Grossman's sealer; **Table 10.1**). A number of potentially more harmful ingredients such as paraformaldehyde, mercury compounds, and corticosteroids have also been added to zinc oxide–eugenol sealers, but these have generally been deleted from the formulas recommended for use today.

The *advantages* of sealers with a zinc oxide–eugenol base are that they have a certain body and therefore readily fill the spaces between the gutta-percha points and the root canal wall. These sealers provide a bacteria-tight seal and, in general, do not shrink. The *disadvantages* of the zinc oxide–eugenol sealers are primarily their solubility in tissue fluids and a certain toxicity. The toxicity is caused by free eugenol that is always present in freshly mixed materials (**Fig. 10.7**). Gradually, the eugenol release diminishes, so that in the long term these sealers are well tolerated. The free eugenol in the freshly mixed materials gives the sealer a temporary antibacterial effect which may conceivably be beneficial. While eugenol is a well-known allergen, there are very few clinical observations or reports of allergic manifestations in conjunction with the use of zinc oxide–eugenol-based root canal sealers. On the contrary, a tremendous body of clinical experience indicates that from a biological point of view, these materials may be used safely.

The *solubility* of the zinc oxide and eugenol sealers when influenced by tissue fluids may be beneficial when there is an excess of material out-

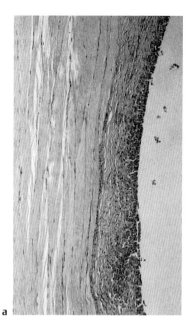

a

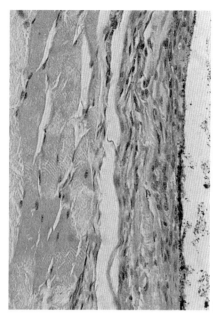

b

Fig. 10.7 Tissue reaction to zinc oxide–eugenol root canal sealer.
a After 8 days, a moderate inflammatory reaction is seen in the tissue adjacent to the material.
b After 6 months, the inflammatory reaction has subsided.

side the root canal in the periodontal tissues. However, the sealers dissolve within the root canal as well (**Figs. 10.6**, **10.8**). Thus, during retreatment of teeth filled with the silver point technique, partial or complete disappearance of the zinc oxide–eugenol-based sealer is a routine finding, as is a stained, corroded silver point, often completely loose in the root canal. *When gutta-percha is used as the core material, a chemical bond forms between the zinc oxide in the gutta-percha point and the eugenol in the sealer.* The stability of the zinc oxide–eugenol-based sealers is, therefore, considerably better when used with gutta-percha than with silver. Still, the solubility of the materials is a drawback, and they should only be used in as small amounts as possible to "glue" the gutta-percha points to the root canal wall.

Sealers based on gutta-percha or natural resins, or both. Pure gutta-percha dissolved in chloroform is a smooth, sticky paste which is referred to as *chloropercha*. Chloropercha has been used as a root canal sealer and commercial products are still available. However, when the solvent of the chloropercha has evaporated, the end product will be gutta-percha, which has no sealing properties and will shrink greatly after having been dissolved in the organic solvent. Chloropercha is, therefore, not suitable as a root canal sealer.

Kloroperka N-O is a root canal sealer which attempts to resolve the disadvantages of regular chloropercha. In this product, the powder consists of 50% zinc oxide, 20% gutta-percha, and 30% natural resins and, when mixed with chloroform, makes a material with many good characteristics. The addition of the natural resins makes Kloroperka N-O very sticky, also after the chloroform has evaporated. It is also relatively tissue compatible. However, Kloroperka N-O shrinks markedly after setting, which means that the material can only be used in extremely small amounts as a glue between the gutta-percha points and the root canal wall. Long-term follow-up studies have shown favorable results of endodontic treatment with Kloroperka N-O used as the sealer. However, in a recent prospective comparative clinical study, it was found to be inferior to zinc oxide–eugenol-based and epoxy resin–based sealers, and its usefulness in modern endodontics may be questionable.

A sealer which enjoys a certain popularity is a 15% solution of colophony, a natural resin, in chloroform. This solution is commonly referred to as *resin chloroform*. It is sticky and provides a bacteria-tight seal if the root canal is completely and three-dimensionally filled with gutta-percha. This is obtained by softening gutta-percha points in the resin chloroform with the inherent possibilities of subsequent shrinkage of the root canal filling. Long-term follow-up studies have shown favorable results of endodontic treatment with the resin chloroform method. However, it is a very technique-sensitive method and its usefulness as a routine method in modern endodontics is questionable.

Sealers based on synthetic resins. Two commercial products of this type will be mentioned: Diaket and AH Plus. *Diaket* is mixed from a fine powder consisting mainly of zinc oxide and bismuth phosphate and a viscous liquid which contains a polyketone compound and dissolved vinyl polymers. It sets by a chelation of zinc with the polyketone in the liquid. Freshly mixed Diaket is thick, extremely sticky, and therefore somewhat difficult to insert into the root canal. However, it seals the root canal effectively, does not shrink, and is rather insoluble in tissue fluids. After setting, Diaket is extremely difficult to remove from the canal and, if used, should always be combined with gutta-percha points. However, *Diaket has marked toxic and tissue-irritating effects* and by comparison with other available materials, the rationale for using Diaket is questionable.

AH Plus is a two-component paste–paste root canal sealer based on epoxyamine resin chemistry. Equal volumes of the two pastes are mixed together when used. This gives a material with a creamy, homogenous consistency which is easily applied to the root canal. It adapts well to the root canal wall, and when used in small amounts with gutta-percha provides adequate long-term stability and a bacteria-tight seal of the canal.

In contrast to a previous epoxy resin sealer (AH26), AH Plus does not release formaldehyde during the setting process. Tests in large animals have shown that the new material is well tolerated by the periapical tissues. However, since AH Plus contains epoxy resins or amines, it may cause sensitisation in susceptible persons. The material should, therefore, not be used in patients allergic to these components. Still this is a question of contact allergy and as long as the material is used in the root canal only, adverse reactions will be extremely rare.

Sealer utilizing dentin adhesive technology (Epiphany). Epiphany is a dual-cure, hydrophilic resin sealer to be used with the Resilon core material described above. Product advertising states that the Resilon/Epiphany system is more effec-

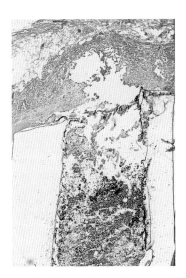

Fig. 10.8 Zinc oxide and eugenol-based root canal sealer in teflon cup implanted in the mandible of a dog. After 30 days it is evident that the sealer has caused an inflammatory reaction in the adjacent tissue and that the material in the cup is partly dissolved and washed out.

tive than traditional gutta-percha/sealer combinations in that it utilizes a resin obturating material and an adhesive resin sealer, creating a monoblock of dentin/adhesisive/sealer/obturating material in the root canal. This is, however, doubtful in that to obtain a true monoblock, unpolymerized resin must be available in both materials to achieve co-polymerization, and there is no unpolymerized resin in Resilon. Epiphany has a creamy, homogenous consistency and is easily applied to the root canal. It adapts well to the root canal wall, and when used with Resilon provides a seal of the canal.

Materials with Assumed Therapeutic Effect

Over the years, attempts have been made to substitute meticulous chemomechanical instrumentation and disinfection of the root canal by obturation of the canal with materials with a long-lasting, preferably permanent antiseptic effect. Pastes containing formaldehyde or iodoform have been widely used. Some products also contain heavy metals such as mercury compounds for disinfection and lead oxide for radiographic contrast. Also, the addition of corticosteroids to root canal filling materials has been popular, probably with a view to controlling postoperative symptoms.

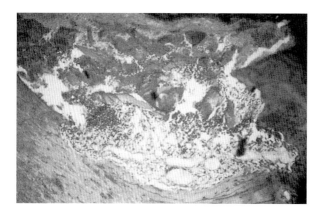

Fig. 10.9 Tissue reaction to paraformal-dehyde-containing root canal cement. After implantation in bone, the material has caused sequestrum formation and necrosis.

The physical properties of these materials vary, but common to all of them is that, from a biological point of view, they are unacceptable as root canal filling materials. Rather than having a therapeutic effect, the results of experimental studies indicate that the materials are highly toxic and tissue-irritating and may maintain a chronic inflammation and cause tissue necrosis and the formation of bone sequestra (**Fig. 10.9**).

Formaldehyde-containing materials also have a pronounced and irreversible neurotoxic effect, and clinical reports of paresthesia associated with the use of such materials in endodontic treatment are numerous. Moreover, most active ingredients in these materials are potent allergens. Admittedly, at present there may be no ideal root canal filling material. However, there is no reason to make the situation worse by adding unfavorable ingredients to already less-than-perfect materials.

Root canal sealers containing calcium hydroxide are available. These materials have been made in an attempt to benefit from the desirable biological effects of calcium hydroxide, especially its antibacterial effect and its ability to induce hard-tissue formation. However, calcium hydroxide works by the release of hydroxyl and calcium ions, and if it is going to have a therapeutic effect, it cannot possibly be a stable component of a root canal sealer. Still, two commercial products will be mentioned, CRCS and Sealapex.

CRCS is basically a zinc oxide–eugenol-based sealer in which the powder contains 16% calcium hydroxide and the liquid 20% eucalyptol. In animal experiments this sealer has proved to be slightly more tissue irritating than a conventional zinc oxide–eugenol sealer, but apparently with comparable stability and sealing ability. Thus,

CRCS may be suitable as a root canal sealer. However, it is unlikely that the material has a therapeutic effect, as the pH of freshly mixed CRCS is less than 9. A pH of 11 and above has been associated with the desirable effects of calcium hydroxide.

Sealapex is a polymeric material which allegedly contains and/or releases calcium hydroxide. The formula for Sealapex has changed since its in-

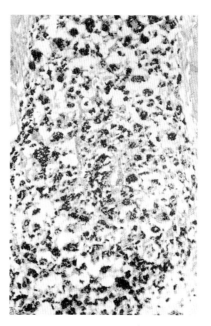

Fig. 10.10 Tissue reaction to calcium hydroxide-containing root canal sealer (Sealapex). The material has caused a severe macrophage reaction. It is transported away and is seen in cells and tissues at a distance from the site of implantation.

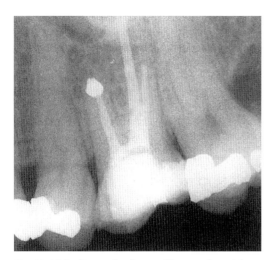

Fig. 10.11 Radiograph of a maxillary molar with a retrograde amalgam filling in the mesiobuccal root and periapical healing

troduction, but characteristic for the material is that it induces a severe macrophage reaction in adjacent tissues. Thus, in addition to being dissolved by tissue fluids like most sealers, it is also phagocytized and transported away by cells (**Fig. 10.10**). However, in a 1-year, in-vivo leakage study, when the material was used in small quantities together with gutta-percha points, it showed a sealing ability comparable with other commonly used sealers. Still, a number of cases have been observed where the Sealapex material has com-

pletely disappeared from the root canal, leaving the nonsealing gutta-percha in the canal. No evidence is available as to a possible therapeutic effect of the material.

Retrograde Filling Materials

A retrograde root filling should seal the root canal bacteria-tight. In principle, the root canal may be filled from the retrograde position with the same materials that are used for orthograde canal obturation. However, in the clinical situation this may be difficult or even impossible because of difficult access to the root canal. The practical approach, therefore, will often be to prepare and fill a retrograde cavity in the end of the root to improve upon the seal of an existing root canal filling or to provide a bacteria-tight seal on its own.

A retrograde filling is an implant and should consist of a material or materials that tolerate the intimate contact with tissue and tissue fluids for long periods of time without being washed out, dissolved, or resorbed. Because of this, *silver amalgam* has been the material of choice for retrograde fillings for many years (**Fig. 10.11**). Amalgam restorations show initial marginal leakage and do not provide a seal of a cavity until corrosion products have formed in the gap between the filling and the cavity wall. This initial marginal leakage may be effectively prevented by the application of a copal varnish to the cavity prior to the insertion of the amalgam (**Fig. 10.12**). *A cavity varnish, therefore, should be routinely used before the placement of a retrograde amalgam filling.* However,

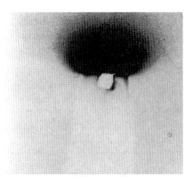

a

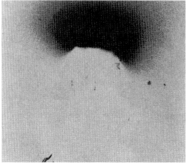

b

Fig. 10.12
a Root with a retro-grade cavity filled with amalgam. Marginal leakage is evi-denced by the penetration of a radioactive isotope between the filling and the cavity walls.

b Root with a retrograde cavity filled with amalgam after the application of a copal varnish to the cavity. The layer of varnish has effectively prevented marginal leakage of the radioactive isotope.

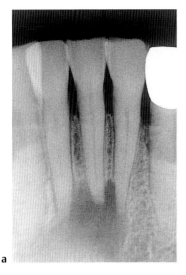

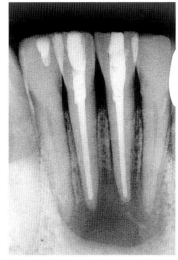

Fig. 10.13
a **Mandibular incicors with asymptomatic apical periodontitis.** *Staphylococcus aureus* is part of the infecting flora and there is no response to long-term calcium hydroxide combined with systemic penicillin plus metronidazole treatment.
b The teeth are root filled.
c Apicoectomy with retrograde fillings (IRM-cement) is performed.
d Complete periapical repair at the 6-month control.

a

b

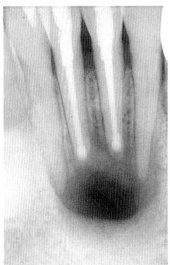

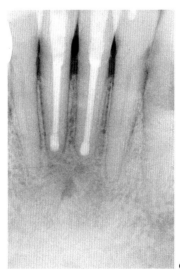

c

d

mainly because of its mercury content, amalgam more and more is regarded as being an unacceptable material in spite of its rather favorable physical properties. Thus, its use as a retrograde filling material when it is implanted into the body simply is prohibited in some countries.

Other materials that are used for retrograde fillings are the *reinforced zinc oxide–eugenol cements*, *Super EBA* and *IRM* (**Fig. 10.13**). Super EBA consists of 60% zinc oxide, 30% alumina, and 10% natural resin which is mixed with a liquid consisting of 37% eugenol and 63% orthoethoxybenzoic acid. IRM consists of 80% zinc oxide and 20% methyl methacrylate and is mixed with eugenol. These cements give a bacteria-tight seal of retrograde cavities. However, it was feared that they would deteriorate over time when left in contact with tissue and tissue fluids. This fear may seem to be mostly unfounded, in that long-term follow-up studies have shown the materials to hold up well for many years. *Cavit* (see p.167) gives a reliable retrograde seal as well, and again long-term follow-up studies suggest that this material also holds up over time when in contact with tissue. *Mineral trioxide aggregate* (MTA) is a material proposed for retrograde root filling. This material has been exposed to a variety of tests and seems promising.

Further Reading

Brodin P. Neurotoxic and analgesic effects of root canal cements and pulp protecting dental materials. Endod Dent Traumatol 1988;4:1–11.

Dorn SO, Gartner AH. Retrograde filling materials: a retrospective success-failure study of amalgam, EBA and IRM. J Endod 1990;16:391–393.

Lee YC, Yang SF, Hwang YF, Chuch LH, Chung KH. Microleakage of endodontic temporary restorative materials. J Endod 1993;19:516–520.

Leonard JE, Gutman JL, Guo IY. Apical and coronal seal of roots obturated with a dentine bonding agent and resin. Int Endod J 1996;29:76–83.

Leonardo MR, Silva LAB, Almeida WA, Utrilla LS. Tissue response to an epoxy resin-based root canal sealer. Endod Dent Traumatol 1999;15:28–32.

Ørstavik D, Mjör IA. Usage test of four endodontic sealers in Macaca fasicularis monkeys. Oral Surg Oral Med Oral Pathol 1992;73:337–344.

Peutzfeldt A, Asmussen E. Influence of eugenol-containing temporary cement on efficacy of dentin-bonding systems. Eur J Oral Sci 1999;107:63–69.

Pitt Ford TR, Andreasen JO, Dorn SO, Kariyawasam SP. Effect of various zinc oxide materials as root-end fillings on healing after replantation. Int Endod J 1995;28:273–278.

Schwartz RS. Adhesive dentistry and endodontics. Part 2: bonding in the root canal system – the promise and the problems: a review. J Endod 2006;32:1125–1134.

Seltzer S, Green DB, Weiner N, DeRenzis F. A scanning electron microscope examination of silver cones removed from endodontically treated teeth. Oral Surg Oral Med Oral Pathol 1972;33:589–605.

Shipper G, Ørstavik D, Teixeira FB, Trope M. An evaluation of microbial leakage in roots filled with a thermoplastic synthetic polymer-based root canal filling material (Resilon). J Endod 2004;30:342–347.

Spångberg L. Biological effects of root canal filling materials. The effect on bone tissue of two formaldehyde-containing root canal filling pastes. Oral Surg Oral Med Oral Pathol 1974;38:934–944.

Staehle HJ, Spiess V, Heinecke A, Mülle HP. Effect of root canal filling materials containing calcium hydroxide on the alkalinity of root dentin. Endod Dent Traumatol 1995;11:163–168.

Tay FR, Pashley DH. Monoblocks in root canals: a hypothetical or tangible goal. J Endod 2007;33:391–398.

Tronstad L, Barnett F, Flax M. Solubility and biocompatibility of calcium hydroxide-containing root canal sealers. Endod Dent Traumatol 1988;4:152–159.

Tronstad L, Trope M, Doering A, Hasselgren G. Sealing ability of dental amalgams as retrograde fillings in endodontic therapy. J Endod 1983;9:551–553.

Tronstad L, Wennberg A. In vitro assessment of the toxicity of filling materials. Int Endod J 1980;13:131–138.

Versiani MA, Carvalho-Junior JR, Padilha MI, Lacey S, Pascon EA, Sousa-Neto MD. A comparative study of physicochemical properties of AH Plus and Epiphany root canal sealants. Int Endod J 2006;39:464–471.

Wennberg A, Ørstavik D. Adhesion of root canal sealers to bovine dentine and gutta-percha. Int Endod J 1990;23:13–19.

11
Endodontic Techniques

Technically, endodontic treatment of teeth comprises three major phases that may be of equal importance for the outcome of the treatment. The three phases are:
— preparation for treatment,
— root canal instrumentation,
— root canal obturation.
In the last decade it has become common practice to use an operating microscope during the various phases of endodontic treatment. (**Fig.11.1**). The microscope offers magnification, but almost as important, it gives excellent light directly through the lenses into the access cavity. This gives the operator tremendous advantages, especially in difficult cases, and in straight root canals it is possible to observe the canal all the way to the apical foramen.

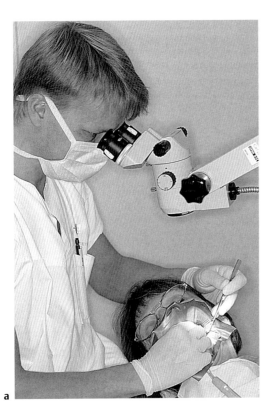

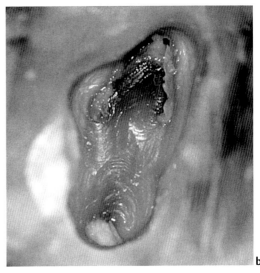

Fig. 11.1
a **Operating microscope in use during root canal instrumentation.**
b Pulp chamber floor of maxillary molar photographed through the microscope. A certain magnification and the direct light into the access cavity make it easier to locate and instrument the canals.

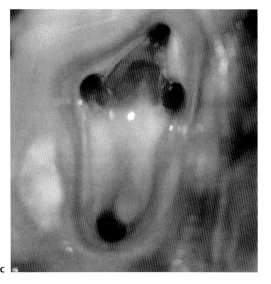

c

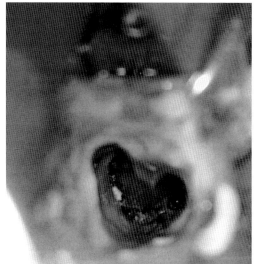

d

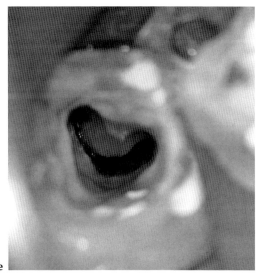

e

Fig. 11.1
c Four canals instrumented.
d Pulp chamber floor of tooth with apparent irregular root canal anatomy.
e During instrumentation it became evident that the tooth had a C-shaped canal that was effectively prepared with relative ease using the microscope.

Preparation for Treatment

Preparation for treatment entails the establishment of the root canal to be treated in an aseptic field of operation. It consists of the preparation of an adequate access cavity, the secure placement of a rubber dam, and disinfection of the rubber dam, the tooth, and the pulp chamber.

Access Cavity
The objective of the access cavity is to provide as unobstructed an access to the root canal(s) of the tooth as possible. When mishaps occur during the instrumentation and obturation phases of the treatment, they can most frequently be attributed to an inadequately or incorrectly prepared access cavity. The most common mistake is an access opening that has been made too small. As a result, canals are missed or the manipulation of the root

canal instruments is unnecessarily hindered by the cavity walls. Also, tissue may be left behind in the coronal pulp, especially in the pulp horns, leading to discoloration of the tooth. On the other hand, tooth structure should not be removed indiscriminately since that would lead to an unnecessary weakening of the tooth and would complicate the restorative procedures. The access cavity should expose the entire pulp chamber, including the pulp horns. In addition, cusps may have to be reduced to provide proper access to certain canals or to prevent uncontrolled fractures if they are weak.

Before the preparation of the access cavity begins, *a good radiograph* of the crown of the tooth, taken with a long-cone paralleling technique, is studied (**Fig. 11.2**). Especially the distance from an occlusal or incisal point of reference to the roof of the pulp chamber is noted. This distance may be marked on the bur to be used for the penetration of the crown to the pulp. Carious dentin is always removed, and fillings and restorations which might prevent a direct view to the root canals are removed as well. Also, *all undermined cusps are reduced at this time* in order to prevent crown-root fractures which might jeopardize the treatment of the tooth.

For the actual penetration to the pulp chamber, *a long-shank round carbide bur* is used in a low-torque ultraspeed handpiece. A long-shank bur is not necessarily used because of the distance to be penetrated, but more because it allows for better visibility and a better possibility of angling the

bur correctly in relation to the long axis of the tooth. Porcelain crowns are penetrated by standard-length, round, diamond-coated burs and the access cavity is then finished with the long-shank carbide bur. When the penetration to the pulp has been achieved, the roof of the pulp chamber is removed by pulling strokes with the bur from the chamber in an occlusal or incisal direction (**Fig. 11.3**). In this way the entire pulp chamber is exposed without overhangs of occlusal tooth substance and without danger of perforations laterally or in the furcation region. The coronal pulp tissue, vital or necrotic, is then removed. A round bur no. 2 may be used with advantage to ensure complete removal of tissue in the pulp horn areas of incisor teeth.

A *double-ended endodontic explorer* (DG-16) which offers two angles of probing is then used to locate the orifices of the root canals on the floor of the pulp chamber. The use of the explorer will also indicate whether the access cavity is adequate or whether, as is often the case, a cavity wall has to be flared more or a cusp be cut to improve the access to the canals. Often it will be evident clinically and radiographically that a root canal is calcified in the orifice area. The microscope is then extremely useful. Sometimes a rigid explorer may be used to penetrate the calcified material. Other times a long-shank bur is used to remove hard tis-

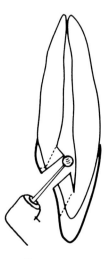

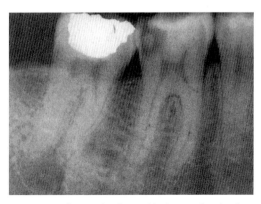

Fig. 11.2 Radiograph of mandibular teeth. The distance between the occlusal surface and the roof of the pulp chamber should be determined prior to the preparation of an endodontic access cavity.

Fig. 11.3 Diagram illustrating penetration of the pulp chamber with a bur. The roof of the pulp chamber is then carefully removed with outward pulling strokes of the bur.

sue to expose the canal. Since the exact location of the root canal is not always known, the bur is used with careful shaving motions in the orifice area. The explorer is used at frequent intervals in an effort to break through the calcified tissue. Exact placement of a 37% phosphoric acid gel for 60 seconds on the calcified orifice may be helpful as well. *The access cavity preparation is complete when the root canals have been located and are accessible for treatment.*

The access cavity is prepared prior to the application of a rubber dam to ensure maximal visibility of the teeth and the relationship between their crowns and roots. This will prevent root perforations and is especially important during the location of the root canal orifices. However, *all subsequent treatment is carried out aseptically with the use of a rubber dam.*

Rubber Dam

A rubber dam is placed on a tooth to be treated endodontically mainly for three reasons:

1) to obtain a field of operation that can be disinfected,
2) to protect the patient from accidentally aspirating or swallowing a root canal instrument, and
3) to protect the patient from the effect of irrigating solutions and other drugs during the treatment.

In addition, there are other advantages with the use of a rubber dam. It makes the treatment faster and, in many ways, less difficult in that it physically eliminates any interference from the oral environment.

Normally, only the tooth to be treated is exposed through a hole in the rubber dam (**Fig. 11.4**). A medium-weight dam will give a good seal around the tooth, usually without the use of a dental floss ligature. A wide variety of clamps are available to hold the rubber dam in place (**Fig. 11.5**), and the use of clamps with wings allows a rapid application of the rubber dam. A rubber dam frame of a radiolucent material that can be left in place during the taking of radiographs should be used (**Fig. 11.4**). The frame should also make it possible to *cover the nose of the patient* to prevent contamination of the field of operation by nasal microorganisms.

If the tooth to be treated is severely broken down, it may be practical to restore it temporarily before the root canal treatment begins. This is also

done to strengthen the tooth, but mainly to facilitate the placement of a well-sealing rubber dam. A quick and adequate method, if enough retention

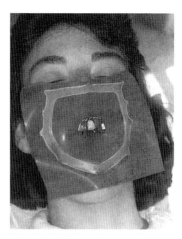

Fig. 11.4 Rubber dam applied to a maxillary central incisor for endodontic treatment. Only the tooth to be treated is exposed and the rubber dam is held in place by a clamp placed on this tooth and the use of a rubber dam frame. Note that the patients's nose is covered by the rubber dam. This is imperative in order to maintain a bacteria-free field of operation. (The frame is outside the rubber dam for demonstration purposes only.).

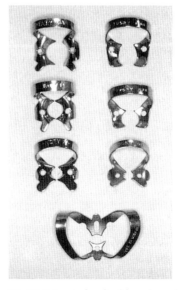

Fig. 11.5 Example of rubber dam clamps. A wide variety of clamps are available for most clinical situations.

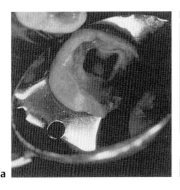
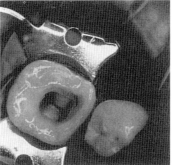

a

b

Fig. 11.6
a Deep mesial cavity making it difficult to obtain effective isolation of the tooth with a rubber dam.
b Cavity is acid-etched, and a mesial wall is fabricated by means of light-cured resin. A dry field of operation is now readily obtained.

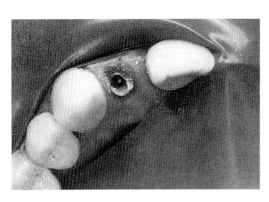

Fig. 11.7 Endodontic treatment of a severely broken down maxillary lateral incisor. The rubber dam is attached to neighboring teeth and although not ideal, protects the patient and helps establish a dry, clean field of operation. However, great care must be taken during the use of root canal irrigants and other medicaments in such situations.

is available, is to restore the tooth with a resin after acid-etching the remaining tooth structure (**Fig. 11.6**). In such instances the pulp chamber may be filled with tightly packed cotton pellets to prevent the resin from blocking the root canal orifices and to facilitate an easy recapitulation of the access cavity. In severely broken-down molar teeth, an orthodontic band may be useful to ensure asepsis. The band must fit snugly at the cemental–enamel junction and should be about 2 mm high to allow an adequate hold for the rubber dam clamp and easy access to the root canals. The floor of the chamber is again packed with hard cotton pellets and the band is filled with zinc oxiphosphate cement and cemented to the tooth. When the cement has set, the cotton pellets are removed, the access cavity is recapitulated, and the preparation is redefined as needed. If the

tooth is fractured at the gingiva, a slight gingivectomy, preferably using electrosurgical instruments to prevent bleeding, may make it possible to apply an adequate rubber dam. In such instances it is also possible to apply the rubber dam to teeth adjacent to the one to be treated (**Fig. 11.7**).

Special considerations in the preparation of access cavities in the various groups of teeth are discussed in Chapter 12.

When the rubber dam has been applied and the tooth to be treated is effectively sealed from the oral environment, *an aseptic field of operation* is established. The access cavity, the tooth, and the rubber dam are disinfected by effective surface-active agents, usually chlorhexidine or iodine preparations combined with hydrogen peroxide or ethanol.

Root Canal Instrumentation

At this time, the instruments used for the preparation of the access cavity and the application of the rubber dam are removed, and *a tray with sterile instruments to be used for the root canal instrumentation is made available* (**Fig. 11.8**).

Length determination. Regardless of technique used, step-back or crown down, hand instruments or motorized instruments, before the actual instrumentation begins the length of the root canal is determined. A small K-file, most often no. 15, is introduced into the canal to a level near the apex of the root and a radiograph is taken (**Fig. 11.9**). The apical level of instrumentation is determined based on the location of the tip of the file in relation to the apex of the root as seen in the radiograph. The length of instrumentation from an occlusal or incisal point of reference, i.e., the working length, is then calculated. *Please note that it is the apex of the root that most often serves as the radiographic landmark and not the apical foramen or apical constriction.* The reason for this is that the apex of the root is almost always distinguishable in a radiograph, whereas the foramen rarely is. Obviously, in the few instances when the apical foramen is actually seen radiographically, it should be used to determine the working length.

Electronic devices are available to determine the location of the apical foramen of teeth. The use of these so-called *electronic apex locators* is based on the hypothesis that the electrical resistance between the periodontal ligament and the oral mucosa is virtually constant. The instrument is calibrated by measuring the resistance between the gingival crevice and the lip. An endodontic instrument attached to the crevice electrode is then inserted into the root canal until the same electrical resistance is registered. It is then assumed that the tip of the instrument has reached the periodontal ligament at the apical foramen.

With clinical practice the electronic apex locator may become a valuable aid in routine endodontics, but even more so in special clinical situations when the radiographic image of the root apices is unclear, when there is suspicion of a root perforation or root fracture, when radiographs are contraindicated, etc. In addition, the instrument offers an excellent opportunity for quick and, if needed, frequent checks on whether the correct working length is actually maintained during the instrumentation phase of the treatment. The electronic apex locator has a definite place in modern endodontic therapy.

Extirpation of the pulp.   When the working length has been established, the pulp of vital teeth is removed. A K-type instrument with as large a diam-

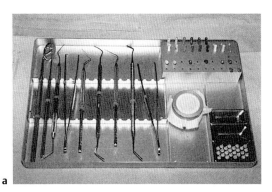

a

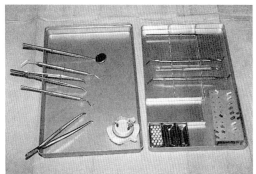

b

Fig. 11.8

a Practical endodontic tray. It contains hand instruments needed during the aseptic phase of the treatment as well as a holder with root canal instruments. The hand instruments: mirror, explorer, pair of pliers, endodontic explorer (DG16), periodontal probe, root canal spreader (D11), spoon excavator (31 L), plastic instrument (Glick no. 1),

curved, heavy anatomical pliers. The root canal instruments: K-files (size 15 – 80), Hedstrom files (size 15, 20, 30, 40, and 50), finger spreaders (size B and D).

b The lid of the tray is used as a work surface. The tray itself should remain sterile throughout the treatment. The anatomical pliers are used to move instruments from the tray to the lid.

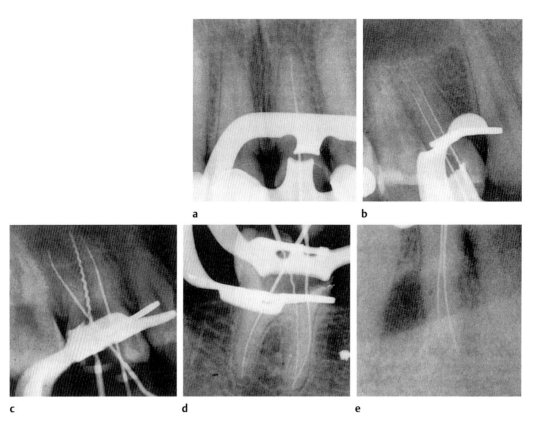

a   b

c   d   e

Fig. 11.9 a–e Radiograph to determine the tooth length of various types of teeth. In multirooted teeth and especially in roots with more than one canal it is advantageous to use different types of root canal instruments to readily determine which canal is

which. In these radiographs, Hedstrom files are consistently used in palatal and lingual canals and K-files in buccal canals. Roots with more than one canal must be exposed at an angle (usually about 15°) to separate the canals in the radiographs.

eter as possible is introduced into the canal *to the predetermined apical level of instrumentation*. The instrument is then rotated as much as possible in contact with the root canal wall in an effort *to sever the pulp at this level*. If this is successful, the pulp may come out in one piece and a pulp stump with a clean-cut wound is left behind in the root canal (**Fig. 11.10**). If it is not successful, the pulp tissue will instead be removed in bits and pieces during the subsequent instrumentation of the canal.

In nonvital teeth with ischemic necrosis, the pulp may be extirpated using the same method. However, in teeth with liquefaction necrosis of the pulp, there is usually so little tissue left in the root canal that an extirpation as such is not feasible. Rather, the tissue remnants will be removed during chemomechanical instrumentation.

Chemomechanical instrumentation. *The principles and goals of the instrumentation phase of endodontic treatment are the same regardless of instruments or technique used* (see Chapters 5 and 6). However, the actual preparation of the canal may vary, depending on, among other things, the preferred obturation technique.

Step-Back Preparation

With the step-back technique, the diameter of the root canal at the apical level of instrumentation is kept as small as possible to resist extrusion of filling material beyond the canal. In addition, the apical part of the canal is given a *moderately tapered form* in an attempt to retain the obturating materials within the canal. Further coronally, the canal is flared as much as necessary according to the anatomy of the canal and to facilitate the obturation of the canal. The flare of the canal is especially pronounced with the use of thermoplasticized gutta-percha obturation techniques which require the insertion of rather large and rigid instruments to the apical region of the canal (see p. 191).

The degree of instrumentation most apically in the root canal is determined by the size of the first K-file that binds in the canal at the apical level of instrumentation. The canal is then enlarged an additional two instrument sizes at this level. This means that if a no. 15 file binds, the canal is enlarged to a size 25. The last file used most apically, in this instance no. 25, is called the *master apical file*. The apical taper is then accomplished by a step-back use of instruments of increasing sizes (**Fig. 11.11**). *Between each change of file, the full length of the canal is recapitulated with the master apical file.* Further coronally, the canal is then flared with hand or engine-driven instruments to give it the desired continuous tapered shape.

The step-back technique can be used in all teeth. However, if the root canal is wide apically so that little natural resistance is offered, a more definite shelf may have to be prepared in the canal wall to help prevent overfilling during the obturation phase. Also, when the step-back technique is used, it must be remembered that *the root canal in many teeth is considerably wider in a buccolingual than in a mesiodistal direction*. The first instrument that binds will do so in the narrowest part of the canal, and an enlargement of two to three instrument sizes, which most often will mean 0.10–0.15 mm, may not be enough to reach the walls at the widest part of the canal. Thus, *tissue commonly is left behind apically with the step-back technique*, especially on the lingual aspect of the root canal wall (**Fig. 11.12**).

Apical Box Preparation

An important result of morphometric studies of the root canals of human teeth is that apically the canals may be wider than assumed and should be enlarged more than has commonly been done—in some groups of teeth, like the incisors, considerably more (see Chapter 12). The *apical box preparation technique* was developed with this information in mind. With this technique, one attempts to give the apical 2–5 mm of the root canal a *cylindrical shape* rather than the tapered shape of the step-back technique (**Fig. 11.13**). In this way

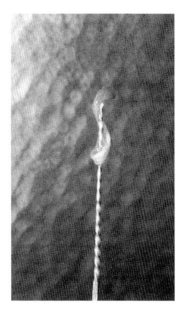

Fig. 11.10 Pulpectomy. The pulp has been severed in the apical area of the root canal by means of a reamer and is removed in one piece.

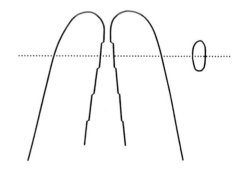

Fig. 11.11 Diagram illustrating the step-back preparation of a root canal. A moderately tapered form of the apical end of the root canal is obtained by a step-back use of instruments of increasing size. No attempt is made to obtain a circular shape of the canal, which usually remains wider in a buccolingual direction than in a mesiodistal direction.

it is hoped one can obtain clean walls consistently in the important apical part of the root canal. K-type instruments are used with filing and rotary cutting actions, stainless steel files sizes 08–20, and nickel-titanium files sizes 25 and up. Further coronally, the canal is flared to a continuous taper with Hedstrom files or engine-driven instruments as with the step-back technique.

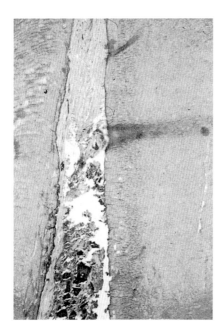

Fig. 11.12 Buccolingual longitudinal section of the apical area of the root canal of a pulpectomized tooth instrumented with the step-back technique. The pulp has been nicely severed, but since the root canal is wider buccolingually than mesiodistally, the buccal and lingual walls are not well instrumented and pulp tissue is left behind on the lingual wall (hematoxylin-eosin).

The apical part of the root canal is opened up with a K-file used with filing motions until the file moves freely in the canal. The file is then rotated with its tip at the exact working length to begin making a shelf in the root canal wall. The next size file is introduced into the canal with twiddling motions until the tip is again *at the exact apical level of instrumentation.* The instrument is then carefully rotated or, if necessary, used with filing strokes first until it can safely be rotated at the desired apical level. The preparation of the apical part of the canal continues systematically with filing and reaming actions until the canal is enlarged two to three instrument sizes. The canal is then flared, beginning with a Hedstrom or engine-driven file *one size smaller* than the last instrument used apically. The patency of the apical part of the canal is checked at regular intervals during the flaring of the coronal part of the canal.

When the flare is considered adequate, the preparation of the apical part of the canal is completed with K-type hand or engine-driven instruments, again mainly with rotary cutting actions. *In this way, a shelf is prepared in the root canal wall at the apical-most level of instrumentation* (**Fig. 11.13**). However, due to the noncutting tip of modern root canal instruments, the apical shelf will not be abrupt, but rather have a sloping form (**Fig. 6.11**). Still, *the shelf constitutes an effective*

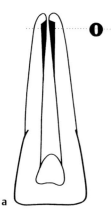
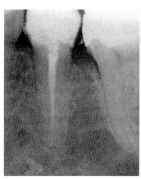
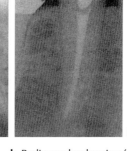

Fig. 11.13
a Diagram illustrating differences in the shape of an apical root canal after step-back and apical box preparation. With the apical box preparation technique, an attempt is made to give the apical root canal a circular shape.

b Radiographs showing (left) a mandibular premolar with step-back preparation and (right) the contralateral tooth with apical box preparation of the root (final reamer no. 70). Note that the two methods differ only in the preparation of the apical part of the canal. The enlargement and flare of the canals further coronally are similar.

apical stop against which a master gutta-percha point of the same size as the final apical instrument can be seated. Also, since the final apical instrumentation is carried out with rotary cutting actions, the apical part of the root canal will, if at all possible, have taken on the shape of a cylindrical box.

The *degree of apical enlargement* is determined by the size, shape, and form of the root of the tooth as seen in preoperative radiographs. However, *since root canals often are widest in the buccolingual direction, which normally cannot be evaluated in radiographs, information on the size and shape of the root canals in the various groups of teeth is utilized as well* (see Chapter 12).

The preparation of a cylindrical apical box with a sufficient diameter can be accomplished with great regularity in all groups of teeth (see Chapter 12). Theoretically, the technique presents the greatest problems in teeth with thin oval roots because in such roots the canal is usually ribbon-shaped. However, studies have shown that ribbon-shaped canals become more circular near the apex of the root, so that at least the apical 1–2 mm of the canal may usually be given a cylindrical shape, even in such teeth. Traditionally, it might also have been difficult to attain a cylindrical box apically in teeth with severely curved roots. However, with the availability of the flexible nickel-titanium instruments, this is not a serious problem at present.

Crown Down Preparation

With the *crown down preparation technique* the root canal is instrumented in the direction from the canal orifice to the apical foramen with progressively smaller instruments. In other words, this technique works contrary to traditional techniques in which the instrumentation in principle starts apically and is carried out with progressively larger instruments in a coronal direction. The crown down technique has never had a large following, among other things because the root canal often became blocked by dentin chips and other instrumentation debris as the instrumentation proceeded in an apical direction. However, with the availability of engine-driven nickel-titanium instruments this suddenly changed and when these instruments are used, crown down preparation of the root canal is nearly a must.

Root canal instrumentation with engine-driven nickel-titanium instruments. The engine-driven nickel-titanium instruments are in reality *drills* that remove root dentin on their way into the root canal and not as they are removed from the canal. This is the main reason why it is practical to begin the instrumentation at the canal orifice and proceed in an apical direction when using these instruments.

To minimize the working torque of the continuous rotating instruments, they should be designed so that they do not prepare the root canal in its entire length, but only a fourth or a third of the canal at a time. (**Fig. 11.14**). This is achieved by using a sequence of instruments with varying tapers and sizes (see p. 163). Thus, the first instrument to be used may be 19 mm long, size 40, with an 0.10 mm taper. This instrument opens up the orifice of the canal, removes dentin overhangs and flares the coronal 2–3 mm of the canal. The second instrument may be 19 mm as well, size 35, and with a 0.08 mm taper. This instrument will penetrate an additional 2–4 mm into the canal. The third instrument should be 25 mm long, size 30, with a 0.06 taper. Depending on the root canal anatomy, this instrument may reach the apical level of instrumentation, or it may stop 1–3 mm from the final level. A fourth instrument 25 mm long, size 25, with a 0.04 or 0.02 mm taper is then used. This instrument will reach the working length. A canal with a continuous taper has now been obtained. An apical box may then be prepared using instruments with taper 0.02 mm and sizes 30 and up as needed

The engine-driven rotary nickel-titanium instruments are used with a light hand and according to the *woodpecker method*, i.e., with a pecking motion removing a little at a time. Each instrument should only be used as long as it moves forward. When the resistance is such that the instrument no longer advances, it should immediately be removed from the canal and the instrumentation should continue with the next file in the sequence. In other words, *these instruments must not be used stationary in the canal and they must not be forced in an apical direction.* A saying goes that "each instrument should only take what the canal will give." When used this way, the root canal is instrumented quickly and with a high degree of safety using engine-driven instruments. However, cyclic fatigue is a factor and the instruments wear with use. Thus, after five to seven

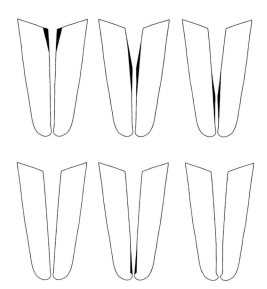

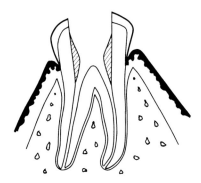

Fig.11.15 Diagram showing the elimination of the cervical curve of a root canal by removing the overlying coronal dentin. This greatly facilitates the instrumentation around an apical curve of the canal.

Fig. 11.14 Diagram indicating crown down preparation of the root canal as performed with engine-driven nickel-titanium instruments. In order to reduce working torque and instrument breakage, only part of the canal is instrumented at a time, beginning at the canal orifice and proceeding in an apical direction.

cases an instrument should be discarded even though it might still look good.

Instrumentation of Curved Root Canals

The guidelines for root canal instrumentation as outlined are valid for curved canals as well. However, there are certain special rules to follow in order to avoid operational mishaps due to added technical difficulties in such canals.

A root canal may be curved both coronally (cervically) and apically. Regardless of instruments or technique used, it is then important to eliminate one of the curves, i.e., the curve in the cervical area, before the actual instrumentation of the canal begins (**Fig.11.15**). This greatly reduces the stress on the root canal instruments and improves the safety of curved canal instrumentation. With straight line access and the use of *flexible nickel-titanium instruments*, the apical curve can be instrumented effectively and safely. With rounded, noncutting tips the nickel-titanium instruments follow the original canal space and work centered in the canal even when the canal is curved. The instruments are used with filing and combined filing–reaming motions with the under-

standing that working around a curve is a severe strain on the instruments. The instrumentation should therefore be carried out with special care and gentleness and even severely curved roots may then be successfully prepared.

The engine-driven rotary nickel-titanium instruments work well in curved canals and may be used using the technique described above in these canals too (**Fig.11.16**). Only be aware of the fact that the working torque when using these instruments increases with increasing taper of the instruments. Thus, instruments with taper 0.02 mm may be used with advantage in severe cases. An instrument used in a severely curved part of the canal should be discarded and not used again.

Stainless steel instruments are rigid and above certain sizes will not follow the original root canal space when used in curved canals. Steel instruments, therefore, have to be *precurved* so that they match the curve of the canal. With careful use of precurved steel instruments, curved canals may be successfully instrumented (**Fig.11.16**). However, mishaps are not uncommon. Because of the rigidity of the instruments, the inner side of the curve may be straightened until the root is perforated or stripped. The strip perforation in theory may be avoided by so-called outer curve filing, i.e., the precurved files are manipulated by bending the handle so that their effect is mainly on the outer curve of the canal. This is especially important in mesial roots of lower molars where the dentin toward the furcation and interradicular area that forms the inner curve of the canal may be as thin as 0.2 mm. Also, if the instruments are

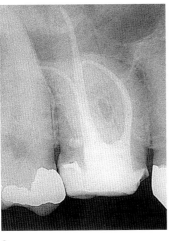

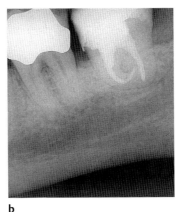

b

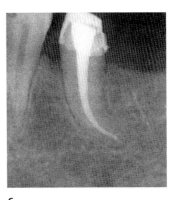

c

a

Fig 11.16

a Radiograph of maxillary molar with severely curved buccal roots. Since the curves are not sharp (large radius), the root canals can be instrumented with the flexible engine-driven nickel-titanium instruments in a routine fashion.

b Mandibular molar with severely curved mesial root. Although the curve is very sharp (small radius), the root canal was instrumented with engine-driven nickel-titanium instruments (apical box size 35). However, in this type of canal, great care must be taken to reduce the working torque and to work centered in the canal (0.02 mm tapered instruments; reduced speed; frequent change of instruments).

c Radiograph of a mandibular premolar with a curved root. The root canal has been prepared with an apical box and final *steel* reamer no. 70.

not meticulously precurved to match the curvature of the canal, the apical part of the canal may be straightened and transported away from the original canal space, or the root may be perforated in this area (**Figs. 13.5**, **13.6**, **13.7**). Preferably steel instruments should not be used in curved root canals.

Numerous techniques have been developed to obturate the root canal bacteria-tight. The most commonly used techniques are discussed below.

Root Canal Obturation with Silver Points

Silver points are used in combination with a sealer to fill the root canal. The silver points are available in standardized sizes, which makes point selection easier than before. Still, the points are completely incompressible and may readily bind in the canal to give an incorrect clinical feel of a good apical fit. Thus, if *silver points are used, the root canal should always be prepared with a cylindrical apical box.*

When an acceptable fit is established clinically and radiographically, the silver point is marked at the level of an occlusal or incisal reference point, usually a cusp or the incisal edge of the tooth. The point is then removed and sealer is applied to the canal walls by means of a hand-held lentulo, a paper point, or the like, and the silver point is slowly reintroduced into the canal to the predetermined level. During the insertion, the point acts as a piston to press the sealing material in an apical and lateral direction.

By these relatively simple procedures, a good three-dimensional filling and seal of the root canal are achieved, provided that the sealer used has acceptable dimensional stability (**Fig. 11.17**). However, *as the sealer breaks down under the influence of tissue fluids, the silver point will become exposed to the tissue fluids and corrosion will occur* (**Fig. 10.6**). Also, dissolution of the sealer may result in leakage, reinfection of the root canal, and often a direct oral–apical communication through the

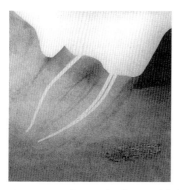

Fig.11.17 Radiograph of a mandibular molar with silver point root canal fillings at the 5-year control. Normal periapical conditions are seen.

canal. It may take a considerable amount of time for the sealing material to break down if the silver point was well adapted. Failures of silver point-treated teeth, therefore, are often seen several years after the endodontic treatment is completed (**Fig.11.18**).

The use of the silver point technique is becoming less and less accepted throughout the world. It is described here because of its considerable traditional importance.

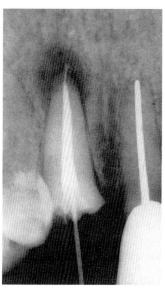

a

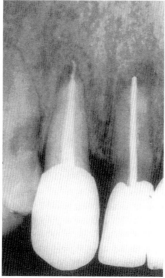

b

Fig. 11.18
a Radiograph of a maxillary lateral incisor 8 years following root canal filling with the silver point technique. The periapical conditions are normal.
b Three years later, i. e., 11 years following obturation of the root canal, apical root resorption and an apical radiolucency are observed.

Root Canal Obturation with Gutta-Percha Points

Gutta-percha points are used to fill the root canal in various ways and with different techniques. The most important techniques are the dipping technique, the thermoplasticized gutta-percha techniques, the lateral condensation technique, and the standardized technique. In addition, a combination of two or more of these techniques is used advantageously in many clinical situations.

The Dipping Technique
The dipping technique is based on gutta-percha's property of becoming soft when dipped in chloroform, eucalyptol, or other organic solvents. When softened and forced into the root canal, a gutta-percha point may be given the exact three-dimensional form of the root canal space. Unfortunately, the dipping technique has been advocated by some for use without a sealer. This is a misconception, probably due to the fact that the surface of a gutta-percha point has a certain stickiness in the

softened condition. However, as stressed above (see p.169), gutta-percha alone cannot seal the root canal. When the solvent has evaporated, the point loses its stickiness and gaps will develop between the point and the root canal wall. Thus, *the use of a sealer is mandatory with all gutta-percha techniques.* Traditionally, the dipping technique has been used with resin-based chloropercha-like sealers like Kloroperka N-O or simply resin chloroform. However, all types of sealers may be used.

With the dipping technique the root canal should be prepared so that it either has a continuous tapered preparation or it should have a definite apical shelf in the root canal wall (apical box preparation). A master point is then selected which is two to three sizes larger in diameter than the final apical instrument, and the point should stop in the canal 2–3 mm short of the working length. This is checked radiographically and the master point is marked in this position at the level of an occlusal or incisal reference point. A second mark is used to indicate the distance the point has to be introduced further into the canal to reach the apical level of instrumentation.

The master point is then removed and a sealer is applied sparingly to the walls of the root canal. Subsequently, the master point is dipped in chloroform for about 5–10 seconds, depending on the size of the point. It is quickly reintroduced into the canal and firmly pushed in an apical direction until the second mark is at the occlusal point of reference, indicating that the gutta-per-

cha point has reached the correct apical level. Since the gutta-percha is soft, the master point will now have taken on the three-dimensional shape of the root canal apically, and this part of the canal will be sealed. In the wider coronal parts of the canal, accessory points dipped in sealer are inserted next to the master point, and by lateral condensation the canal is filled completely with gutta-percha. If the condensation is successful, a homogenous and bacteria-tight obturation of the root canal is achieved (**Fig. 11.19**).

The dipping technique is basically simple and straightforward. However, as with all soft gutta-percha techniques, overfilling of the canal will occur, especially if the master point is softened too much. In addition, there may be problems with shrinkage of gutta-percha when the material has been softened in chloroform (**Fig. 11.20**).

Thermoplasticized Gutta-Percha Techniques

These techniques use *heat-softened gutta-percha* and, as with the dipping technique, *the goal is to achieve a bacteria-tight, three-dimensional filling of the root canal by softening the gutta-percha.*

The warm gutta-percha technique. With this technique, the gutta-percha is heated inside the root canal by means of hot hand instruments, so-called *heat carriers.* The root canal is given a continuous tapered shape, although the coronal parts of the canal are widened somewhat more than is the case with most techniques in order to facili-

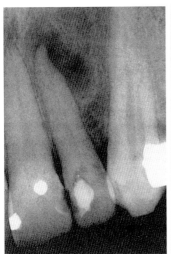
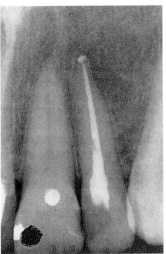

Fig. 11.19
a **Radiograph of a nonvital maxillary lateral incisor with apical periodontitis.**
b Resolution of the periapical lesion is evident at the 2-year control. The root canal was obturated with the dipping technique. The slight overfilling of the canal is not an uncommon occurrence with this technique.

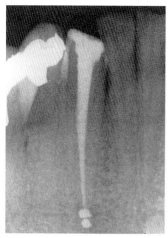
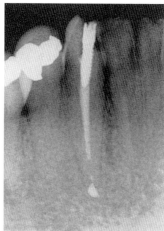

a
b

Fig.11.20
a Radiograph of a mandibular canine with the root canal obturated by means of the dipping technique.
b At the 6-month control, the gutta-percha in the apical area of the root canal as well as part of the overfilling have disappeared, in all likelihood because of excessive softening of the material in chloroform.

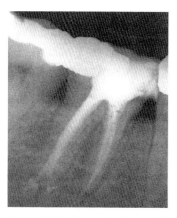

Fig. 11.21 Radiograph of a mandibular molar with root canals obturated with the warm gutta-percha technique. The wide preparation as seen in the distal canal may be necessary to facilitate the use of root canal pluggers in the apical area. Note the filling of the apical accessory canal and the slight overfilling which are commonly seen with this technique.

tate the use of the rather large and rigid instruments required for the heating and condensation of the gutta-percha. Because of its greater flare, a nonstandardized (accessory) point is used as the master point. The pointed tip is cut off so that the point stops in the canal about 2–3 mm short of the working length. The master point is removed and a sealer is applied to the root canal wall. The use of a zinc oxide–eugenol-based sealer is recommended. The master point is then reintroduced into the canal and seared off at the canal orifice with a hot plastic instrument, and a cold root ca-

nal plugger is used to condense the warm gutta-percha at the orifice of the canal in an apical direction. A heat carrier is then heated with a gas flame until it is red hot and is introduced 3–4 mm into the gutta-percha in the canal and quickly withdrawn. The warm gutta-percha is again condensed in an apical direction by means of cold root canal pluggers. This procedure is repeated to a level 5–6 mm short of the working length when it is assumed that the apical part of the canal is filled three-dimensionally with gutta-percha.

Since the root canal is sealed coronally during the vertical condensation of the gutta-percha, considerable apical and lateral hydraulic forces are generated. As a result, the root canal sealer is often seen to be forced into lateral and accessory root canals when this technique is used (**Fig.11.21**). If a root canal post is required, the obturation of the canal is considered completed when the apical 5–6 mm are filled. If not, additional sealer is applied to the wall of the coronal part of the canal and pieces of gutta-percha, 3–4 mm long, are heated and condensed vertically in the canal until the entire space is filled.

The warm gutta-percha technique is an ambitious technique. Its advantage is meant to be that *the root canal system with lateral and accessory canals* is more completely obturated when using this technique than with other more traditional techniques. Since the technique requires vertical condensation of softened gutta-percha, it is rather difficult to control and, as with the dipping technique, overfillings of the root canal are commonly seen. No long-term follow-up studies of the re-

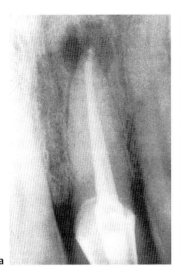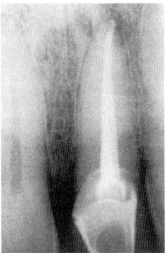

a   b

Fig. 11.22
a Radiograph of a maxillary incisor with the root canal obturated with the injection-molded gutta-percha technique. A slight extrusion of gutta-percha is seen in spite of apical box preparation of the root canal.
b Periapical repair is evident.

sults obtained with the warm gutta-percha technique have been published.

The injection-molded gutta-percha technique. With this technique, the gutta-percha is heated outside the mouth until it flows (about 160 °C) and by means of a pressure syringe is injected into the root canal after a sealer has been applied to the root canal wall. The injection needle has to be brought as close to the apical level of instrumentation as possible, and at least to the apical third of the canal. By slowly pulling the needle back while the gutta-percha is being injected, the entire root canal can be filled virtually in seconds (**Fig. 11.22**).

Obviously, shrinkage of the gutta-percha occurs when the material is heated to such temperatures. To counteract the shrinkage as much as possible, only 2–3 mm of the canal should be filled at a time. A continuous condensation force is then exerted on the gutta-percha during the cooling of the material, which takes about 2 minutes. A new portion of soft gutta-percha is then added and again it is held under pressure until cooled. In this way the entire root canal is filled step by step.

This is, again, a method dealing with softened gutta-percha being vertically condensed in the root canal. The method is difficult to control and both overfilled and incompletely filled canals occur regularly (**Fig. 11.23**). For this reason, the method is also used with an unsoftened master gutta-percha point, which, when placed in the

root canal, will block the apical opening of the canal. Injection-molded gutta-percha is then used to fill those parts of the canal that are traditionally filled by accessory points and lateral condensation. Moreover, the injection technique has shown some promise in the obturation of blunderbuss canals of immature teeth after an apical mineralized barrier has been created by means of long-term calcium hydroxide treatment (see p. 120). On the whole, the suitability of the injection-molded

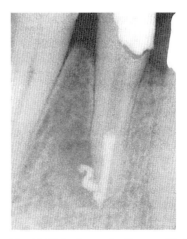

Fig. 11.23 Radiograph of a mandibular premolar with the root canal obturated with the injection-molded gutta-percha technique. The method is difficult to control, and without a good apical stop, severe extrusion of material readily occurs.

gutta-percha technique greatly depends on whether the foraminal area of the root canal is plugged or not prior to the actual filling of the canal. No data on long-term results with this technique are available.

Thermomechanical condensation techniques. Efforts have been made to soften gutta-percha inside the root canal by friction heat from rotary or vibratory instruments. Functioning systems have been developed and are commercially available. However, these systems are all technique-sensitive and difficult to control. In addition, frequent fractures of the instruments in the canal appear to be a problem. At this time it is difficult to foresee a breakthrough in obturation technique in this area.

Lateral Condensation Technique

The purpose of the lateral condensation technique is to fill the root canal three-dimensionally and bacteria-tight with gutta-percha and a sealer *without softening the gutta-percha with chemicals or heat*. In this way, the conceivable problems with shrinkage of softened gutta-percha are prevented, as are many of the difficulties of controlling the apical level of the root canal filling. The root canal is prepared with a continuous taper. A master gutta-percha point of the same size as the master apical file is selected and placed in the canal to the working length. The placement of the master point is controlled radiographically, and necessary adjustments are made. The master point is then marked at the level of an occlusal or incisal reference point and is removed from the canal. A sealer is applied sparingly to the canal wall or the master point is coated with the sealer before being reinserted into the canal to the correct apical level *without being softened*. A spreader, for example, a finger spreader no. B, is then introduced into the canal, ideally to the level of or near the apical end of the master point. The spreader is carefully moved back and forth to create space for an accessory gutta-percha point. In the process, the master point is forced laterally against the root canal wall and is deformed to match the shape of the root canal, hence the term "lateral condensation" of gutta-percha. An accessory point is selected to fit into the space made by the spreader. The spreader is then removed, the accessory point is dipped in sealer and quickly introduced into the canal to the level of the tip of the spreader, and importantly, *without being softened*. The spreader is used again in the same fashion, this time to the same level or to a level slightly coronally to the tip of the first accessory point, and a second point is coated with sealer and inserted. This sequence is repeated until the apical part of the root canal is filled three-dimensionally with gutta-percha. In the coronal flared part of the canal, larger spreaders and larger accessory points may be used to speed up the obturation procedure until the canal is completely filled with gutta-percha. *And importantly, since the material was not softened, the root canal filling will be dimensionally stable* (**Fig. 11.24**).

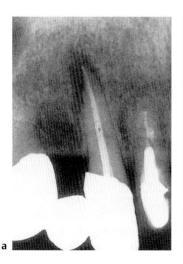 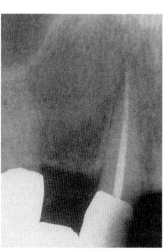

Fig. 11.24
a Radiograph of a maxillary canine with apical periodontitis treated with the step-back/lateral condensation technique.
b At the 5-year control, there is resolution of the periapical lesion and the root canal filling is dimensionally stable.

a

b

This is an excellent technique when mastered. However, lateral condensation of gutta-percha in the apical part of the root canal is far from an easy procedure. In order to obtain a three-dimensional filling of the apical area of the canal with gutta-percha, the unsoftened points have to be deformed and given the shape of the canal by effective use of the spreader. This is difficult and the apical part of the canal may be filled mostly with sealer if the technique of lateral condensation is not fully mastered. Then, gradually as the sealer dissolves under the influence of tissue fluids, the obturation of the canal may be incomplete. Because of this, attempts have been made to improve upon the technique by using electrically heated spreaders during the lateral condensation. The gutta-percha is then softened by the heat and the immediate fill of the canal may be improved. However, as discussed above, heated and softened gutta-percha is bound to shrink and the long-term seal of the canal may be affected by the shrinkage.

Standardized Endodontic Technique

The standardized technique was made possible through the development of the standardized root canal instruments and the standardized gutta-percha points. It is based on morphometric studies of the roots and root canals of human teeth and the findings that a cylindrical apical box may be prepared in the canal of most teeth in all groups of teeth. An *unsoftened gutta-percha master point* of the same size as the diameter of the apical box will then fit in the apical part of the canal, in principle like a cork in a bottle (**Fig. 11.25**).

In developing this technique, the fact has been taken into account that other possibly more ambitious techniques may suffer from shrinkage of the gutta-percha or will often be single-point techniques without an optimal matching of the gutta-percha point to the shape and size of the apical part of the root canal. With the standardized technique, the principle of a single point plus sealer obturating the apical part of the root canal has been accepted, and the challenge of the technique then is to prepare the canal so that this becomes feasible and will give long-term results that are at least as good as or better than other accepted techniques.

The root canal is prepared according to the apical box technique (**Figs. 11.13**, **11.25**). A standardized gutta-percha master point is then selected which is of the same size as the final instrument used with a rotary cutting action in the preparation of the apical box of the root canal. It should

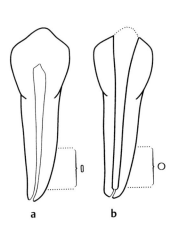
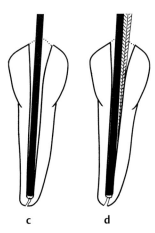

Fig. 11.25 Diagram illustrating technical principles of endodontic treatment with the standardized technique.

a Tooth with a root canal, usually with an oval shape in the apical area.

b Apical area of the canal prepared to take on a circular shape (apical box preparation).

c Unsoftened gutta-percha master point with the same diameter and form as the last-used reamer introduced into canal. The master point should fit apically like a cork in a bottle.

d Apical area of the canal sealed by the master point plus sealer. Further coronally, additional accessory gutta-percha points are used to complete the obturation of the flared part of the canal.

be remembered that the standardization of the gutta-percha points is less accurate than the standardization of the metallic instruments so that a few points may have to be tried before one is found that can be seated at the correct apical level of instrumentation, giving the desired resistance to dislodgment which is commonly referred to as tug back. The final placement of the master point is controlled radiographically (**Fig. 11.26**),

and necessary adjustments based on the radiographic findings may be made at this point. When the fit and placement are found to be right, the master point is marked at an occlusal or incisal point of reference and is removed. A sealer is then placed sparingly on the root canal wall or the master point is coated with the sealer. The master point is then reinserted into the canal to the working length *without being softened*. If the point does

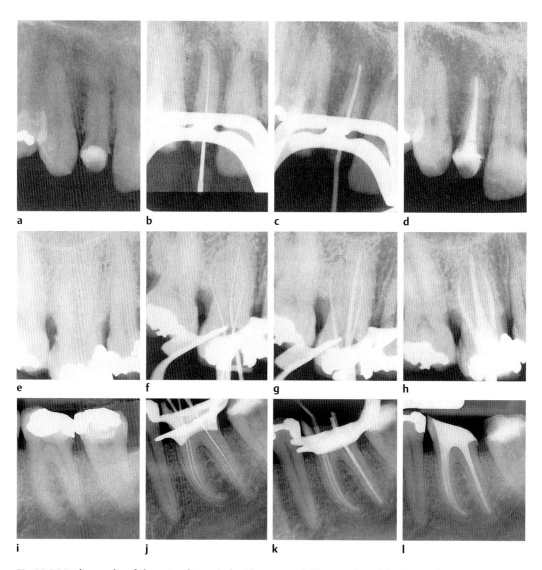

Fig. 11.26 Radiographs of three teeth treated with the standardized technique.
a, e, i Preoperative radiographs.
b, f, j Tooth length radiographs.

c, g, k Master point trial radiographs.
d, h, l Postoperative radiographs. Note the degree of apical enlargement in the various roots as well as the excellent technical control of the method.

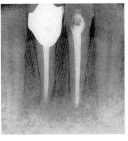
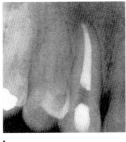
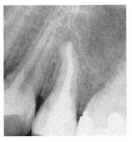
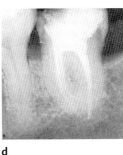

a   b   c   d

Fig.11.27 Radiographs of teeth treated with the standardized technique.
a Mandibular incisors with narrow roots and wide root canals (apical box size 70).
b Maxillary canine with a curved, wide root canal (apical box size 80).

c Maxillary premolar with S-shaped root and wide root canal (apical box size 90).
d Mandibular molar with a severely curved mesial root (apical boxes size 35).

not reach the desired apical level, it is removed from the canal and a K-type instrument of the same size as the master point is used to clear the root canal, most often from dentin chips that may have become dislodged during application of the sealer. *Please note that when appliyng this technique the final position of the master point in the root canal should not be affected by subsequent vertical or lateral condensation. It must, therefore, be placed exactly in its correct position before accessory points are inserted and condensed in the flared part of the canal.*

When satisfied that the master point is optimally placed, a spreader is introduced alongside the master point to determine the apical level to which the first accessory point should reach. The flared part of the canal is then filled with accessory gutta-percha points dipped in sealer, and since the apical seal is provided by the master point a much less agressive lateral condensation than described for the lateral condensation technique is required (**Figs. 11.25, 11.26**).

An *important advantage* of the standardized technique is the systematization offered by a standardized instrumentation and obturation system. The technique is easy to comprehend and especially the obturation phase is simple compared to most other methods. *Overfilling rarely occurs and long-term follow-up studies show that the root canal fillings remain dimensionally stable.*

Possible drawbacks of the standardized technique are related to the instrumentation phase of the treatment in that the apical part of the root ca-

nal is prepared wider than is commonly seen with other techniques in order to ensure a clean canal and to obtain the desired cylindrical apical box. Canals which may create problems for the standardized technique are especially found in mandibular incisors, maxillary first premolars, and maxillary lateral incisors. Still, with a proper understanding of root canal anatomy, the standardized technique will be an effective and safe method even in these teeth (**Fig. 11.27**). Excellent long-term results in all groups of teeth are reported with the standardized technique.

Two-Step and Other Techniques

Occasionally during endodontic treatment there will be teeth with special problems where the routine methods have to be modified. In some instances, such as in teeth where the root canal divides into two canals in the middle or apical third of the root or in teeth with internal resorption, *a technique in which the tooth is filled in two steps may be practical* (**Fig. 11.28**).

In teeth where the canal divides, both canals are prepared according to the technique used. Thereafter one of the canals is obturated. When this is completed, a heated root canal instrument is brought to the level where the root canal divides and the gutta-percha is removed coronally to this level. The second apical canal and the main canal are then filled in the customary way.

Similarly, *in teeth with internal resorption* the root canal apical to the resorption defect is filled first with the routine technique used (**Fig. 11.29**).

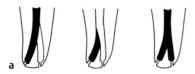

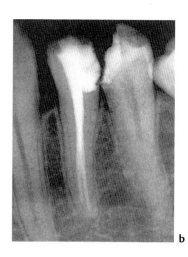

Fig. 11.28

a Diagram illustrating the obturation of a root canal in which the apical half of the root is split. If the main canal is not wide enough for both apical canals to be filled simultaneously, one canal is filled first. The gutta-percha is then burned away with a hot root canal instrument at the level where the canal divides. Then the main canal and the second apical canal are filled.

b Radiograph of an endodontically treated mandibular premolar in which the root canal divides in the apical half of the root.

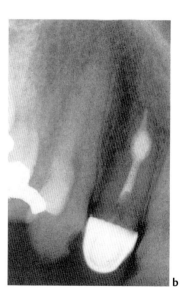

Fig. 11.29

a Diagram illustrating the obturation of a root canal with an internal resorption lacuna. The root canal apical to the resorptive defect is filled in the normal manner. The gutta-percha is then removed to the apical floor of the resorption lacuna and the lacuna is filled by means of vertical condensation of softened gutta-percha.

b Radiograph of an endodontically treated maxillary lateral incisor with internal resorption.

The gutta-percha points are then seared off at the apical level of the resorption lacuna. Thereafter, the resorption defect and the coronal part of the canal are filled *by vertical condensation of softened gutta-percha* without risk of overfilling the canal.

In teeth with incomplete root formation, the diameter of the root canal may be wider than the largest size gutta-percha point available. In such teeth it may be a good alternative to customize a master point to fit the root canal. This is done by heating several gutta-percha points in warm water and rolling them between two glass slabs until they become one point with a diameter slightly larger than that of the canal to be filled.

The surface of the customized point is then again carefully softened in warm water and the point is inserted into the root canal to the working length. The point is moved slightly up and down in the canal, and after hardening is removed. Sealer is then applied to the canal and the customized point is reinserted to seal the apical part of the canal. Coronally, necessary accessory points are added under lateral condensation in the normal way. *If the canal is blunderbuss-shaped, the apical end of the customized point is softened over an alcohol flame.* It is then introduced into the canal and carefully but firmly forced toward the apical hard-tissue barrier so that the gutta-percha fills the apical undercuts in three dimensions (**Fig. 11.30**). To minimize the shrinkage of the softened gutta-percha, a continuous force is exerted on the gutta-percha point during the material's cooling period (2 minutes).

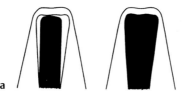

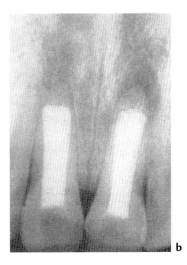

Fig. 11.30

a Diagram illustrating the obturation of an apexified immature tooth with a root canal in the shape of a blunderbuss. A gutta-percha point which fits the major part of the root canal is fabricated. The point is removed, sealer is applied to the canal, the end of the gutta-percha point is softened, and the point is firmly forced against the apical hard-tissue barrier so as to fill the apical undercuts in three dimensions.

b Radiograph of endodontically treated maxillary incisors with blunderbuss-shaped root canals.

Root Canal Obturation with Adhesive Technique

The use of resin-based enamel/dentin adhesives has become routine in operative dentistry. As a result, marginal leakage in conjunction with bonded restorations is greatly reduced. However, true adhesive restorative materials do not exist at present, and the bonding is due to micromechanical retention of the resinous material to the tooth.

The Resilon/Epiphany technique. As described earlier in Chapter 10, the Resilon/Epiphany system was specifically developed as root canal filling materials to be used with an adhesive technique. Resilon is the obturating material that comes in standardized and accessory points and tablets, and Epiphany is the sealing material that is supposed to bond both to dentin and to Resilon. The materials handle easily, and may be used with any obturating method.

Epiphany is used like a two-step, self-etching adhesive. An acidic primer is applied to the root canal to demineralize the surface layer of the root dentin. The primer is dried by air blasts and paper points to remove the volatile carrier (ethanol), and the dual-cure Epiphany is applied. The Resilon obturating material is then inserted, and an immediate coronal seal is obtained by light-curing the coronal aspect of the root filling. In the canal, the Epiphany sealer will self cure within 45 minutes to seal the entire canal.

The results of experimental as well as clinical studies suggest that normal, good results are obtained with the Resilon/Epiphany system (**Fig. 11.31**). However, any added benefits from the attempted bonding of the sealer to the root canal wall are not obvious, and bacterial leakage has been found to occur at the same rate and speed with Resilon/Epiphany as, for instance, with gutta-percha/AH Plus. Conceivably, this may be due to problematic but rather normal conditions in the root canal. Remnants of tissue fluids, irrigation solutions, and alcohol from the primer will all adversely affect the bond. The use of sodium hypochlorite will leave an oxygen-rich surface layer in the root canal, which results in reduced bond strength. Then there is polymerization shrinkage of the resin sealer. Unfortunately, resins in thin layers like the sealer in a root canal generate very high forces from polymerization contraction. The contraction force may exceed the bond strength of the resin adhesive to dentin, resulting in gap formation. A deterioration of the resin bond with time is also documented, and loss of bond strength is

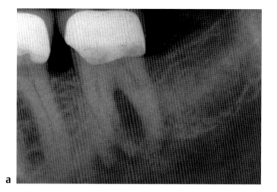

a

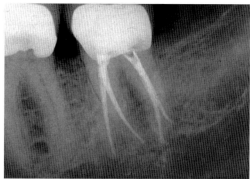

c

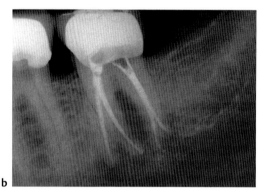

b

Fig. 11.31
a Radiograph of mandibular molar with four roots and symptomatic apical periodontitis. Four root canals are instrumented, irrigated, and packed with calcium hydroxide paste.
b After 4 weeks the patient is asymptomatic and the root canals are treated and obturated according to the Resilon/Epiphany system.
c At the 6-month control, periapical repair is evident.

detected as early as after 3 months. Clearly, adhesive obturating materials ought to have a greater potential than traditional materials to achieve a true bacteria-tight seal of the root canal. The Resilon/Epiphany obturating system may well represent the type of materials that are needed. However, the technique to obtain a strong and lasting bond between the sealer and the root canal dentin should be improved.

Root Canal Obturation with Pastes

Materials mixed from a powder and a liquid into a paste that constitute the sole material for obturation of the root canal are available on the market. The paste materials may be introduced into the canal by means of lentulo spirals or by injection. At first glance this may seem to be a simple and attractive technique, but in reality it is not. Overfilling of the canal is the rule, not the exception. The homogeneity of the root canal filling is often not satisfactory, and the canal is often inadequately sealed in spite of overfilling. Some of the pastes will shrink after setting, and most of them are soluble in tissue fluids. From the point of view of physical properties, the resin-based pastes Diaket and AH26 (see p. 173) are the most interesting materials. However, the fact that these materials are almost impossible to remove from the root canal after setting is reason enough for them not be used other than in conjunction with gutta-percha.

Regenerative Endodontics

Regenerative endodontics is the creation and delivery of tissues to replace diseased, missing, or traumatized pulp tissue. During the past 100 years, numerous attempts have been made to develop so-called biological obturation techniques, i.e., techniques aimed at inducing hard-tissue closure of the root canal or ingrowth of new connective tissue into the canal from the periapical area. Well known in this regard are the experiments from the first half of last century with calcium hydroxide as a permanent root filling material. The idea behind these experiments was that if the root canal were filled with calcium hydroxide, a precipitation of calcium salts would occur that might ultimately cause a complete obturation of the canal.

However, since calcium hydroxide dissolves in tissue fluids rather rapidly, an obturation of the root canal obviously did not take place. Still, *it was learned from these experiments that calcium hydroxide indeed has a hard tissue–inducing effect.* This effect is presently being utilized in many areas of modern endodontic therapy, in pulp capping and pulpotomies, in apexigenesis and apexification treatment of teeth with incompletely formed roots, and in the treatment of perforation and resorption defects in the root (**Figs. 5.8**, **6.18**, **8.18**).

More recently, interesting animal experiments have been reported in which *a gel of collagen and biologically active chemicals* was applied in the root canal. With this method, both ingrowth of tissue and apical and intra-canal calcifications have been observed. Probably the most interesting experiments in this regard, however, are the attempts *to induce ingrowth of new connective tissue into the root canal by means of a blood clot.* In these experiments the root canal is instrumented through the apical foramen, but otherwise prepared in the normal way. Periapical bleeding is then provoked and when the canal is filled with blood, it is sealed bacteria-tight at a distance from the apex. In vital teeth, new connective tissue or a "new pulp" forms routinely in the canal if infection of the blood clot is prevented (**Fig. 5.23**). The findings of these experiments have already been adopted clinically; after a pulpectomy, the root canal is now consistently filled to a level 1–3 mm short of the radiographic apex, even if the entire pulp has been extirpated. The unfilled space apical to the root filling will then be filled automatically with tissue fluids and blood which will become organized into new connective tissue. In nonvital teeth, new connective tissue is seen only in exceptional cases, possibly because of inadequate infection control in the clinical situation. However, recent reports of an aggressive use of antibiotics locally in the root canal before inducing the bleeding show interesting and promising results.

The interesting results achieved with calcium hydroxide, the blood clot, and other experiments of this type have resulted in considerable enthusiasm, and regenerative endodontics is presently a hot issue, especially in the research laboratory, but also in the clinic. Therefore, there is every reason to believe that present endodontic techniques may change in the future. *Until then, however, the goal must be to achieve a bacteria-tight seal of a clean, bacteria-free root canal with biologically acceptable materials.*

Further Reading

Alster D, Feilzer AJ, de Gee AJ, Davidson CL. Polymerization contraction stress in thin resin composite layers as a function of layer thickness. Dent Mater 1997;13:146–150.

Ari H, Yasar E, Belli S. Effects of NaOCl on bond strengths of resin cements to root canal dentin. J Endod 2003;29:348–351.

Banchs F, Trope M. Revascularization of immature permanent teeth with apical periodontitis: new treatment protocol? J Endod 2004;30:196–200.

Baumann MA. Das RaCe-System. Ein vielversprechender neuer Ansatz für die Wurzelkanalaufbereitung mit Nickel-Titan Feilen. ZWR 2001;110:1–9.

Baumgartner G, Zehnder M, Paqué F. *Enterococcus faecalis* type strain leakage through root canals filled with gutta-percha/AH Plus or Resilon/Epiphany. J Endod 2007;33:45–47.

Benner MD, Peters DD, Grower M, Bernier WE. Evaluation of a new thermoplastic gutta-percha obturation technique using ^{45}Ca. J Endod 1994;20:315–319.

Chueb L-H, Huang T-J. Immature teeth with periradicular periodontitis or abscess undergoing apexogenesis: a paradigm shift. J Endod 2006;32:1205–1213.

Conner DA, Caplan DJ, Teixeira FB, Trope M. Clinical outcome of teeth treated endodontically with a nonstandardized protocol and root filled with Resilon. J Endod 2007;33:1290–1292.

Dalat DM, Spångberg LSW. Comparison of apical leakage in root canals obturated with various gutta-percha techniques using a dye vacuum tracing method. J Endod 1994;20:315–319.

Fan B, Wu M-K, Wesselink PR. Leakage along warm gutta-percha fillings in the apical canals of curved roots. Endod Dent Traumatol 2000;16:29–33.

Flath RK, Hicks ML. Retrograde instrumentation and obturation with new devices. J Endod 1993;19:2–10.

Glosson CR, Haller RH, Brent Dove S, del Rio CE. Comparison of root canal preparations using NiTi-hand, NiTi engine-driven and K-flex endodontic instruments. J Endod 1995;21:146–151.

Gutmann JL, Rakusin H. Perspectives on root canal obturation with thermoplasticized injectable gutta-percha. Int Endod J 1987;20:261–270.

Hammad M, Qualtrough A, Silikas N. Extended setting shrinkage behaviour of endodontic sealers. J Endod 2008; 34: 90–93.

Hasimoto M, Ohno H, Sano H, Kaga M, Oguchi H. In vitro degradation of resin–dentin bonds analyzed by microtensile bond test, scanning and transmission electron microscopy. Biomaterials 2003;24:3795–3803.

Hörsted P, Nygaard-Östby B. Tissue formation in the root canal after total pulpectomy and partial root filling. Oral Surg Oral Med Oral Pathol 1961;14:83–91.

Karr NA, Baumgartner JC, Marshall JG. A comparison of gutta-percha and Resilon in the obturation of lateral grooves and depressions. J Endod 2007;33:749–752.

Kerekes K, Tronstad L. Long-term results of endodontic treatment performed with a standardized technique. J Endod 1979;5:83–90.

Kobayashi C, Suda H. New electronic canal measuring device based on the ratio method. J Endod 1994;20:111–114.

Leonardo MR, Barnett F, Debelian GJ, de Pontes Lima RK, Bezerra da Silva LA. Root canal adhesive filling in dogs' teeth with or without coronal restoration: a histopathological evaluation. J Endod 2007;33:1299–1303.

Martin H. Ultrasonic disinfection of the root canal. Oral Surg Oral Med Oral Pathol 1976;42:92–99.

McComb D, Smith DC. A preliminary scanning electron microscopic study of root canals after endodontic procedures. J Endod 1975;1:738–742.

Molven O, Halse A, Grung B. Surgical management of endodontic failures: indications and treatment results. Int Dent J 1991;41:33–42.

Murray PE, Garcia-Godoy F, Hargreaves KM. Regenerative endodontics: a review of current status and call for action. J Endod 2007;33:377–390.

Schilder H. Filling root canals in three dimensions. Dent Clin North Am 1967;11:723–744.

Short JA, Morgan LA, Baumgartner JC. A comparison of the canal centering ability of four instrumentation techniques. J Endod 1997;23:503–508.

Tronstad L. Den standardiserte teknikk for endodontisk behandling. In: Ondontologi' 81. Copenhagen: Munksgaard 1981, pp 21–32.

Walton RE. Histologic evaluation of different methods of enlarging the pulp canal space. J Endod 1976;2:304–311.

Wildey WL, Senia S. A new root canal instrument and instrumentation technique. Oral Surg Oral Med Oral Pathol 1989;67:189–192.

Yared GM, Ben Dagher FE. Influence of apical enlargement on bacterial infection during treatment of apical periodontitis. J Endod 1994;20:535–537.

12
Dental Morphology and Treatment Guidelines

The root canal system of human teeth may be extremely complex. Still, in spite of the irregularities, all groups of teeth have a general pattern in their root canal morphology. *Virtually all teeth have main root canals and it is the main canals that we instrument and obturate during endodontic treatment.* Lateral and accessory canals are influenced by irrigants and antiseptics, and *only in rare instances will the outcome of the treatment depend on whether an accessory canal is actually obturated or not.* This is the case even if an endodontic lesion clearly originates from a lateral root canal. *If adequate chemomechanical instrumentation and disinfection are carried out and the main root canal is filled, the lateral periodontitis will heal even if the lateral canal is not filled* (**Fig.12.1**). This is an extremely important concept in endodontics, and without this concept, root canal treatment has no logical foundation. Therefore, the root canal morphology of the teeth as it pertains to clinical endodontic therapy will be discussed.

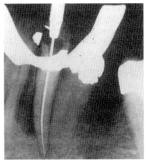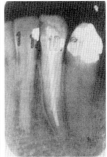

Fig. 12.1
a **Radiograph of a nonvital mandibular canine with lateral periodontitis.**
b At the 2-year control there is resolution of the lateral radilucent lesion. Note that a possible lateral canal going to the lesion has not been instrumented or obturated.

Maxillary Central Incisor

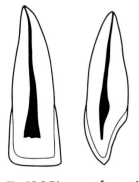

Average length of the tooth:		22.5 mm
Number of roots:		1 (100%)
Number of root canals:		1 (100%)
Lateral root canals:		Occasional
Apical root canal delta:		Frequent
Apical foramen	0–1 mm from apex:	80%
	1–2 mm from apex:	20%
Diameter of the root canal	1 mm from apex:	0.3–0.45 mm
	2 mm from apex:	0.35–0.7 mm
	3 mm from apex:	0.4–0.8 mm
	5 mm from apex:	0.45–0.9 mm
Recommended apical enlargement (master point):		60–80

Fig. 12.2 Diagram of a maxillary central incisor: Buccal, proximal, and incisal view.

Treatment Guidelines
The access cavity is prepared with long-shank round burs and the point of entry is on the palatal surface of the tooth, slightly incisal to the singulum. The bur is held at an angle of about 30° to the long axis of the tooth and the long shank is helpful in aligning the bur correctly. When an opening to the pulp chamber has been achieved, the access cavity is enlarged mainly with outward strokes of the bur to reflect the size and shape of

the pulp chamber (see p.179). It is very important to include the pulp horns in the cavity so that all tissue and discolored dentin are removed to prevent discoloration of the tooth. A round bur no.2 is used for this purpose. Also, the root canal has a definite cervical constriction that should be re-moved before the actual root canal instrumentation begins. This is done with a long, tapered, diamond-coated bur, a Gates-Glidden, or similar bur. The apical part of the root canal is circular in shape and a circular apical box may be readily prepared in this tooth.

Maxillary Lateral Incisor

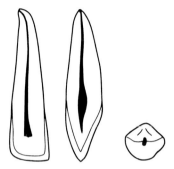

Average length of the tooth:		22 mm
Number of roots:		1 (99.9 %)
Number of root canals:		1 (99.9 %)
Lateral root canals:		Occasional
Apical root canal delta:		Frequent
Apical foramen	0 – 1 mm from apex:	90 %
	1 – 2 mm from apex:	10 %
Diameter of the root canal	1 mm from apex:	0.3 – 0.6 mm
	2 mm from apex:	0.35 – 0.8 mm
	3 mm from apex:	0.4 – 1 mm
	5 mm from apex:	0.4 – 1 mm
Recommended apical enlargement, straight canal:		60 – 80

Fig. 12.3 Diagram of a maxillary lateral incisor: Buccal, proximal, and incisal view.

Treatment Guidelines
The access cavity is prepared with long-shank, round burs as described for the maxillary central incisor. *The lateral incisor typically has a wide root canal in a narrow root.* Thus, the diameter of the canal in the apical 5 mm of the root is generally wider than both in the maxillary central incisor and the maxillary canine. However, the most apical part of the canal has a fairly round shape, so that a circular apical box may be prepared in lateral incisors. *Still, it must be understood that the canal of these teeth should be enlarged considerably more in the apical area than would normally be expected judging by the size of their roots.*
The root of the maxillary lateral incisor is frequently curved apically, *often in a palatal direction* so that the curve may not be apparent in a radiograph immediately. Although the curved canals are generally narrower than the canals in lateral incisors with straight roots, they are still wide and may be difficult to instrument adequately. *As a result, historically speaking, endodontic treatment of the maxillary lateral incisor has failed more than in any other tooth.* However, the use of flexible nickel-titanium instruments has made it easier to instrument wide, curved canals without perforations, canal transportation, or other mishaps.

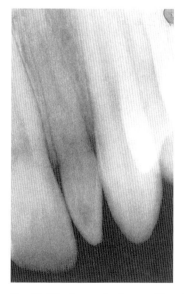

Fig. 12.4 Radiograph of a maxillary lateral incisor with enamel invagination in a 16-year-old.

Enamel invagination and dens in dente occur most often in the maxillary lateral incisor (**Fig. 12.4**). These malformations may allow penetration of bacteria to the pulp and endodontic treatment of these teeth will frequently be necessary. The practical approach will depend on the clinical and radiographic findings and the degree of irregularities of the tooth. Often a surgical intervention with retrograde fillings to support the best possible orthograde obturation of the root canals will be necessary.

Maxillary Canine

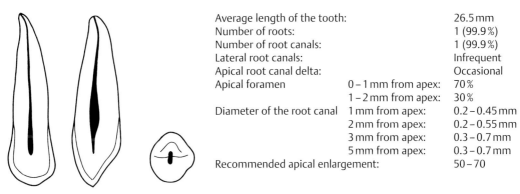

Average length of the tooth:		26.5 mm
Number of roots:		1 (99.9 %)
Number of root canals:		1 (99.9 %)
Lateral root canals:		Infrequent
Apical root canal delta:		Occasional
Apical foramen	0–1 mm from apex:	70 %
	1–2 mm from apex:	30 %
Diameter of the root canal	1 mm from apex:	0.2–0.45 mm
	2 mm from apex:	0.2–0.55 mm
	3 mm from apex:	0.3–0.7 mm
	5 mm from apex:	0.3–0.7 mm
Recommended apical enlargement:		50–70

Fig. 12.5 Diagram of a maxillary canine: Buccal, proximal, and incisal view.

Treatment Guidelines

The access cavity is prepared with long-shank, round burs as described for the maxillary central incisor. The maxillary canine is the longest tooth in the dentition and teeth 30 mm and longer are occasionally seen. The root canal is straight and circular in shape and only a very slight apical curvature of the root is sometimes seen. A circular apical box may be readily prepared, and this tooth lends itself exceptionally well to treatment with the standardized technique. On extremely rare occasions, the maxillary canine may have two root canals.

Maxillary First Premolar

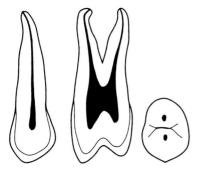

Average length of the tooth:		20.6 mm
Number of roots:		1 (19 %); 2 (80 %); 3 (1 %)
Number of root canals:		1 (4 %); 2 (95 %); 3 (1 %)
Lateral root canals:		Infrequent
Apical root canal delta:		Infrequent
Apical foramen	0–1 mm from apex:	95 %
	1–2 mm from apex:	5 %

Diameter of the canal in teeth with

	3 canals	2 canals	1 canal
1 mm from apex:	0.15–0.2 mm	0.15–0.7 mm	0.5 mm
2 mm from apex:	0.15–0.2 mm	0.2–1 mm	0.7–1.2 mm
3 mm from apex:	0.15–0.35 mm	0.2–0.9 mm	0.7–1.2 mm
5 mm from apex:	0.25–0.35 mm	0.25–1 mm	0.8–1.2 mm

Recommended apical enlargement in teeth with 1 canal: 50–70
Recommended apical enlargement in teeth with 2 canals: 35–50
Recommended apical enlargement in teeth with 3 canals: 35

Fig. 12.6 Diagram of a maxillary first premolar: Buccal, proximal, and occlusal view.

Treatment Guidelines

The maxillary first premolar has, as a rule, two root canals. The pulp chamber is elongated in a buccopalatal direction and the orifices of the canals are located slightly centrally to the buccal and lingual cusp tips. The access cavity is prepared with a long-shank, round bur directed at the long axis of the tooth with the point of entry in the middle of the occlusal central groove. When the pulp chamber has been penetrated, the bur is used in the normal manner with outward strokes to remove the tooth structure overhanging the pulp chamber. The shape of the floor of the pulp chamber will usually indicate the number of canals. If one canal is present, it is located centrally in the tooth. If two canals are present, they are usually further apart, i.e., further buccally and palatally than perhaps would be expected. Teeth with three canals have two buccal canals and one palatal canal. Most maxillary first premolars have a distinct concavity in the mesial root surface, in-

creasing the risk of mesiocervical perforations during access preparation. The cusps of this tooth are often weakened when endodontic treatment is indicated, and their height should be reduced or they should be strengthened with a bonded restoration prior to endodontic treatment to prevent uncontrolled crown-root fractures.

The root canals of the maxillary first premolar vary considerably in width, and the variations are not necessarily related to the diameter ot the root. Endodontically, this is a difficult tooth, and more failures are found with it than with any other tooth except the maxillary lateral incisor. To improve upon this, it is necessary to understand and accept how wide the apical part of the root canals can be in the maxillary first premolar and to instrument them accordingly. This requires both patience and skills in the narrow and often curved roots of this tooth. However, a circular apical box can most often be prepared and the use of flexible nickel-titanium instruments is helpful.

Maxillary Second Premolar

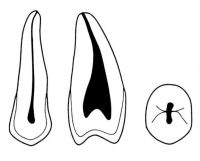

Average length of the tooth:			21.5 mm
Number of roots:			1 (90%); 2 (9%); 3 (1%)
Number of root canals:			1 (75%); 2 (24%); 3 (1%)
Lateral root canals:			Infrequent
Apical root canal delta:			Infrequent
Apical foramen	0–1 mm from apex:		75%
	1–2 mm from apex:		25%

Diameter of the canal in teeth with

	3 canals	2 canals	1 canal
1 mm from apex:	0.1 mm	0.3–0.35 mm	0.2–0.7 mm
2 mm from apex:	0.1–0.25 mm	0.3–0.7 mm	0.25–0.7 mm
3 mm from apex:	0.2–0.35 mm	0.3–1.1 mm	0.4–1.2 mm
5 mm from apex:	0.2–0.35 mm	0.3–1.1 mm	0.4–1.2 mm

Recommended apical enlargement in teeth with 1 canal: 40–70
Recommended apical enlargement in teeth with 2 canals: 35–50
Recommended apical enlargement in teeth with 3 canals: 35

Fig. 12.7 Diagram of a maxillary second premolar: Buccal, proximal, and occlusal view.

Treatment Guidelines

The maxillary second premolar usually has one root and one root canal. The pulp chamber is elongated in a buccopalatal direction, and the access cavity is prepared as described for the maxillary first premolar. The coronal part of a single root canal is ribbon-shaped. It tapers off and takes on a circular form in the apical third of the root. In about 10–15% of the teeth, a single canal splits

into two canals in the apical 3–4 mm of the root. When two canals are present, their orifices are located buccally and palatally, centrally to the cusp tips, as in the maxillary first premolar. The two canals may occasionally join apically, but as a rule they have separate apical foramina. When three canals are present, two are located buccally and one palatally. These canals are narrow and may be difficult both to locate and to instrument. Otherwise, the maxillary second premolar is easier to instrument than the first premolar, also when two canals are present, and in most instances the canals can be given a circular form in the apical area.

Maxillary Molars

Maxillary First Molar

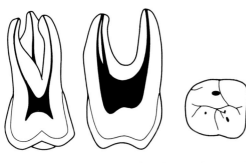

Average length of the tooth:	20.8 mm
Number of roots:	2 (15%); 3 (85%)
Number of root canals:	3 (60%); 4 (40%)
Lateral root canals:	Occasional
Apical root canal delta:	Infrequent

Fig. 12.8 Diagram of a maxillary first molar: Buccal, proximal, and occlusal view.

Maxillary Second Molar

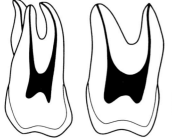

Average length of the tooth:	20 mm
Number of roots:	1 (1%); 2 (19%); 3 (80%)
Number of root canals:	1 (1%); 2 (2%); 3 (57%); 4 (40%)
Lateral root canals:	Occasional
Apical root canal delta:	Infrequent

Fig. 12.9 Diagram of a maxillary second molar: Buccal, proximal, and occlusal view.

Mesiobuccal Root of Maxillary Molars

Number of root canals:		1 (60%); 2 (40%)
Number of apical foramina:		1 (85%); 2 (15%)
Apical foramen 0–1 mm from apex:		80%
Apical foramen 1–2 mm from apex:		20%
Diameter of canal in roots with	2 canals	1 canal
1 mm from apex:	0.1–0.4 mm	0.2–0.6 mm
2 mm from apex:	0.1–0.5 mm	0.2–0.8 mm
3 mm from apex:	0.15–0 mm	0.35–1 mm
5 mm from apex:	0.15–0 mm	0.35–1 mm
Recommended apical enlargement in roots with 1 canal:		35–50
Recommended apical enlargement in roots with 2 canals:		35–45

Distobuccal Root of Maxillary Molars

Number of root canals:		1 (100%)
Apical foramen:	0–1 mm from apex:	75%
	1–2 mm from apex:	25%
Diameter of the canal:	1 mm from apex:	0.15–0.4 mm
	2 mm from apex:	0.15–0.55 mm
	3 mm from apex:	0.15–0.6 mm
	5 mm from apex:	0.2–1.2 mm
Recommended apical enlargement:		40–60

Palatal Root of Maxillary Molars

Number of root canals:		1 (100%)
Apical foramen:	0–1 mm from apex:	80%
	1–2 mm from apex:	20%
Diameter of the canal:	1 mm from the apex:	0.15–0.4 mm
	2 mm from apex:	0.2–0.8 mm
	3 mm from apex:	0.2–0.9 mm
	5 mm from apex:	0.2–1.2 mm
Recommended apical enlargement:		60–100

First molar

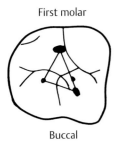

Buccal

Fig. 12.10 Diagram illustrating the location of the root canal orifices in a maxillary first molar.

Second molar

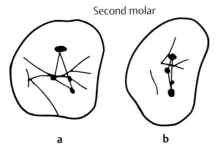

a   b

Fig. 12.11
a Diagram illustrating the location of the root canal orifices in a maxillary second molar. As compared to the first molar, the distobuccal canal has "moved" in a mesiopalatal direction.
b In molars with narrow pulp chambers, the orifices of all four canals may be located on a more or less straight line between the mesiobuccal and palatal canals.

The palatal root may have two canals in molars with fused roots. However, clinically, the second palatal canal will appear as the distobuccal canal.

Treatment Guidelines
The pulp chamber of the maxillary molars is generally located in the mesial two-thirds of the crown (**Fig. 12.10**). The access cavity is prepared with long-shank, round burs and the point of entry is the mesio-occlusal central groove ot the tooth. The orifice of the main mesiobuccal canal is located slightly palatally to the mesiobuccal cusp tip. The orifice of the palatal canal is found central–palatally in the mesial two-thirds of the crown. When a second mesiobuccal canal is present, its orifice will be seen near the main mesiobuccal canal on a straight line between this canal and the palatal canal. The distobuccal canal is located slightly distally to the midline between the mesial and distal surfaces of the crown and somewhat more palatally than the mesiobuccal canal. The pulp chamber has a triangular base with the canal orifices located in the corners of the triangle. In molars with their roots grouped closely together, as is most often seen in second molars, the orifice of the distobuccal root canal will have "moved" in a mesiopalatal direction along a line perpendicular to the line between the mesiobuccal and palatal canals (**Fig. 12.11**). In second molars with extremely narrow pulp chambers, the distobuccal

canal may have moved so far mesially and palatally that the orifices of all four canals are located on a more or less straight line between the mesiobuccal and palatal canals. If the mesiobuccal cusp is weak, or if a crown restoration is planned subsequent to the endodontic treatment, this cusp should always be cut prior to treatment. This will greatly improve the visibility of the access cavity and facilitate the root canal instrumentation and obturation phases of the treatment.

As indicated above, the mesiobuccal root of about every other maxillary molar has two canals. The coronal part of the canal located furthest buccally is fairly wide and this canal is readily located. The orifice and coronal part of the second mesiobuccal canal may be extremely narrow, and as a result this canal is often overlooked in the clinical situation. Still, the success rate of endodontic treatment of this root is good, conceivably because the two canals in most instances have a common apical foramen. Obviously, all maxillary molars should be examined for a second mesiobuccal canal. Circular apical boxes may be prepared in most mesiobuccal roots, regardless of the presence of one or two canals.

The distobuccal root is generally straight and has one canal with a near-circular shape in the apical area. The distobuccal root canal is exceptionally well suited to being instrumented with a circular apical box.

The palatal root is most often straight, but may curve in a buccal direction in its apical part. This may not be readily detected radiographically. The palatal root canal is wide and appears to present few problems during the instrumentation phase. However, the canal may be ribbon-shaped and may be wider apically than is clinically apparent. Apical foramina with a largest diameter of more than 3 mm have been observed in mature teeth. However, most often, the palatal canal decreases in size in the apical 2–5 mm of the root and it takes on a circular shape in this area. Still, the apical part of the canal should be instrumented as wide as the diameter and a possible buccal curvature of the root allow. A circular apical box is then usually attained.

Maxillary Third Molar
As is known, the morphology of the third molar varies considerably and is rather unpredictable. However, this tooth may also be well developed and may appear clinically and radiographically as a first or second molar. In these instances, the data for the first and second molars may be used for the third molar as well. If the third molar has an extremely irregular form, it may or may not be possible to perform adequate endodontic treatment of the tooth. This decision will have to be made based on the actual clinical and radiographic findings in each individual tooth.

Mandibular Incisors

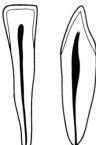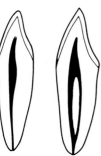

Average length of the central incisor: 20.7 mm
Average length of the lateral incisor: 21.7 mm
Number of roots: 1 (100 %)
Number of root canals: 1 (60 %); 2 (40 %)
Number of apical foramina: 1 (99 %); 2 (1 %)
Lateral root canals: Occasional
Apical root canal delta: Infrequent
Apical foramen   0–1 mm from apex: 90 %
　　　　　　　　1–2 mm from apex: 10 %
Diameter of the root canal: 1 mm from apex: 0.15–0.7 mm
　　　　　　　　　　　　2 mm from apex: 0.3–1 mm
　　　　　　　　　　　　3 mm from apex: 0.3–1 mm
　　　　　　　　　　　　5 mm from apex: 0.3–1.3 mm
Recommended apical enlargement in teeth with 1 canal: 35–60
Recommended apical enlargement in teeth with 2 canals: 35–50

Fig. 12.12 Diagram of mandibular incisors: Buccal, proximal, and incisal view.

Treatment Guidelines

The access cavity is prepared with long-shank, round burs. The point of entry is the central area of the lingual surface of the crown. When two canals are present, there is a buccal and *lingual canal with the lingual canal peripheral in the root.* The access cavity, therefore, must be enlarged in a cervical direction to expose the lingual canal orifice. Also, it is often necessary to enlarge the access cavity in an incisal direction, even to a point where the incisal edge is broken, to facilitate adequate access to the root canals. Special attention is given to the pulp horns and a round bur no. 2 is used to clean these areas of the crown.

Apart from the fact that the mandibular central incisor is somewhat smaller than the lateral incisor, the teeth are quite similar. This applies to their root canal system as well. The root canal is ribbon or hour glass shaped, or two canals may be present *that almost without exception join in a common apical foramen.* Endodontically, the mandibular incisor is a difficult tooth with a rather high failure rate. The lingual canal is often overlooked, usually because of an inadequate access cavity. In teeth with two canals, the apical part of the canals may be given a cylindrical shape. In roots with a single canal, the apical part of the canal will usually be ribbon-shaped and much wider in a buccolingual direction than has generally been assumed. A longitudinal filing technique, therefore, should be used all the way to the working length. It is important in these teeth to pay special attention to the buccal and lingual walls of the canal because of its wide buccolingual diameter. A master point as large as possible (depending on the mesio-distal diameter of the canal) is then used, but lateral condensation to the working length may be necessary in these teeth.

Mandibular Canine

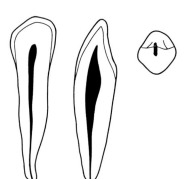

Average length of the tooth:	25.6 mm
Number of roots:	1 (98 %); 2 (2 %)
Number of root canals:	1 (94 %); 2 (6 %)
Lateral root canals:	Infrequent
Apical root canal delta:	Infrequent
Apical foramen 0 – 1 mm from apex:	95 %
1 – 2 mm from apex:	5 %
Diameter of the root canal 1 mm from apex:	0.1 – 0.5 mm
2 mm from apex:	0.2 – 0.6 mm
3 mm from apex:	0.2 – 0.7 mm
5 mm from apex:	0.2 – 1.3 mm
Recommended apical enlargement:	40 – 70

Fig. 12.13 Diagram of a mandibular canine: Buccal, proximal, and incisal view.

Treatment Guidelines

The access cavity is prepared with long-shank, round burs. The point of entry is the central area of the lingual surface, and the bur is held at a 30° angle to the long axis of the tooth until it has penetrated to the pulp chamber. The access cavity is then enlarged in an incisal direction to facilitate the location of a lingual second root canal, which, if present, splits off from the main canal in the midroot area and usually joins the main canal again 1 – 5 mm from the apical foramen. Only occasionally do the two canals end in separate foramina, and two roots in this tooth is an infrequent occurrence. Thus, as a rule, the second canal does not influence the size and shape of the main root canal near the apex where the canal has a circular shape and can readily be given the shape of a circular apical box.

Mandibular First Premolar

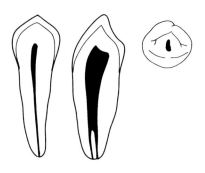

Average length of the tooth:	21.6 mm
Number of roots:	1 (100 %)
Number of root canals:	1 (75 %); 2 (20 %);
	3 or more (5 %)
Lateral root canals:	Occasional
Apical root canal delta:	Occasional
Apical foramen 0 – 1 mm from apex:	80 %
1 – 2 mm from apex:	20 %
Diameter of the root canal 1 mm from apex:	0.1 – 0.35 mm
2 mm from apex:	0.2 – 0.5 mm
3 mm from apex:	0.2 – 0.7 mm
5 mm from apex:	0.2 – 1.6 mm

Recommended apical enlargement in teeth with 1 canal: 50 – 70
Recommended apical enlargement in teeth with 2 canals: 35 – 50

Fig. 12.14 Diagram of a mandibular first premolar: Buccal, proximal, and occlusal view.

Treatment Guidelines

The access cavity is prepared with long-shank, round burs. The point of entry is slightly buccal to the central occlusal groove. *The crown of the mandibular first premolar often tilts in a lingual direction so that the occlusal surface has a lingual inclination.* This must be taken into account during access cavity preparation or a buccal root perforation may occur. For the same reason, the buccal cusp may have to the reduced to allow adequate access to the root canals.

The mandibular first premolar most often has one straight root canal from the pulp chamber to the apical foramen. Five percent of these teeth have two uninterrupted root canals. The orifices of the canals are then situated buccally and lingually on the pulp chamber floor. In 15 % of these teeth, a second canal branches off from the main canal in a buccal or lingual direction in the middle or apical area of the root. The occurrence of a split root canal is suggested radiographically when the image of the canal suddenly decreases dramatically in width or seemingly disappears (**Fig. 12.15**). Locating and instrumenting the branching second canal may be difficult. A stainless steel K-file with a curved tip should be used to probe the root canal wall in the area where the split appears to have taken place before any instrumentation of

the canal is done. If the second canal is located, it should be opened up and instrumented first, and the patency of this canal should be constantly checked during the instrumentation of the main canal. With regard to shape and size of the root canals of the mandibular first premolar, they can readily be given a cylindrical shape apically.

Mandibular first premolars that have three, four, and even five root canals are occasionally seen.

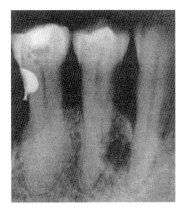

Fig. 12.15 Radiograph of mandibular premolars. A split in the root canal in the apical half of the root is indicated by the disappearance of the canal in the radiograph.

Mandibular Second Premolars

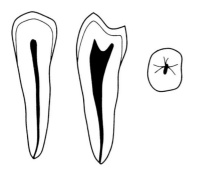

Average length of the tooth:	21.5 mm
Number of roots:	1 (100%)
Number of root canals:	1 (89%); 2 (10%); 3 (1%)
Lateral root canals:	Occasional
Apical root canal delta:	Occasional

Apical foramen	0–1 mm from apex:	65%
	1–2 mm from apex:	30%
	2–3 mm from apex:	5%
Diameter of the root canal 1 mm from apex:		0.2–0.4 mm
	2 mm from apex:	0.2–0.5 mm
	3 mm from apex:	0.2–0.5 mm
	5 mm from apex:	0.2–0.7 mm

Recommended apical enlargement in teeth with 1 canal: 40–70
Recommended apical enlargement in teeth with 2 canals: 35–50

Fig. 12.16 Diagram of a mandibular second premolar: Buccal, proximal, and occlusal view.

Treatment Guidelines

The access cavity is prepared as described for the mandibular first premolar. The lingual tilt of the crown occurs in this tooth as well, although the lingual cusp is more developed than in the first premolar, reducing the lingual inclination of the occlusal surface. A split of the root canal below the pulp chamber floor is seen, but much less frequently than in the mandibular first premolar. On the whole, the mandibular second premolar is a tooth that gives few endodontic problems. The root canal is narrow in the apical area of the root and a cylindrical apical box can readily be prepared.

Mandibular Molars

Mandibular First Molar

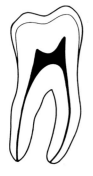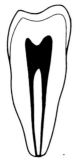

Average length of the tooth:	21 mm
Number of roots: 3 (2%):	2 (98%)
Number of root canals:	4 (7%); 3 (80%); 2 (13%)
Lateral root canals:	Occasional (furcation)
Apical root canal delta:	Frequent (mesial root)

Fig. 12.17 Diagram of a mandibular first molar: Buccal, proximal, and occlusal view.

Mandibular Second Molar

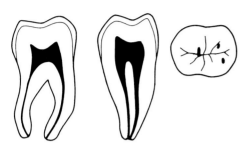

Average length of the tooth:	20 mm
Number of roots: 3 (1%):	2 (84%); 1 (15%)
Number of root canals:	4 (7%); 3 (77%); 2 (13%); 1 (3%)
Lateral root canals:	Occasional (furcation)
Apical root canal delta:	Frequent (mesial root)

Fig. 12.18 Diagram of a mandibular second molar: Buccal, proximal, and occlusal view.

Mesial Root of Mandibular Molars

Number of root canals:		1 (13%); 2 (87%)
Number of apical foramina:		1 (40%); 2 (60%)
Apical foramen	0–1 mm from apex:	80%
	1–2 mm from apex:	20%
Diameter of canal	1 mm from apex:	0.15–0.4 mm
	2 mm from apex:	0.2–1 mm
	3 mm from apex:	0.2–1.9 mm
	5 mm from apex:	0.3–2.8 mm
Recommended apical enlargement:		35–45

Distal Root of Mandibular Molars

Number of root canals:		1 (93%); 2 (7%)
Number of apical foramina:		1 (97%); 2 (3%)
Apical foramen	0–1 mm from apex:	65%
	1–2 mm from apex:	35%
Diameter of the root canal	1 mm from apex:	0.25–0.6 mm
	2 mm from apex :	0.25–1 mm
	3 mm from apex:	0.35–1.8 mm
	5 mm from apex:	0.4–2.6 mm
Recommended apical enlargement in teeth with 1 canal:		60–80
Recommended apical enlargement in teeth with 2 canals:		40–60

Treatment Guidelines

The pulp chamber of the mandibular molar is located in the mesial two-thirds of the crown. The access cavity is prepared with long-shank, round burs and the point of entry is the mesial aspect of the central occlusal groove of the tooth. The orifice of the mesiobuccal canal is located directly underneath the tip of the mesiobuccal cusp, and this cusp should be reduced in height, if at all possible, to facilitate the locating and instrumentation of the mesiobuccal canal. The mesiolingual canal is located between the lingual cusp and the central occlusal groove. In second molars, a rib-bon-shaped common orifice for the two mesial canals may be present. The distal canal is located centrally in the tooth slightly distal to the buccal groove. When one distal canal is present, the floor of the pulp chamber has an approximately triangular shape with the three canals in the corners of the triangle. A rhomboidal shape of the pulp chamber floor either indicates a severely ribbon-shaped distal canal or two separate canals with their orifices at the distal corners of the floor.

The root canal morphology of the mesial root of mandibular molars is extremely irregular and quite unpredictable from one tooth to the next

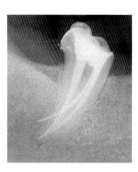

Fig. 12.19 Radiograph of mandibular molar with unusual root canal anatomy. The mesio-lingual and the distal root canals meet apically in a joint apical foramen.

(**Fig. 12.19**). If one canal is present, it may be ribbon or hour glass shaped and difficult to instrument. When two canals are present, they are usually connected by multiple bridges of tissue of varying widths. Also, the apical foramen may be ribbon-shaped with a largest diameter which is larger than the smallest diameter of the root. Still, one or two main root canals can always be recognized clinically, and in 40% of the roots, they end apically in one apical foramen, mostly in the second molar. Careful but determined use of Hedstrom files on the buccal and lingual canal walls is helpful during the debridement of these canals. Also, the mesial wall should be fairly vigorously instrumented with an outer-curve filing technique. However, the distal wall of the mesial canals must be treated with great care, first, because the root in this area is extremely thin, and second, because the distal wall borders on the inner curve of the canal since this root always curves in a distal direction. It is advantageous to use nickel-titanium instruments in curved root canals. Because of their flexibility, these instruments follow the curve and work centered in the canal. In spite of the irregularities of the root canal system of the mesial root of the mandibular molar, the success rate of endodontic treatment of this root is excellent. A cylindral apical box may be prepared in most instances, and a final instrument no. 35 is usually adequate (**Fig. 11.26**).

In contrast to the mesial root, the distal root of the mandibular molar has a fairly uniform canal morphology. In most instances, one central canal with a circular shape apically is present. In some instances, the canal is ribbon-shaped coronally and it can be difficult with clinical means to determine whether the canal continues as a single canal to the foramen or whether it divides in the apical area. The rule then is that, when in doubt, a ribbon-shaped canal should always be prepared as if it were two separate canals, one distobuccal and one distolingual. Two master points are used and inserted from the peripheral corners of the canal and the rest of the ribbon is filled with accessory points and lateral condensation.

Mandibular Third Molar

The mandibular third molar is often well developed and the information given above for the mandibular first and second molars may then be utilized for the third molar as well. If the tooth has an irregular morphology, modifications in technique will have to be introduced as needed in the actual clinical situation.

Further Reading

Kerekes K, Tronstad L. Morphometric observations on the root canals of human incisors. J Endod 1977;3: 24–29.

Kerekes K, Tronstad L. Morphometric observations on the root canals of human premolars. J Endod 1977; 3:74–79.

Kerekes K, Tronstad L. Morphometric observations on the root canals of human molars. J Endod 1977;3: 74–79.

Trope M, Elfenbein L, Tronstad L. Mandibular premolars with more than one root canal in different race groups. J Endod 1986;12(8):343–345.

Vertucci F. Root canal anatomy of human permanent teeth. Oral Surg Oral Med Oral Pathol 1984; 58: 589–597.

Yang Z-P, Yang S-F, Shay J-C, Chi C-Y. C-shaped root canals in mandibular second molars in a Chinese population. Endod Dent Traumatol 1988; 4: 160–163.

13
Endodontic Complications

Complications not provoked by the operator may occur during endodontic treatment. However, more often they are the result of deviations from the accepted principles of endodontic treatment.

The most common complications that occur during the various phases of endodontic treatment are discussed below.

Incomplete Analgesia

Is is often difficult to obtain complete local analgesia when treating inflamed pulps. The reason for this appears to be that commonly used local anesthetics like lidocaine have an inadequate effect on the C-fibers of the pulp. These fibers are activated and participate in the transmission of pain when the pulp is inflamed. However, *unlike lidocaine, a local anesthetic like eugenol affects both A- and C-fibers*. When applied liberally to exposed dentin and left for 1–2 minutes, eugenol will in most instances penetrate into the pulp in concentrations sufficient to have an analgesic effect on pain mediated by both A- and C-fibers. As a result, the pulp can be exposed with minimal pain. However, the effect of the eugenol is limited to only a small area of the pulp tissue immediately subjacent to the cavity. An *intrapulpal injection* of 0.2–0.4 mL of lidocaine or similar is, therefore, given under pressure when exposure of the pulp has been obtained. The pressure potentiates the effect of the drug and adequate anesthesia of the pulp is routinely obtained with this technique.

The intrapulpal injection is rather painful and it is important that the patient is informed beforehand about what is going to happen and why it is necessary. However, the effect of the intrapulpal injection is so profound that the patient will soon understand the benefits of enduring a short moment of pain when, as a result, further treatment is performed without symptoms.

Access Cavity

It may appear that the majority of operational mishaps and complications during endodontic treatment either occur during the preparation of the access cavity or arise from the fact that the access cavity is not given a proper size or form. The most common mistake is that the access cavity is too small (**Fig. 13.1**). This leads to entrapment of tissue, especially in the pulp horn areas of the crown, and to discoloration of the tooth. It also leads to difficulties in locating the canal orifices, and canals may readily be missed. In addition, if the access opening is not adequate, the root canal instruments may be improperly guided by the walls of the access cavity, increasing the risk of root perforations. Remember that the root canal orifices in a tooth with more than one canal are in the peripheral corners of the floor of the pulp chamber.

The *reduction of cusp height* is often beneficial in improving access to a root canal. Weak cusps should always be cut or reduced, also to prevent crown or crown-root fractures. Such fractures are often untreatable and in most instances could have been prevented if a cusp were cut in conjunction with the access cavity preparation.

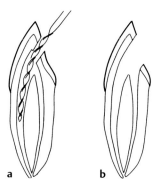

Fig. 13.1
a **Diagram illustrating the effect of an access cavity that is too small.** The lingual canal cannot be located and will be missed.
b Correct access cavity. The root canal orifices are visualized and both canals can be instrumented.

Perforations from the Pulp Chamber

A common complication during access cavity preparation is *perforation of the root with a bur* (**Fig.13.2**). This usually occurs because the operator has not studied the dimensions and form of the crown and pulp chamber of the tooth and the direction of its roots. A good radiograph taken with the paralleling technique is helpful in this regard.

Due to the limited length of the shank of the bur, *perforations from the pulp chamber will be in the cervical area of the tooth, either laterally or in*

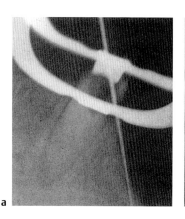

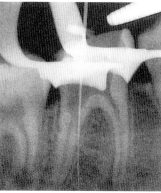

Fig. 13.2 Radiographs of teeth with root perforations with burs during attempts to locate root canal orifices.
a Lateral perforation.
b Furcation perforation. The rubber dam has caused the operator to lose his sense of direction and it should not have been applied until the root canal was located.

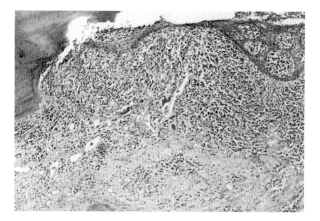

Fig. 13.3 Section from a tooth with unsuccessful treatment of a furcation perforation. The bone in the furcation area has resorbed and granulomatous tissue is present. The inflammation has resulted in the development of a periodontal pocket, and epithelium has grown down from the sulcus and is covering the tissue in the furcation (hematoxylin-eosin).

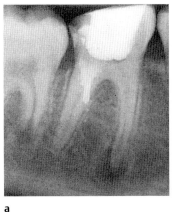
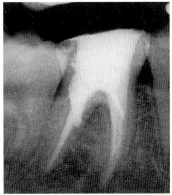
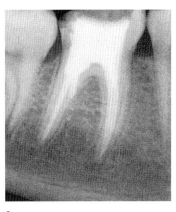

a   b   c

Fig. 13.4 Radiographs showing treatment of the tooth in Fig. 13.2b.

a The perforation canal is filled with material(s) forming a bacteria-tight seal. The pulp chamber is then sealed and the patient is dismissed.

b The endodontic treatment is completed at the second visit when the material in the perforation canal has set so that the seal is not disturbed.

c One-year control. Normal interradicular and periapical conditions are observed.

the furcation region. The lateral perforations should, if at all possible, be exposed surgically and restored like a class 5 cavity. A furcation perforation, on the other hand, if restorable, has to be repaired from the pulp chamber. In principle, the materials that are used for retrograde root canal fillings can be used for this purpose, and success or failure will depend on whether or not it is possible to seal the perforation and to prevent an infection becoming established in the periodontal tissues (**Fig. 13.3**). *Therefore, time is of the essence and if a furcation perforation occurs, it should be repaired immediately.*

The treatment is done aseptically. The pulp chamber is cleansed with sterile saline or anesthetic solution and the bleeding is stopped with sterile cotton pellets and paper points. A material which gives a bacteria-tight seal is then carefully packed into the perforation cavity (**Fig. 13.4**). If the opening to the periodontal ligament is wide, it is advantageous to pack calcium hydroxide against the periodontal tissues as a matrix against which the material may be condensed. In this way, the impingement of the material on the periodontium may be somewhat limited. When the perforation has been sealed, the access cavity is immediately closed and the treatment is not continued until a following visit.

Root Perforations

Apical Perforations

Root perforations may also occur during the instrumentation of the root canal. They usually occur in the apical third of curved roots at the outer-curve aspect of the root (**Fig. 13.5**). *There are three main reasons for this perforation: An inadequate access cavity, failure to precurve a rigid steel root canal instrument, especially if it also has an active tip, and the use of too large an instrument too quickly to reach the working length.* Often it is a combination of two or all three of these mistakes. However, with the availability of flexible nickel-titanium instruments with noncutting tips today, perforations of curved roots fortunately have been greatly reduced.

When a perforation has been diagnosed, an effort has to be made to get back into the root canal using a small (no. 8 – 15), sharply curved K-file and liberal amounts of a chelating agent (ethylenediamine tetraacetic acid, EDTA). If the original canal is found, it is instrumented in the normal fashion and is filled, ignoring the perforation. Tissue fluids and blood will then fill the perforation canal and if a bacterial infection was prevented or has been

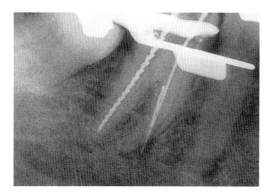

Fig. 13.5 Radiograph of a mandibular molar with apical perforation at the outer-curve aspect of the mesial root during instrumentation.

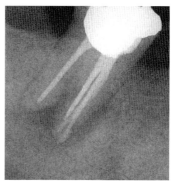

Fig. 13.7 Radiograph of a mandibular molar with apical perforation at the outer-curve aspect of the mesial root. In this instance it was possible to regain access to the root canal apically to the perforation so that it could be instrumented. Perforation canal and root canal were then obturated.

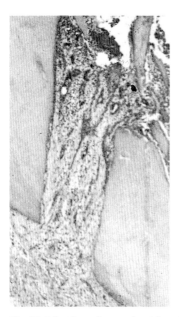

Fig. 13.6 Section of a tooth with apical root perforation. Connective tissue from the periodontal ligament has grown into the perforation canal (hematoxylin-eosin).

eliminated, will be organized to new connective tissue (see pp. 98, 99) (**Fig. 13.6**).

However, if the perforation canal is 3 mm or longer, it should be filled like a branching root canal (**Fig. 13.7**). This may be extremely difficult. An electronic apex locator is useful in such instances to aid in determining the exact location of the root surface. As a basis for the obturation attempt, it must be understood that overfilling is almost in-

evitable because of the tubal shape of the canal without the slightest indication of an apical stop. A gutta-percha point is selected which gives some tug back 1 mm from the root surface as indicated by the apex locator. The gutta-percha point is then marked at an occlusal point of reference, taken out, coated sparingly with a sealer, and reinserted into the canal to the predetermined level. It is immediately seared off with a hot K-type instrument at the entrance to the perforation canal and smoothed against the root canal wall so as not to interfere with the obturation of the canal proper.

The treatment approach described above often fails because of technical difficulties. Attempts have been made, therefore, to treat root perforations long term with calcium hydroxide *to obtain a hard-tissue barrier at the perforation opening* (**Fig. 13.8**). However, for reasons not fully understood, a hard-tissue barrier forms less readily on the lateral aspects of the root than at the apical foramen, and a considerably longer induction period is needed. This method, therefore, will in most instances not be practical. On the other hand, a surgical approach may save the tooth if the perforation is in an area of the root where it can be surgically exposed. A cavity encompassing the perforation opening is then prepared into the root and filled with materials used for obturation of retrograde cavities (**Fig. 13.9**).

Special problems arise if the original root canal cannot be renegotiated after the root is perforated.

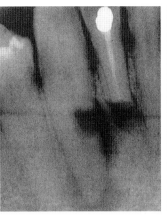 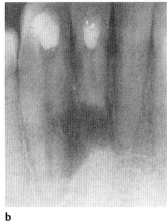

a

b

Fig. 13.8

a Radiograph of a mandibular canine with lateral perforation of the root since apicoectomy of the neighboring lateral incisor.

b Following treatment with calcium hydroxide for 26 months, a hard tissue barrier has formed, bridging the lateral perforation defect.

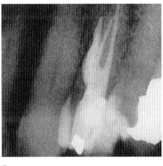 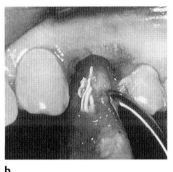

a

b

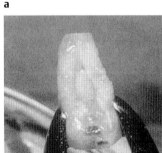 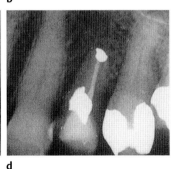

c

d

Fig. 13.9

a Radiograph of a maxillary premolar with root perforation and massive extrusion of root filling materials through the perforation opening. Retreatment: Intentional replantation.

b The tooth is carefully extracted and immersed in sterile physiological saline.

c The extruded materials are removed, and a cavity encompassing the perforation opening is restored with a copal varnish and amalgam.

d One-year control. Normal periradicular conditions are observed.

If the perforation has occurred in an area 1–4 mm from the apex of a vital tooth, the root canal should be instrumented and filled to a level 1 mm short of the perforation opening (use an apex locator), ignoring the uninstrumented apical part of the root canal. This approach may be tried in nonvital teeth as well, but here the only chance of success is if the infection in the uninstrumented apical part of the root canal can be eliminated (**Fig. 13.10**). In other words, the tooth is treated as if the inaccessible part of the main root canal were a lateral canal inaccessible to instrumentation. Long-term calcium hydroxide treatment is the method of choice in these teeth since calcium hydroxide with its continuous disassociation in the tissue fluids and its long-lasting antibacterial effect renders a most effective influence on bacteria in the areas of the root canal system which are inaccessible to the instruments. However, this treatment approach may be unsuccessful. A surgi-

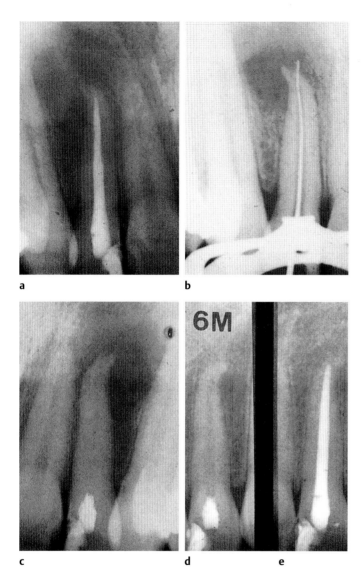

a

b

c   d   e

Fig. 13.10
a **Radiograph of an endodontically treated maxillary lateral
 incisor with symptomatic apical periodontitis.**
b During retreatment, an apical
 perforation of the root became
 evident.
c Long-term calcium hydroxide
 treatment was initiated.
d After 6 months, resolution of the
 periapical lesion has occurred.
e The root canal was then obturated short of the site of the apical perforation.

cal approach with removal of the uninstrumented part of the root is then usually the method of choice (**Fig. 13.11**).

Lateral Perforations

As with the apical perforations, a perforation of the lateral aspects of the root most often occurs because of inadequate access to the root canal and, consequently, an improper guidance of the root canal instruments. Also, the use of rigid (steel) instruments in curved roots may lead to a straightening of the canal with a strip perforation at the inner curve of the root (**Fig. 13.12a**). The *strip perforation* is, because of its large size and irregular shape, an especially serious complication and commonly leads to loss of the root or extraction of the tooth.

Otherwise, lateral root perforations should be treated as described for the perforations in the apical area of the root. An effort should always be made to regain access to the root canal. If that is accomplished, the tooth should be treated in the normal fashion (**Fig. 13.12b**). If the root canal cannot be instrumented apically to the perforation

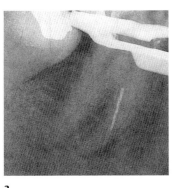
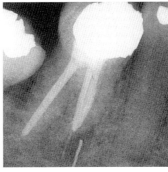
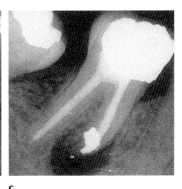

a   b   c

Fig. 13.11
a Radiograph of a mandibular molar with apical perforation of the mesial root and a fractured instrument in the root canal. The root canal apical to the perforation could not be negotiated.

b The mesial root canals were filled short of the perforation opening.
c The uninstrumented part of the root as well as the instrument fragment were removed surgically. A retrograde filling was placed.

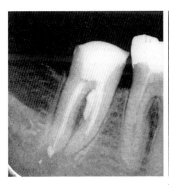
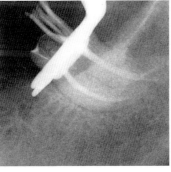

a   b

Fig. 13.12
a Radiograph of a mandibular molar with technically very inadequate endodontic treatment. The distal root is underinstrumented and overfilled. The mesial root is instrumented short and has a large strip perforation at the inner curve of the root to the furcation.
b Mandibular molar with an extremely curved distal root. A lateral perforation has occurred at the outer curve of the root. The root canal and the perforation canal were obturated.

site, a common approach is to remove the perforated root. In the case of a very important single-rooted tooth, an attempt may be made to surgically expose the perforation area of the root and to instrument and obturate the inaccessible part of the root canal through the perforation opening. However, in most instances such teeth will have to be extracted.

Post Perforations

Root perforations often occur when preparing the space for root canal posts. The reason for this mishap most often is that the direction of the root is misjudged during the use of large and rigid burs to remove gutta-percha and enlarge the canal enough to receive the post.

Post perforations are usually too large to be treated from the root canal. If possible they should be surgically exposed and sealed from the outside (**Fig. 13.13**). The post should be cemented in the root canal prior to the surgical operation so that extruded cement may be removed and other irregularities corrected. The perforation opening should be sealed with a material used for retrograde root filling.

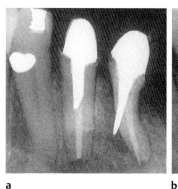
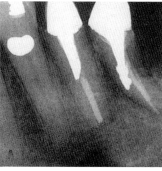

a   b

Fig. 13.13
a Radiograph of a mandibular second premolar with root perforation and protrusion of a root canal post into periodontal tissues.
b The perforation site was surgically exposed, the post reduced, and the perforation opening sealed with amalgam and copal varnish. Periradicular repair is evident.

Obliterated Root Canal

Obliteration of the root canal is a common and quite annoying occurrence in many teeth in need of endodontic treatment. It may be observed in a rather generalized fashion in elderly patients; otherwise it occurs as a sequel to long-standing chronic pulpal inflammation or traumatic injuries of the teeth. In luxated and avulsed teeth, the obliteration of the root canal occurs in an unpredictable and irregular fashion as a metaplastic formation of hard tissue throughout the revascularized tissue in the canal. In other instances, the root canal obliterates by apposition of hard tissue on the root canal walls, usually leaving a thin string of pulp tissue centrally in the canal. It is important to understand that this string of pulp tissue can be so narrow that it may not be visible in radiographs or, in other words, *a tooth which appears radiographically to have a completely obliterated root canal clinically may exhibit a patent canal where a no. 8 or 10 K-file can be inserted to the working length without any hindrances.* In other instances, the root canal may be obliterated clinically as well, either fully or partially. A partial obliteration is often found in the orifice area of the canal as a result of secondary dentin formation to caries, abrasion, or other external irritation, but may occur at any level.

If the obliteration is apical, the canal should be instrumented and obturated as far as it is patent and no heroic efforts should be made to penetrate the apical calcified tissue. The prognosis for this treatment approach is good (**Fig. 13.14**). If the obliteration is coronal in the canal, the calcified tissue may be penetrated by an endodontic explorer or removed by a bur. Burs may also be used for a complete penetration of obliterated canals in teeth with straight roots. This will be required especially in traumatized incisors with calcified canals, as about 20% of such teeth develop endodontic problems over time. When this procedure is planned, the access cavity should be larger than normal to allow light to enter, and the use of a fiberoptic light is beneficial as well. If available, a microscope should be used. The calcified material in the root canal usually is of a different color than primary dentin. It is often darker, but may also stand out because it has a glass-like appearance. *The difference in color is the most important guidance during the penetration of a calcified root with a bur.* In addition, radiographs are taken at different angles to ensure that the direction of the drilling appears proper. Liberal amounts of a chelating agent (EDTA) are used for irrigation and the canal is frequently probed with small K-files to ascertain whether a canal lumen might be located (**Fig. 13.15**). If not, the drilling is continued until the apical area of the root has been reached. If this is not considered possible, teeth with obliterated root canals may be treated surgically with retrograde fillings as a last resort (**Fig. 6.30**). However, it must then be remembered that even if a root canal is clinically and radiographically obliterated, there will always be necrotic tissue in microscopic spaces in the root. This tissue may harbor bacteria, and leakage of bacterial products may occur in spite of the retrograde filling and cause the treatment to fail (**Fig. 6.31**).

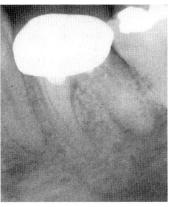
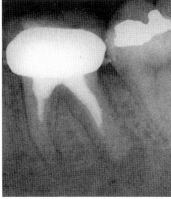
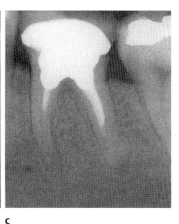

a   b   c

Fig. 13.14

a **Radiograph of a pulpotomized mandibular molar with apical radiolucency at the distal root.**

b The tooth was retreated, but because of apical obliteration, the root canals could not be negotiated to the desired apical levels. After 4 weeks of calcium hydroxide treatment, the instrumented parts of the root canals were obturated.

c Ten-month control. Resolution of the periapical lesion is observed, indicating that, in this instance, it was possible to obtain a bacteria-free root canal system in spite of what might appear to be inadequate instrumentation of the root canal.

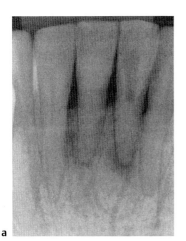
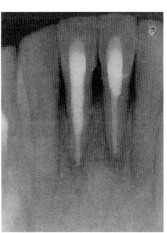

a   b

Fig. 13.15

a **Radiograph of mandibular incisors with symptomatic apical periodontitis and obliterated root canals.**

b The root canals could be located and instrumented to the desired apical levels after initial penetration to different levels of the roots with round burs run at slow speed.

Fracture of an Instrument

If an instrument fractures in the root canal during instrumentation, it should be removed if at all possible. However, a fracture usually occurs because the tip of the instrument is wedged in the canal and is twisted off. It is, therefore, in general extremely difficult to remove instrument fragments. The microscope is again of inestimable value in that the fragment usually can be seen in the canal (**Fig. 13.16**). An attempt may then be made to work a second instrument alongside the fragment. This can be done with steel K-files with active tips (**Fig. 13.16**) or preferably with special

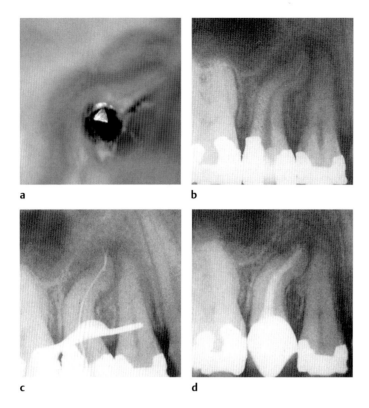

a

b

c

d

Fig. 13.16

a Root canal with broken in-strument photographed through microscope. The focus is adjusted so that the fragment is in focus. Being able to see the fragment makes it easier to remove it.

b Radiograph of a nonvital maxillary premolar with an S-shaped root and apical periodontitis. An instrument has fractured and the fragment is situated in the apical end of the canal.

c A second instrument has been worked alongside the fragment and an effort is made to create a space next to it. The fragment may then be loosened and irrigated out of the canal.

d One-year control. Nearly complete resolution of the periapical lesion is seen.

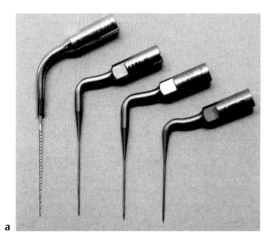

a

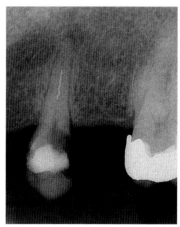

b

Fig. 13.17

a Vibratory tips energized by an ultrasonic unit designed for the removal of instrument fragments inside the root canal. The K-file-like instrument to the left is used to remove dentin and create space adjacent to the broken instrument. If the

fragment does not come out during this procedure, one of the bland tips (that does not remove dentin) may be introduced into the canal to vibrate the instrument until it is loose.

b Radiograph of maxillary premolar with broken instrument in root canal.

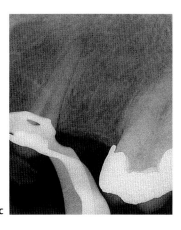

c

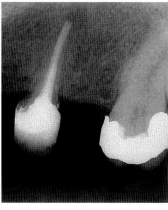

d

Fig. 13.17
c Instrument fragment is removed using vibratory tips in
a.
d Since the fragment could be
removed, the root canals were
instrumented and obturated in
routine fashion.

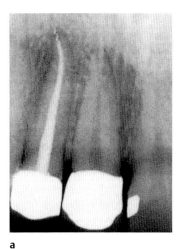

a

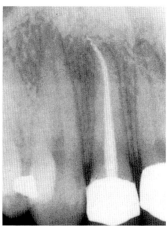

b

Fig. 13.18
**a Radiograph of a maxillary in-
cisor with a fragment of a
lentulo protruding through
the apical foramen.** A slight
apical radiolucency is evident.
The fragment could not be removed and the root canal was
obturated to a level slightly
short of the radiographic apex.
b At the 1-year control, resolution
of the apical radiolucency is observed. This is an example that
an instrument impinging on the
periodontal tissues might not
have to be surgically removed if
the mishap occurred at a stage
of the treatment when the root
was already bacteria-free.

nickel-titanium K-file-like instruments which are
ultrasonically energized (**Fig. 13.17**). If it has been
possible to create space next to the fragment, the
vibrating action of an ultrasonic tip may dislodge
the broken instrument and it will come out with
the irrigation solution used (EDTA). However,
sometimes we must be content if we can fill the
canal adjacent to or past the instrument fragment.
Unfortunately, even that will not be possible in
many instances and the canal is then filled to the
broken instrument (**Fig. 13.18**). This may have a
negative effect on the success rate of the treatment, especially if the fracture occurs in nonvital,
infected teeth. Apicoectomy, preferably with removal of the fragment through the apical end of
the root canal and retrograde fillings, may then be
the treatment of choice.

Adverse Reactions to Medicaments

Local Tissue Irritation

Certain antiseptics used in the root canal, especially aldehydes and phenol derivatives, distinguish poorly between bacterial cells and tissue cells. *They may, therefore, cause a chemically-induced inflammation in the periapical tissues with exudation into the root canal.* This situation is often referred to as a "weeping canal" and is annoying in that the apical part of the canal cannot be dried properly. Also, the chemically-induced periapical exudation may be mistakenly diagnosed as an infectious apical periodontitis, and in order to eliminate the alleged infecting bacteria, steadily stronger medicaments may be used.

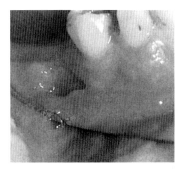

Fig. 13.19 Tissue necrosis in the oral vestibule following inadvertent injection of sodium hypochlorite through the apical foramen of the adjacent tooth.

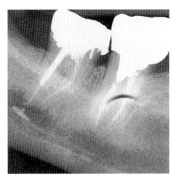

Fig. 13.20 Radiograph showing root canal filling material in mandibular canal after endodontic treatment of a mandibular second molar. The material contained formaldehyde and the patient has paresthesia of the lower right lip area.

Clearly, this will make the situation worse. The right therapy is a discontinuation of the use of the tissue-irritating antiseptics followed by 2 – 3 weeks of calcium hydroxide in the root canal. The chemically-induced exudation will then have stopped and the root canal can be dried and obturated.

Other medicaments which are safe when used correctly may cause severe tissue damage under unfortunate circumstances. If the needle gets wedged in the root canal during irrigation with sodium hypochlorite so that the medicament is injected beyond the foramen and into the periapical tissues, necrosis of the periodontal ligament, alveolar bone, and even oral mucosa may develop (**Fig. 13.19**). This condition is extremely painful, and the patient must be on a moderate to strong analgesic regime for several days. Also, an antibiotic should be given to prevent an infection of the damaged tissues. In addition, sodium hypochlorite and especially chloroform may cause burns of the gingiva and mucosa if there is a leak in the rubber dam during endodontic treatment. These wounds may look bad and be painful, but they are superficial and much less serious than the reaction which occurs when a toxic medicament is injected beyond the apex of the tooth.

Neurotoxic Reactions

Neurotoxicity of a medicament or of an active ingredient of a material may cause special problems in endodontics because a major nerve trunk, the mandibular nerve, may be affected to such an extent that its function is permanently impaired (**Fig. 13.20**). A large number of reports on paresthesia of this nerve exist. Most of the incidents have occurred after use of root filling materials that contain formaldehyde. *Formaldehyde is a potent neurotoxin and its neurotoxic effect is irreversible.* Only in isolated instances have patients regained nerve function after surgical removal of excess material contacting the nerve.

Many other substances used in endodontics have a certain neurotoxic effect as well. Of the medicaments that have a place in modern endodontics, *chloroform* and *eugenol* should be mentioned. However, in contrast to formaldehyde, the neurotoxic effect of even high concentrations of these drugs appears to be reversible.

Allergic Reactions

Although many substances which are potent allergens are used during endodontic treatment, allergic reactions are extremely rare. The few reports that exist deal with allergic reactions to iodine (in patients with whom iodine preparations have been used as an intracanal medicament), to an epoxy resin root canal sealer, and to eugenol. The reactions are characterized by pain similar to that of a flare-up and often by a rash which may be generalized or located in the vicinity of the treated tooth. The therapeutic approach is to remove the medicament or material and thoroughly irrigate the root canal and fill it with calcium hydroxide. The reaction will then quickly subside.

Only one report on an allergic reaction to eugenol or a eugenol-containing material has been published. This is rather astonishing since eugenol is known to be a potent allergen and conceivably hundreds of millions of root canals have been filled using eugenol-containing sealers. However, the reaction we are discussing here is *contact allergy*, and the contact area between the root filling materials and the periapical tissues is of course minute. On the other hand, when zinc oxide and eugenol-containing pastes are used as, for instance, periodontal packs in contact with larger areas of exposed tissue, allergic reactions to eugenol are not uncommon.

Overfilling of the Root Canal

Overfilling of the root canal has taken place when the materials used for obturation of the canal impinge on the periodontal tissues. The materials in the tissue will have an irregular form and may mechanically cause an inflammatory reaction. Also, macrophages will try to remove the material or at least smooth off the sharp edges to eliminate the mechanical irritation. In addition, any toxic or allergenic influences of a material intended for use in the root canal are potentiated because of the increased tissue-material contact outside the canal.

The inflammatory reaction caused by a material is often visible radiographically as a narrow radiolucent zone develops around the material. However, if reasonably biocompatible materials are used, in most instances they will heal in (**Fig.13.21**). Especially gutta-percha is well tolerated by the tissues, and the sealers, which may be tissue irritating, usually dissolve or are resorbed. Occasionally overfilling may cause long-lasting symptoms or paresthesia. Surgical removal of the material may then be attempted. Similarly, if root resorption is seen in conjunction with overfilling of the canal, an apicoectomy with removal of the material may be the treatment of choice (**Fig.13.22**).

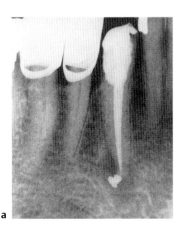
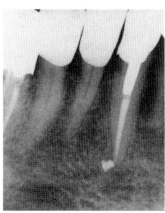

a

b

Fig. 13.21
a **Radiograph of a mandibular canine with apical periodontitis.** The root canal has been obturated with a soft gutta-percha technique and gutta-percha has been extruded beyond the apical foramen.
b At the 3-year control, resolution of the periapical lesion is evident. The extruded material has healed into the periapical tissues.

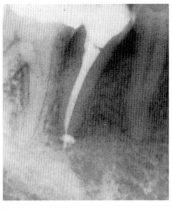 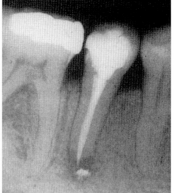 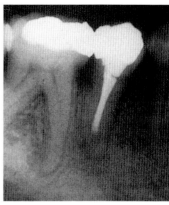

a   b   c

Fig. 13.22
a Radiograph of a mandibular premolar. The root canal was obturated with a soft gutta-percha technique and extrusion of material beyond the apical foramen has occurred.

b At the 6-month control, apical resorption of the root is observed.
c Following apicoectomy and removal of the material in the tissue, periapical healing has occurred.

Vertical Root Fractures

Teeth with vertical fractures of the root with communication between the oral cavity and the periodontium cannot be treated permanently and must be extracted (**Figs. 2.34, 13.23**). Many heroic methods have been tried to save such teeth, for instance extracting them, gluing the two halves together with a variety of glues and cements, and then replanting them in the socket. However, the seal is quickly broken and the fracture line will again be a major portal of entry for saliva and oral microorganisms. For shorter periods of time, i.e., for a few months, teeth with vertical fractures

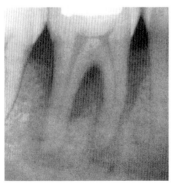 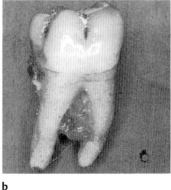 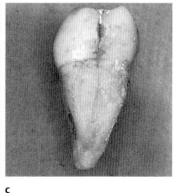

a   b   c

Fig. 13.23
a Radiograph of a mandibular molar with periradicular radiolucencies because of a vertical fracture of the tooth.
b The extracted tooth with granulation tissue in the furcation.

c The vertical fracture in the mesiodistal plane as seen in the extracted tooth has served as a portal of entry for bacteria to the periodontal tissues.

may be kept in the mouth without symptoms by packing calcium hydroxide into the root canal. The long-lasting antibacterial effect of calcium hydroxide and its continuous and slow dissolution into the fracture line is beneficial in that it prevents ingrowth of bacteria. However, when the calcium hydroxide paste is washed out, it must be renewed or an exacerbation will soon occur. Thus, as indicated above, a permanent approach to the treatment of this condition is presently not available.

Further Reading

Åkerblom A, Hasselgren G. The prognosis for endodontic treatment of obliterated canals. J Endod 1988;14: 565–567.

Benenati FW, Roane JB, Biggs JJ, Simon JH. Recall evaluation of iatrogenic root perforations repaired with amalgam and gutta-percha. J Endod 1986;12:161–166.

Brodin P. Neurotoxic and analgesic effects of root canal cements and pulp protecting dental materials. Endod Dent Traumatol 1988;4:1–11.

De-Deus G, Reis C, Brandão C, Fidel S, Fidel RAS. The ability of Portland cement, MTA, and MTA Bio to prevent through-and-through fluid movement in repaired furcal perforations. J Endod 2007;33: 1374–1377.

Hammarström L, Pierce A, Blomlöf L, Feiglin B, Lindskog S. Tooth avulsion and replantation—a review. Endod Dent Traumatol 1986;2:1–8.

Hülsman M, Schinkel I. Influence of several factors on the success or failure of removal of fractured instruments from the root canal. Endod Dent Traumatol 1999;15:252–258.

Kahnberg KE. Surgical extrusion of root-fractured teeth—a follow-up study of two surgical methods. Endod Dent Traumatol 1988;4:85–89.

Kerekes K, Tronstad L. Long-term results of endodontic treatment performed with a standardized technique. J Endod 1979;5:83–90.

Kvinnsland I, Oswald RJ, Halse A, Grönningsaeter AG. A clinical and roentgenological study of 55 cases of root perforation. Int Endod J 1989;22:75–84.

Morfis AS. Vertical root fractures. Oral Surg Oral Med Oral Pathol 1990;69:631–635.

Nagai O, Tani N, Kayaba Y, Kodama S, Osada T. Ultrasonic removal of broken instruments in root canals. Int Endod J 1986; 298–301.

Petersson K, Hasselgren G, Tronstad L. Endodontic treatment of experimental root perforations in dog teeth. Endod Dent Traumatol 1985;1:22–28.

Saunders JL, Eleazer PD, Zhang P et al. Effect of separated instruments on bacterial penetration of obturated root canals. J Endod 2004;30:177–179.

Sjögren U, Hägglund B, Sundquist G, Wing K. Factors affecing the long-term results of endodontic treatment. J Endod 1990;16:490–504.

Strindberg LZ. The dependence of the results of pulp therapy on certain factors. An analytic study based on radiographic and clinical follow-up examination. Acta Odont Scand 1956;14:Suppl 21.

Tronstad L, Barnett F, Duran C, Hasselgren G. Tissue response to anodyne medicaments. Oral Surg Oral Med Oral Pathol 1984;58:605–609.

Trope M, Maltz DO, Tronstad L. Resistance to fracture of restored endodontically treated teeth. Endod Dent Traumatol 1985;1:108–111.

Trope M, Rabie G, Tronstad L. Strengthening and restoration of immature teeth with an acid-etch resin technique. Endod Dent Traumatol 1986;1:246–256.

Trope M, Tronstad L. Long-term calcium hydroxide treatment of a tooth with iatrogenic root perforation and lateral periodontitis. Endod Dent Traumatol 1985;1:35–38.

Yared GM, Bou Dagher FE, Machtou P, Kulkarni GK. Influence of rotational speed, torque, and operator proficiency on failure of greater taper files. Int Endod J 2002;35:7–12.

14
Endodontic Retreatment

As discussed above, the results of endodontic treatment are influenced by a number of biological and technical factors like diagnosis, root canal morphology, root canal instrumentation and obturation, and complications during the treatment. Still it should be understood that the underlying reason for failure usually is infection and the influence of bacteria and bacterial components and products on the periapical tissues. Thus, in a study of 60 root filled teeth which were extracted because of apical periodontitis, bacteria were found in the root canal of all teeth (**Fig.14.1**). This finding stresses the importance of obturating the root canal bacteria-tight at all levels and also that the root filling should be protected by a solid, well-fitting coronal restoration. The lack of healing after endodontic treatment may also be due to extraradicular infection that might not respond to conventional treament.

The goal of *endodontic retreatment* is the same as for primary treatment, namely to obtain a bacteria-free tooth with a bacteria-tight root filling and an adequate coronal restoration so that healing may occur and reinfection is prevented. About two-thirds of retreatment cases will heal after renewed conventional treatment. Of the latter, one-third of which mostly comprises treatment-resist-

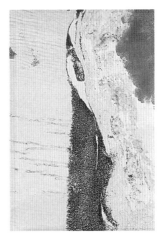

Fig 14.1 Inadequately root filled tooth with large bacterial colony and plaque between root filling material and root canal wall.

ant or refractory cases, again about two-thirds will heal following surgical–endodontic treatment. In addition, the success rate in this group may be improved by adequate systemic antibiotic treatment, preferably following identification of the infecting bacteria.

Indications for Retreatment

Root Filled Teeth with Apical Periodontitis
Epidemiological studies have shown a clear correlation between the technical standard of the root filling and the periapical condition of root filled teeth. Thus, whereas 80–90% of teeth with adequate root fillings have a normal apical periodontium, only about 50% of teeth with inadequate root fillings have a normal periapex. There is no reason to expect that healing of an apical periodontitis occurs if the root filling does not provide an adequate seal of the root canal. Teeth with a technically inadequate root filling and a persisting

apical periodontitis should therefore be retreated (**Fig.14.2**).

If the root filling, as seen radiographically, is technically adequate, an apical periodontitis will usually resolve within a period of 2–3 months to 3–4 years. It is unlikely that a lesion that has not healed after 4 years will heal in the future. Persisting infection will have to be suspected and if pathways of infection like a vertical fracture or a deep periodontal pocket are not diagnosed, chances are that there is coronal leakage or an extraradicular infection and the tooth should be re-

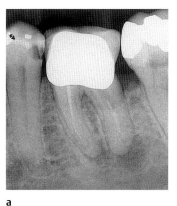
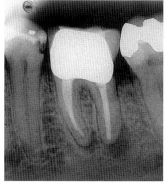
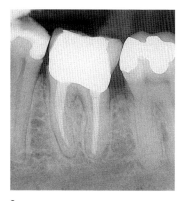

a   b   c

Fig 14.2
a Radiograph of a mandibular molar with inadequate root filling and asymptomatic apical periodontitis.

b The tooth has been retreated conservatively
through the crown.
c Complete periapical repair is evident at the 6-month
control.

treated endodontically. If treatment failure is diagnosed sooner than at the 4-year control, the retreatment should of course be carried out as soon
as the failure is evident.

Teeth without apical periodontitis that appear
to have been treated technically adequately may
also fail, and an apical periodontitis may develop
(**Fig. 6.14**). These teeth should be retreated immediately.

Root Filled Teeth with Normal Apical Periodontium

Teeth with inadequate root fillings but without
clinical or radiographic signs of periapical inflammation represent a problem group. A certain
percentage of these teeth will fail every year, and
in reality all teeth in this group are candidates
for retreatment (**Fig. 14.3**). However, there is no
immediate urgency in treating these teeth that
have no signs of disease and the treatment can
be done over time and if possible when it is convenient for the patient. Often it will be practical

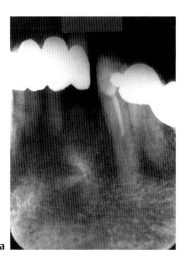
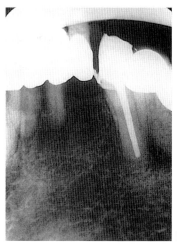

a   b

Fig. 14.3
a Radiograph of a mandibular
canine with root filling material in the coronal half of
the canal. No periapical inflammation is evident.
b The tooth is retreated endodontically in conjunction with
renewing the coronal restoration.

to carry out the endodontic retreatment in conjunction with renewing a coronal restoration. Clearly the patient has to be made aware of the situation, and regular clinical and radiographic controls are necessary.

Retreatment

Before beginning retreatment of a tooth where the primary treatment has failed, it is important to try to find out the reason why it failed: Is the coronal restoration inadequate or lost? Has a root canal been missed? Is the root canal inadequately instrumented? Is the root filling inadequate? Is the problem extraradicular infection? If clear technical deficiencies with the primary treatment are evident, chances are good that the retreatment will be successful (**Fig. 14.2**).

Many of the technical problems that arise during endodontic treatment are due to lacking or poor access to the root canals. The *access cavity* may have been too small or even placed wrongly in the tooth. The retreatment therefore begins with creating coronal conditions so that adequate access to the root canals may be gained.

By far the most root filled teeth today are obturated with gutta-percha and a sealer. If the quality of the root filling is really poor, it may be removed by means of an instrument, for example, a Hedstrom file. If this is not possible, the safest method is to use an organic solvent like chloroform to soften the gutta-percha and then remove it with hand files or (carefully!) with engine-driven, rotary nickel-titanium instruments that are flexible and with a rounded tip so that they follow the root canal well. It will usually be necessary to apply a drop of chloroform to the root canal a couple of times during the procedure.

When the root filling has been removed, the treatment continues following the guidelines for treatment of nonvital teeth as described in Chapter 6. It is important to remember that when the primary treatment has failed, in all likelihood it is because of problems with infection. During retreatment it is therefore important to be extra careful with asepsis and extra vigorous with the antimicrobial treatment. The root canal should be instrumented wide, especially apically, and liberal amounts of sodium hypochlorite should be used for irrigation during and after the instrumentation. The instrumentation phase of the treatment is concluded with a final rinse of the canal with 10 mL ethylenediamine tetraacetic acid (EDTA).

This will remove the smear layer from the root canal wall and hopefully instrumentation debris from root canal deltas and side canals so that an intracanal antimicrobial medicament might have as good an effect as possible.

Like primary treatment of nonvital teeth, retreatment of failed cases routinely is performed in two visits. This is done to provide the opportunity to carry out an effective antimicrobial treatment of the root canal system and the root dentin for a period between the two visits. This is best done by using the long-term calcium hydroxide method. The calcium hydroxide–saline paste is then left in the root canal for 2–3 months. After this time there will usually be clinical and radiographic signs of healing or the periapical lesion might have healed (**Fig. 6.9**). The root canal is then obturated bacteria-tight and a well-sealing temporary filling is inserted in the access cavity.

Treatment-Resistant Cases

If the criteria for root filling are not met at the second visit, one must evaluate whether local treatment of the tooth has been optimal. If the answer is yes, the lack of response to the treatment may be due to extraradicular infection. Studies have shown that even 6 months of calcium hydroxide in the root canal have minimal effect in many of these cases. Systemic antibiotic treatment then appears a logical next step (**Fig. 14.4**). As discussed above, many oral bacteria have developed resistance against certain antibiotics. The type and sensitivity of the infecting bacteria should therefore be determined if at all possible so that an effective antibiotic may be selected. If bacterial identification is not carried out, penicillin is still the drug of choice in the treatment of endodontic infections. In difficult cases it may be combined with metronidazole, which has an especially good effect on anaerobic bacteria. Clindamycin is another effective antibiotic against these infections. Clindamycin may also be used in patients with penicillin allergy.

In long-standing infections with fistulous tracts and leakage through the root canal, enteric

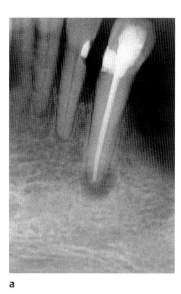

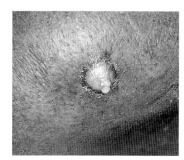

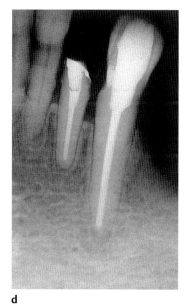

Fig. 14.4

a Postoperative radiograph of mandibular canine with apical periodontitis. The root canal was obturated after instrumentation and 3 weeks of calcium hydoxide treatment.

b After 5 weeks the patient returned with an extraoral fistula near the chin. Retreatment was begun. The root filling was removed and calcium hydroxide was introduced into the canal. After 3 months the fistula had not closed. Bacterial samples were then taken from the root canal and the fistula and, in accordance with the microbiological diagnosis, the patient was given penicillin plus metronidazole for 10 days.

c During this period the fistula closed. The calcium hydroxide treatment continued.

d After another 3 months the periapical lesion had healed and the root canal was obturated.

bacteria and bacteria from the environment may be present in the endodontic lesion. These so-called *superinfections* will as a rule not respond to the antibiotics normally used. However, if the type and sensitivity of the nonoral bacteria can be determined, the "correct" antibiotic may be selected and the lesion may heal (**Fig. 14.5**).

Surgical Retreatment

Surgical removal of the periapical lesion may be effective retreatment of refractory cases (see p. 125). In addition to the lesion, 1–3 mm of the root tip with the apical delta is removed. If the infecting bacteria then are mainly eliminated, the lesion may heal (**Fig. 6.33**). However, all bacteria are most certainly not removed from the periapical area with this method and the treatment may also fail. The success rate of surgical retreatment is greatly improved by combining it with systemic antibiotic treatment as discussed above.

Thus, it is clear from the above that effective antimicrobial treatment has to be part of endodontic retreatment in all instances, regardless of the method used. The clinical situation will have to decide whether the antibacterial treatment should be carried out locally in and at the tooth or by using a combined local/systemic approach.

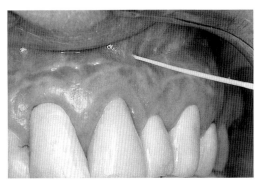

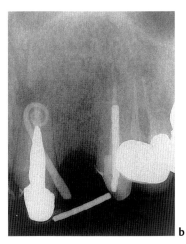

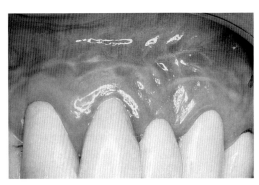

Fig. 14.5
a Gutta-percha point in fistula in vestibule near maxillary left central and lateral incisors. The fistula has persisted for 8 years during which time the patient has been apicoectomized six times. In addition, the lateral incisor is extracted.
b The fistula now seems to originate from the central incisor. Bacterial samples from the fistulous tract showed pure culture of *Pseudomonas aeruginosa*. Ciprofloxacin was given for 4 weeks.
c The fistula closed during this period and at the 2-year control the fistula stayed closed and the patient was free of symptoms.

Further Reading

Allen DE, Newton CW, Brown CE. A statistical analysis of surgical and nonsurgical endodontic retreatment cases. J Endod 1989; 15: 261–266.

Barnett F, Axelrod P, Tronstad L, Graziani A, Slots J, Talbott G. Ciprofloxacin treatment of periapical *Pseudomonas aeruginosa* infection. Endod Dent Traumatol 1990; 4: 132–137.

Dahle UR, Sunde PT, Tronstad L. Treponemes and endodontic infections. Endod Topics 2003;6:160–170.

Edgar SW, Marshall JG, Baumgartner JC. The antimicrobial effect of chloroform on *Enterococcus faecalis* after gutta-percha removal. J Endod 2006;32:1185–1187.

Gatti JJ, Dobeck JM, Smith C, White RR, Socransky SS, Skobe Z. Bacteria of asymptomatic periradicular endodontic lesions identified by DNA-DNA hybridization. Endod Dent Traumatol 2000; 16: 197–204.

Gorni FGM, Gagliani MM. The outcome of endodontic retreatment: a 2-yr follow up. J Endod 2004;30:1–4.

Grung B, Molven O, Halse A. Periapical surgery in a Norwegian county hospital: follow-up findings of 477 teeth. J Endod 1990;16:411–117.

Happonen R-P. Periapical actinomycosis: a follow-up study of 16 surgically treated cases. Endod Dent Traumatol 1986;2:205–209.

Hepworth MJ, Friedman S. Treatment outcome of surgical and non-surgical management of endodontic failures. J Can Dent Ass 1997; 63:364–371.

Kvist T, Reit C. Results of endodontic retreatment: a randomized clinical study comparing surgical and nonsurgical procedures. J Endod 1999;25:814–817.

Molander A, Reit C, Dahlén G, Kvist T. Microbiological status of root filled teeth with apical periodontitis. Int Endod J 1998;31:1–7.

Sunde PT, Olsen I, Debelian GJ, Tronstad L. Microbiota of periapical lesions refractory to endodontic therapy. J Endod 2002;28:304–10.

Sunde PT, Olsen I, Göbel UB et al. Fluorescence *in situ* hybridization (FISH) for direct visualization of bacteria in periapical lesions of asymptomatic root-filled teeth. Microbiol 2003;149:1095–1102.

Sunde PT, Tronstad L, Eribe ER, Lind PO, Olsen I. Assessment of periradicular microbiota by DNA-DNA hybridization. Endod Dent Traumatol 2000;16:191–96.

Sundqvist G, Figdor D, Persson S. Microbiologic findings of teeth with failed endodontic treatment and the outcome of conservative retreatment. Oral Surg Oral Med Oral Pathol 1998;85:86–93.

Tronstad L, Barnett F, Cervone F. Periapical bacterial plaque in teeth refractory to endodontic treatment. Endod Dent Traumatol 1990;6:73–77.

Tronstad L, Barnett F, Riso K, Slots J. Extraradicular en-dodontic infections. Endod Dent Traumatol 1987;3:86–90.

Tronstad L, Kreshtool D, Barnett F. Microbiological monitoring and results of treatment of extraradicular endodontic infection. Endod Dent Traumatol 1990;6:129–136.

Tronstad L, Petersson K. Endodontisk revisjonsbehandling. Tandläkartidn 1995;87:161–170.

Tronstad L, Sunde PT. The evolving new understanding of endodontic infections. Endod Topics 2003;6:57–77.

15

Bleaching of Discolored Teeth

Discoloration of the teeth, especially the anterior teeth, may become a serious aesthetic problem. The problem may be corrected by bleaching the teeth, although the success of bleaching therapy is strongly dependent on the nature of the discoloration.

Discoloration of Teeth

Vital Teeth

Secondary mineralization. Obliteration of the pulp chamber and the tubules of the coronal dentin may occur especially after concussion and subluxation injuries of the teeth. The increased mineralization leads to a loss of translucency of the crown with a yellowish-brownish discoloration. Most often, this type of discoloration is mild and aesthetically not very disturbing. In photographs, however, these teeth may appear dark and it is often because of this that a patient seeks treatment.

Enamel defects. In teeth with enamel hypo-calcifications and hypoplasia, the enamel has defects and may be porous. Stains are readily taken up from the oral cavity in the defective areas, and in teeth with severe anomalies (amelogenesis imperfecta) the results may be aesthetically very disturbing. Severe discolorations are also seen in patients who have been exposed to excessive amounts of fluoride during tooth formation (**Fig. 15.1**). Excessive fluoride intake causes disturbances in the mineralization of the dental tissues, resulting in localized, or in severe cases, generalized porosities and defects in the enamel.

Systemic drugs. The administration of systemic drugs during tooth formation may cause tooth discoloration and severe aesthetic problems. The most dramatic example of this is *tetracycline staining of teeth*. The teeth may be yellow to yellowish-brown or light to very dark gray, depending on the

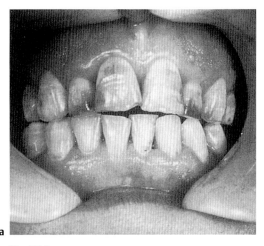
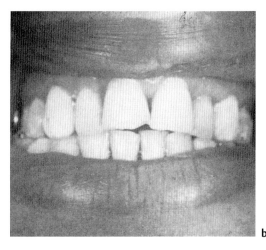

a

b

Fig. 15.1
a Patient with brown discoloration of the teeth due to generalized fluorosis.

b Removal of discolorations is observed following vital bleaching therapy.

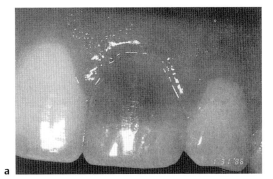

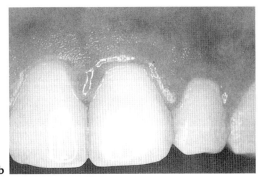

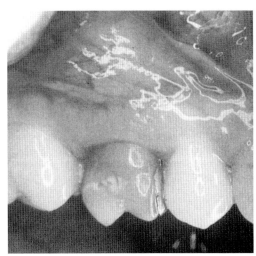

Fig. 15.3 Maxillary molar with a large MOD amalgam restoration. A grayish-bluish discoloration of the entire tooth can be seen.

Fig. 15.2

a Severe bluish-black discoloration of a maxillary left central incisor with necrotic pulp. The discoloration is caused by breakdown products from tissue and blood penetrating into the dentinal tubules.

b Excellent aesthetic results following endodontic treatment, bleaching, and restoration of the access cavity with the acid-etch resin technique.

type of tetracycline used. The discoloration is due to the drug binding to the hydroxyapatite crystals of the area of the tooth which is being formed during the time of the administration of the drug. Because of the age of a child when the incisors are formed, *tetracycline discoloration affects the dentin* more than the enamel. Tetracycline discoloration of teeth is a phenomenon well known to physicians today and the use of this drug in pregnant women and children under 8–9 years of age has virtually stopped.

Other substances, for example, iron, are known to cause a certain discoloration of teeth. However, today this is seen extremely rarely and is not a clinical problem.

Nonvital Teeth

Pulp necrosis. Necrotic tissue is a major cause of tooth discoloration (**Fig. 15.2**). Breakdown products from tissue and especially from blood infiltrate the dentinal tubules and give the tooth a brownish-gray discoloration. Sometimes the discoloration may be very dark, almost bluish-black. Apparently this is due to the formation of an iron sulfide compound in the tubules with iron deriving from the hemoglobin of the blood and the sulfur from bacterial products. It is important to meticulously remove all necrotic pulp tissue during endodontic treatment. For instance, the pulp horns are easily overlooked and necrotic tissue left behind in these areas where the tooth is especially thin will inevitably lead to discoloration.

Endodontic medicaments and materials. Certain medicaments and materials used in endodontic treatment may lead to tooth discoloration. The worst offenders like silver nitrate and silver-containing root canal sealers should be only of historical interest. However, all endodontic materials have to be meticulously removed from the pulp chamber when the root canal has been filled, as they will at least decrease the translucency of the tooth. Also, many materials, like zinc oxide–eugenol cements, have a tendency to darken over time when influenced by light through the enamel and dentin of the tooth.

Restorative materials. Of the restorative materials, the different amalgams may cause tooth discoloration (**Fig. 15.3**). The dentin in contact with the restoration and sometimes the entire crown of the tooth may turn bluish-gray. From an aesthetic point of view, this is an especially displeasing color, and amalgam restorations should never be used in anterior teeth. Thus, it follows that lingual access cavities for root canal treatment should not be obturated with amalgam fillings. This will in-

evitably lead to discoloration of the tooth and logically, but mistakenly, the patient will relate the discoloration to the endodontic treatment. Amalgam discolorations are difficult to correct with bleaching procedures.

Discoloration of teeth in conjunction with filling materials are otherwise seen with *marginal leakage* and the penetration of staining substances from tobacco, coffee, tea, red wine, etc. into the dental tissue. The use of the acid-etch technique with resin-type restorations has greatly reduced this type of discoloration.

Bleaching of Endodontically Treated Teeth

Preparation for Bleaching

If at all possible, a photograph of the patient's teeth should be taken prior to the bleaching procedures (**Fig. 15.2**). The periapical condition of the tooth and the technical quality of the root canal filling are then ascertained radiographically. *If the root canal is not adequately obturated, retreatment is absolutely necessary*, as gases released during

the bleaching procedures may otherwise penetrate into the periapical tissues and cause pain and a flare-up—like situation. *All fillings in the crown of the tooth are removed, as are possible areas of severely discolored dentin, for example, in the pulp horns.* The root canal filling is reduced to a level 1–2 mm apical to the canal orifice and preferably below the level of the gingival margin,

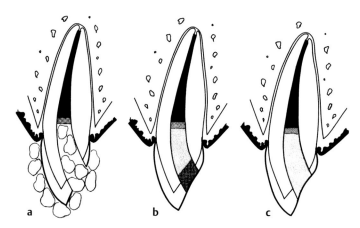

Fig. 15.4 Diagram illustrating bleaching procedures in endodontically treated teeth.

a The root filling is reduced to a level below the gingival margin. All tooth surfaces are acid-etched to make the tooth as pervious to the bleaching agent as possible. Hydrogen peroxide is applied by means of cotton pellets to all tooth surfaces. A heat or light source is used to obtain oxygen release.

b Walking bleach method. Sodium perborate mixed with hydrogen peroxide is sealed into the access cavity by means of a resin-reinforced zinc oxide–eugenol cement.

c Restoration of the tooth following bleaching. All tooth surfaces are again acid-etched and a light-cured unfilled resin is applied. The access cavity is then restored with a composite resin. Sometimes a very light or pink resin in the access cavity may give the best aesthetic results.

and the gutta-percha is covered with a layer of resin-reinforced zinc oxide–eugenol cement to provide an additional seal of the root canal (**Fig. 15.4**). Vaseline is then applied to the gingival tissues of the tooth to be treated and to adjacent teeth. This will help protect the tissue from the bleaching agent. The discolored tooth is then meticulously isolated with a rubber dam and ligated with a waxed dental floss. As always, the rubber dam should cover the patient's nose.

The tooth is then thoroughly sprayed with water and dried with compressed air. A final inspection is carried out and, if necessary, a round bur no. 2 is used to remove remnants of materials and severely discolored dentin and otherwise to freshen up the walls of the access cavity. The entire tooth is then acid-etched for 60 seconds using a 37 % phosphoric acid gel. The gel is placed liberally on the dentin walls of the access cavity as well as on the buccal and lingual enamel surfaces to remove smear layers and otherwise make the tooth as pervious to the bleaching agent as possible. The phosphoric acid is rinsed away with copious amounts of water and the tooth is meticulously dehydrated with compressed air, absolute alcohol, and chloroform. The actual bleaching procedure may then begin.

Bleaching Agents

The bleaching is performed with oxidizing agents: *3 % hydrogen peroxide* is commonly used. Hydrogen peroxide is readily destabilized with heat or light or a combination of the two, and oxygen is released. A special device to heat the hydrogen peroxide in a controlled fashion to the desired temperature level (about 40 °C) is commercially available, as are heat lamps that combine the effects of heat and light. Also, the fiber-optic light sources used for polymerization of light-cured resins may be used with advantage.

Sodium perborate is another powerful oxidizing agent. It is stable in powder form, but when mixed with water will release hydrogen peroxide and oxygen. Sodium perborate mixed with 3 % hydrogen peroxide to a paste is therefore used for bleaching purposes, sealed into the access cavity of the tooth between two dental visits (**Fig. 15.4**). This is called the walking bleach method and is quite effective. The fact that a gas forms when the *walking bleach method* is used can readily be verified clinically if too weak a material (e.g., a paste of zinc oxide and eugenol) is used to seal in the

sodium perborate–hydrogen peroxide mixture in the access cavity. When the patient returns for the second visit, numerous point-size holes will be evident in the temporary filling where the gas has escaped. Also, as mentioned above, if the root canal filling does not adequately seal the canal, the gas may escape to the periapical area causing tenderness to percussion and periapical pain.

Bleaching Procedures

After acid-etching, rinsing, and drying of the tooth, cotton pellets soaked in 3 % hydrogen peroxide are applied to all surfaces of the tooth, including the pulp chamber and the access cavity, as well as the buccal and lingual enamel surfaces (**Fig. 15.4**). Heat or light is then applied. If a heat lamp is used, it is held at a certain distance from the wet cotton pellets. The distance will depend on how hot it is. However, if a hot instrument is used, it must be brought in contact with the cotton pellets on all surfaces of the tooth. The cotton pellets are kept constantly wet by careful but continuous application of hydrogen peroxide with closed cotton pliers. When light activation is used, the procedure should continue for 10–20 minutes. A hot instrument should be used four to five times in the pulp chamber as well as four to five times on each external surface of the tooth.

In most instances, a one-visit bleaching will not be sufficient to reach the desired result. It is practical, therefore, to continue the treatment with the walking bleach method. A paste of sodium perborate and 3 % hydrogen peroxide is then mixed and inserted into the access cavity of the tooth (**Fig. 15.4**). The pulp chamber and the buccal aspect of the access cavity should be filled with the paste, leaving enough space lingually for an adequate 2–3-mm-thick temporary restoration. A resin-reinforced zinc oxide–eugenol cement is usually adequate, but a bonded composite resin restoration may be preferable if the loss of tooth substance is severe.

The patient's next appointment should be in about 1 week. If the color of the tooth is then satisfactory, the tooth is restored (**Fig. 15.4**). If not, the bleaching may continue as described for the first visit or, just as practical, with a second period of walking bleach. As a rule, one to three visits will give a satisfactory result. If after the third visit little or no improvement is evident, the bleaching therapy should be discontinued.

Restoration of the Bleached Tooth

The purpose of the restoration is to replace lost tooth substance and to strengthen the tooth, but also to seal all surfaces of the tooth so that the good aesthetic results obtained by the bleaching procedure may become as permanent as possible (**Fig. 15.2**). The temporary filling and the sodium perborate are meticulously removed and the access cavity carefully cleansed. The tooth is then acid-etched, (including the pulp chamber, the access cavity, and the enamel surfaces) and is restored with a composite resin technique (**Fig. 15.4**). An unfilled resin is first applied to the walls of the access cavity. Compressed air is carefully used to force the resin into the exposed dentinal tubules and the resin is light-cured for at least 60 seconds. Knowing that the resins currently available dar-

ken somewhat over time, a lighter composite resin than suggested by the shade of the tooth is then used to fill the pulp chamber and the internal aspects of the access cavity. A resin of the correct shade is obviously used for restoration of visible cavities. Finally, an unfilled resin is again used to paint the external enamel surfaces of the tooth. The unfilled resin will penetrate into the pits of the enamel resulting from the acid-etching, sealing the surfaces against influences from the oral environment as much as possible. Clearly, the resin on the surface of the tooth will disappear over time from tooth-brushing and wear and tear. However, resin tags will fill the pits of the enamel for some time and add to the external seal of the tooth until the surface is remineralized.

Bleaching of Vital Teeth

Bleaching of vital teeth is a much more doubtful and less predictable procedure than bleaching of endodontically treated teeth. In general it can be said that if the discoloration occurs in the enamel and is not too severe, the condition may be improved by bleaching. Dentin discolorations, on the other hand, are extremely difficult to influence with an external approach and in most instances an apparent improvement due to bleaching turns out to be a temporary success.

Bleaching of Teeth with Enamel Defects

Hypoplasia. Teeth with stained hypoplastic enamel pits most often should not be bleached. Even if a bleaching procedure might have an effect, the hypoplastic defects will soon have picked up staining substances again. A more permanent treatment is to clean out the enamel pits with a round bur no. 1–2, acid-etch the clean defects, and fill them using the acid-etch composite resin technique to create a smooth surface.

Fluorosis. Discolored teeth due to fluorosis, on the other hand, my lend themselves better to a bleaching therapy (**Fig. 15.1**). Vaseline and a rubber dam are applied as discussed above and the discolored areas are etched with 37% phosphoric acid for 60 seconds. The tooth is rinsed with water and the enamel surface dehydrated with alcohol and chloroform. Cotton pellets with 3% hydrogen

peroxide are then repeatedly applied to the stained areas, and heat or light activation of the medicament is carried out for 10–20 minutes. In some instances it may be beneficial to use a fine sandpaper disk or a finishing bur to remove carefully the surface layers of the discolored enamel in conjunction with the bleaching procedures. When the stains have been removed or the result is considered optimal, the treated areas of the tooth surface are again etched with phosphoric acid and an unfilled resin is applied to seal the porous enamel in order to prevent future discolorations as much as possible.

Bleaching of Teeth with Dentin Discolorations

The main reason for dentin discoloration in the last generation has been *systemic use of tetracycline*. Fortunately, this problem has virtually disappeared in recent years and a rather heroic, but in the long-term ineffective, method of external bleaching of such teeth using 30% hydrogen peroxide and strong heat (>52°C) will not be discussed in detail here. More lasting results have been reported by bleaching tetracycline-stained teeth subsequent to endodontic treatment, since this allows direct access to the discolored dentin through the endodontic access cavity. However, this may be characterized as a heroic approach as well in that all anterior teeth will be discolored and in need of endodontic treatment prior to bleaching. Probably a more acceptable treatment approach for the very few patients encountered today with this kind of tooth discoloration would be to use a porcelain veneer–bonding technique to achieve the desired aesthetic results.

Teeth which are discolored because of *excessive mineralization of the coronal dentin and secondary dentin formation in the pulp chamber* may be lightened only following endodontic therapy. The calcified material filling the pulp chamber and the pulp horn areas of the tooth is then removed and the access cavity is restored with a light resin to further improve the result. If this is regarded as an acceptable method for hypermineralized teeth but less so for tetracycline-stained teeth, it is simply because discoloration due to hypermineralization is mostly seen in a single tooth whereas tetracycline discoloration afflicts all teeth.

External bleaching has no appreciable effect on teeth with hypermineralized coronal dentin.

Further Reading

Amato M, Scaravilli MS, Farella M, Riccitiello F. Bleaching teeth treated endodontically: long-term evaluation of cases. J Endod 2006;32:376–378.

Cvek M, Lindvall AM. External root resorption following bleaching of pulpless teeth with hydrogen peroxide. Endod Dent Traumatol 1985;1:56–60.

Friedman S, Rotstein I, Libfeld H, Stabholz A, Heling I. Incidence of external root resorption and esthetic results in 58 bleached pulpless teeth. Endod Dent Traumatol 1988;4:23–26.

Smith JJ, Cunningham CJ, Montgomery S. Cervical canal leakage after internal bleaching procedures. J Endod 1992;18:476–81.

Spasser HF. Simple bleaching technique using sodium perborate. NY State Dent J 1961;27:332–334.

Weiger R, Kuhn A, Löst C. Radicular penetration of hydrogen peroxide during intra-coronal bleaching with various forms of sodium perborate. Int Endod J 1994;27:313–317.

16
Restoration of Endodontically Treated Teeth

Endodontically treated teeth are usually weak because of loss of tooth structure due to caries restorations, access cavity preparation, and necessary and unnecessary flaring of the root canal in the cervical area of the teeth. Also, loss of moisture in the dentin of these teeth allegedly results in a decreased resilience which has been associated with increased likelihood of fracture. Often so much of the coronal tooth structure is lost that it becomes necessary to use the root to obtain the required retention for a restoration, usually in the form of a root canal post. *Thus, endodontically treated teeth may present with two main problems when a restoration is considered, i.e., a reduced strength of the remaining tooth structure and how to obtain the necessary retention for the restoration.*

Strengthening of Endodontically Treated Teeth

Intracoronal Restorations
A root canal post is sometimes used with the purpose of strengthening a nonvital tooth. This is inappropriate. *The preparation of a post space will significantly weaken a tooth, and no known method of restoration will strengthen the tooth sufficiently to match its previous resistance to fracture.*

Thus, a post space should not be prepared in an endodontically treated tooth if this is not absolutely necessary and a root canal post should only be used when needed for retention of a coronal restoration.

The most effective method to strengthen endodontically treated teeth in most clinical situations is to use an acid-etch resin technique to create a bond between the resin in the access cavity and the dentin of the cavity walls. The root filling is removed to a level 1–2 mm below the entrance to the root canal, and the access cavity is meticulously cleaned with small burs; if a eugenol-containing cement has been used the cavity is washed with alcohol. The alcohol is removed with a spray of water and air and the dentin is dried and etched with 37% phosphoric acid for 60 seconds. This removes the smear layer of the dentin as well as the highly mineralized peritubular dentin surrounding the dentinal tubules, leaving a clean dentin surface with wide open dentinal tubules (**Fig. 16.1**). The dentinal tubules are now used for retention of the resin restoration. The access cavity is dried and dehydrated to such a degree that the water in the dentinal tubules is removed. This can readily be done in a nonvital root filled tooth. A lightly filled resin is then applied to the cavity walls, and by means of careful use of compressed air and "con-

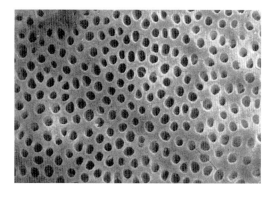

Fig. 16.1 Scanning electron micrograph of an acid-etched dentin surface. The lumina of the dentinal tubules may effectively be used for retention of resin restorations.

densation" with cotton pellets is forced to penetrate into the open dentinal tubules. This results in numerous (hundreds of thousands) resin tags inside the dentin (**Fig.16.2**). When a filled resin then is used to complete the restoration, it not only fills the cavity, but will, because of the resin tags in the tubules of the cavity walls, "hold the tooth together" and increase its strength significantly (**Fig.16.3**). Studies have shown that teeth that are restored in this way have almost the same resistance to fracture as intact teeth. If a metallic restoration is required, the orifice areas of the root canals and the pulp chamber are acid-etched and restored with resin as described above. The gold inlay or the amalgam filling is then placed in the tooth with the resin as the base (**Fig.16.4**). This combined restoration has a strengthening effect the same as if the entire cav-

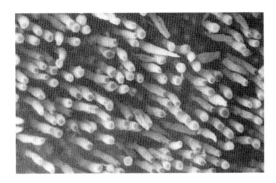

Fig. 16.2 Scanning electron micrograph of resin–dentin interface. The tooth has been dissolved with nitric acid and sodium hypochlorite, exposing the tags of resin that were inside the dentinal tubules. A restoration retained in this way will greatly strengthen the tooth and increase its resistance to fracture.

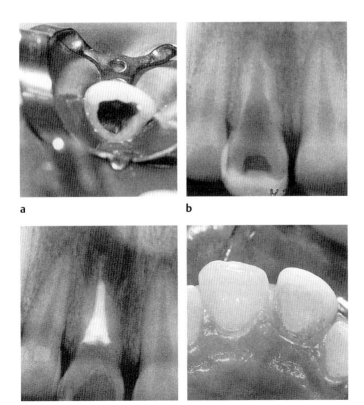

a

b

c

d

Fig. 16.3

a, b **Clinical and radiographic view of a maxillary incisor severely weakened by caries of an endodontic access cavity, pulp chamber, and root canal which were exposed to the oral cavity for 2 years.**

c Endodontic treatment (apexification and arrest of root resorption). The root canal filling ends 1–2 mm below the marginal bone level.

d The lingual cavity is acid-etched and unfilled resin is forced into the exposed dentinal tubules. The cavity is then filled with a composite resin.

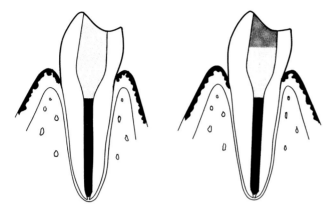

Fig. 16.4 Diagram illustrating intracoronal strengthening and restoration of an endodontically treated premolar. The orifice area of the root canal, the pulp chamber, and the access cavity are acid-etched and restored with the unfilled / filled resin technique. A gold inlay or amalgam filling may then be placed in the tooth with the resin as the base.

ity were restored with the acid-etch resin technique. The type of composite resin used in these intracoronal restorations is of little consequence for the strength of the tooth since it is the lightly filled resin that penetrates the dentinal tubules or, for that matter, the enamel pits if portions of the enamel are included in the retentive area. *The acid-etch resin technique may be used with advantage in all endodontically treated teeth where an intracoronal restoration is planned either to completely restore the tooth or to fill the pulp chamber and part of the cavity, leaving enough space for a final metallic restoration.*

Coronal Restorations

The acid-etch resin technique may also be useful to augment and strengthen existing coronal tooth structure when a crown restoration is planned. Quite often the use of a root canal post may be avoided when this method is used. The coronal 1–2 mm of the root canal should be included in the space to be acid-etched and filled with the resins. However, *no additional flaring or enlarging of the canal should be carried out since this will further weaken the tooth.*

Retention of Prosthetic Appliances in Endodontically Treated Teeth

The need for retention of prosthetic appliances shows wide variations, depending on intermaxillary relations, type of appliance, and position of the tooth in the arch. Thus, the need for retention increases with increasing vertical overbite and increasing cuspal inclinations. Also, the need for retention increases when crowns are used as abutments for fixed or removable partial dentures. The most demanding situations exist when crowns are used as distal abutments in fixed partial dentures with multiple cantilever pontics, or in removable free-end saddle partial dentures connected to their abutment teeth through some kind of precision attachment.

When the need for retention has been established, the retentive capacity of the individual teeth is analyzed. Important in this regard is the volume and shape of the remaining tooth substance. Retention increases with increased interfacial contact areas between crown, cement, and prepared tooth surfaces. However, the most essential factor influencing the retention is not the size of the contacting areas, but the geometry of these areas, such as the angle of convergence between opposing outer surfaces and the relationship between the height of the preparation and its base diameter. In general, sufficient retention is achieved when the angle of convergence is less than 20° and the inner diagonal of the preparation is longer than the base diameter (**Fig. 16.5**). If this cannot be achieved, proximal grooves may be prepared or a root canal post may have to be used for additional retention.

Normally, the need for additional root canal retention through a post can be estimated by comparing the height (mean height) of the remaining coronal dentin and that of an ideally prepared tooth. As a rule of thumb, the required extension

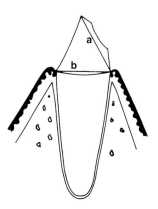

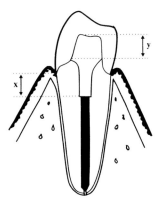

Fig. 16.5 Diagram of a tooth prepared for coronal restoration. Sufficient retention is generally attained when the diagonal of the prepared tooth (**a**) is longer than the diameter of the tooth at the gingival margin (**b**).

Fig. 16.6 Diagram of a tooth with a root canal post to retain coronal restoration. Sufficient retention is usually obtained when the extension of the post into the root canal apically to the gingival margin (X) is the same as the difference between the ideal height of the prepared tooth and the average height of the remaining coronal dentin (Y); (X≥Y).

of a post into the root canal apically to the gingival margin should be the same as the difference between the mean height of the remaining coronal dentin after the preparation and the height of an ideal preparation (**Fig. 16.6**). To avoid unfavorable stress distributions in the root during function, *a root canal post should never end at the level of the alveolar crest*. Its apical end should either be coronal to the crest or extend at least 2 mm beyond the crest level. At the same time, *a root canal post must not extend into the apical third of the canal in order not to disturb the bacteria-tight seal provided by the root canal filling*. With this in mind, there will always be limitations to the retention that can be obtained in a root canal, and if the retentive needs of a favored type of prosthetic appliance cannot be met by the tooth in question, the prosthetic therapy should be altered.

In addition to the length, the retention of a root canal post also depends on the geometry of the canal preparation. The most important factor in this regard is the angle of convergence of the root canal walls. Optimal retention per unit area is obtained when the root canal walls are parallel or nearly parallel and a cylindrical post that fits the prepared canal is used (**Fig. 16.7**). However, as is known, the coronal part of many root canals is ribbon-shaped or ovoid in cross section so that a preparation of the post space with parallel walls may not be possible. In such instances, prefabri-

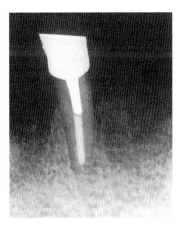

Fig. 16.7 Radiograph of a tooth with post-retained coronal restoration. The post has nearly parallel walls and extends below the marginal bone to the midroot level of the root canal. This post gives excellent retention of the crown without interfering with the bacteria-tight seal of the root canal rendered by the root canal filling.

cated posts preferably should not be used, or at least they should be cemented with a material (acid-etch, composite resin) that will not break down as a luting cement might tend to do under such circumstances.

A root canal post should not be the sole retentive element of a crown. Teeth with posts should be provided with a sufficient circumferential metal collar of the root as well. *In contrast to the root canal post, the metal collar will, in addition to its retentive function, also strengthen the root to a considerable degree.*

Preparation of Root Canal Post Space
When the need for retention has been determined and thereby the apical extension of the root canal post, the post space is prepared. More mishaps occur during preparation of post spaces than probably during any other single endodontic or prosthodontic procedure. The burs which are specially made for this purpose are rigid and have agressive cutting tips and should not be used until the root filling has been removed to the desired level of the canal. A safe and quick method of removing the gutta-percha is to place a drop of chloroform at the orifice of the canal and let it take its effect. Then use an engine-driven flexible nickel-titanium instrument with noncutting tip and taper 0.06 or 0.08 mm as needed. This instrument will follow the canal and remove the gutta-percha or at least prepare a space that works like a directional guide for the burs that subsequently are used to enlarge the canal and give the post space its final form. Using this method the preparation of the post space usually occurs without incidents. If a post is not cemented in the same visit as the post space is prepared, the post space is filled with calcium hydroxide paste and sealed bacteria-tight until the post can be cemented. In this way infection of the post space and the root dentin is avoided.

Cementation of Root Canal Posts
Prior to cementation of the post, the post space is acid-etched to remove the smear layer from the walls of the post space. The cementing agent for routine use is *zinc oxyphosphate cement*. A type of material that has gained some recent popularity is *glass ionomer cements*. However, these materials have not shown superior qualities in comparative tests and little is known about their long-term clinical properties. In wide root canals, as in immature teeth or in ovoid-shaped canals where a cylindrical post will not fit well in the coronal area, an unfilled/filled resin combination should be used for cementation of the post. The resin will fill the voids between the post and the walls of the post space and because of its superior strength in most instances will offer adequate support for the post. It is imperative that the walls of the post space be acid-etched when resins are used for cementation. The wetting ability of a resin is poorer than that of a cement and the dentinal tubules have to be included for retentive purposes.

Further Reading

Glantz P-D, Nilner K. Root canal posts—some prosthodontic aspects. Endod Dent Traumatol 1986;2:231 – 236.

Hansen EK, Asmussen E, Christiansen NC. In vivo fractures of endodontically treated posterior teeth restored with amalgam. Endod Dent Traumatol 1990; 6:49 – 55.

Hansen EK, Asmussen E. In vivo fractures of en-dodontically treated posterior teeth restored with en-amel-bonded resin. Endod Dent Traumatol 1990; 6:218 – 225.

Randow K, Glantz PO. On cantilever loading of vital and non-vital teeth. An experimental clinical study. Acta Odont Scand 1986;44:271 – 277.

Standlee JP, Caputo AA, Hansen EC. Retention of endo-dontic dowels: effects of cement, dowel length, diameter and design. J Prosth Dent 1978;39:400 – 405.

Tronstad L, Asbjørnsen K, Döving L, Pedersen I, Eriksen H. Influence of coronal restorations on the periapical health of endodontically treated teeth. Endod Dent Traumatol 2000;16:218 – 221.

Trope M, Tronstad L. Resistance to fracture of endodontically treated premolars restored with glass ionomer cement or acid-etch composite resin. J Endod 1991;17:257 – 259.

Trope M, Maltz DO, Tronstad L. Resistance to fracture of restored endodontically treated teeth. Endod Dent Traumatol 1985;1:108 – 111.

17
Prognosis of Endodontic Treatment

A number of prognostic studies from many areas of the world have shown the overall success rate of endodontic treatment to be around 90%. Studies which in particular dealt with the results obtained with the standardized technique, found a success rate of 91%. The conceivable influence of a wide variety of biological and technical factors on the outcome of endodontic treatment has been studied, and a fairly clear picture exists at this time as to the relative importance of the various factors.

Age. No difference has been found in the results of endodontic treatment in younger (<35 years) or older (>35 years) patients.

Health. With the exception of patients with AIDS, it has not been found that impairment of general health implies a prognostic risk for endodontic treatment.

Preoperative diagnosis. The overall success rate of endodontic treatment of vital teeth and nonvital teeth without radiographically visible apical periodontitis is 90–95%. The success rate drops by 15–20% in nonvital teeth with apical radiolucencies. The size of the radiolucency tends to be of importance for the prognosis. No difference is seen in the results of endodontic treatment of teeth with asymptomatic apical periodontitis or of teeth with symptomatic apical periodontitis; nor does the presence of a fistula influence the prognosis.

Root canal morphology. Endodontic treatment may be performed with a high degree of success in all groups of teeth. It might seem logical that the results would be better in anterior teeth than in molars where the root canal morphology is more complicated. However, several studies have shown the opposite results, namely that endodontic treatment is more successful in teeth with 3 roots (90%) than in teeth with 2 roots (80%), and better in teeth with 2 roots than in single-rooted

teeth (70%). These rather surprising results are probably due to the fact that the relatively narrow root canals in multirooted teeth are more thoroughly instrumented than the wider canals in single-rooted teeth. The results of a study with the standardized technique, where the apical third of the root canals was enlarged considerably more than in the previous studies, seem to support this hypothesis. In this study the results were the same in molars, premolars, and anterior teeth (91%). However, morphological characteristics of the teeth are mirrored in the results of this study as well: the teeth which in morphometric investigations appeared to be the least suited for the standardized technique had the poorest results (mandibular incisors; maxillary first premolars). The results obtained in maxillary central and lateral incisors were also poorer than one might have expected, probably because, at the time of the treatment, one was unaware of how wide the apical part of the root canal of these teeth really is, and to which size it ought to be enlarged. *Thus, a thorough knowledge of root canal size and morphology clearly is necessary to obtain the best possible results in endodontic treatment.*

Root canal instrumentation. The technical aspects of endodontic treatment have a great influence on the prognosis. A prerequisite for effective disinfection and successful obturation of the canal is adequate instrumentation. It is difficult or nearly impossible by clinical means to determine if the apical part of the root canal is actually adequately instrumented. *With the standardized technique, therefore, an attempt is made to combine radiographic findings and the clinical feel of the operator with a thorough knowledge of the actual width of the apical part of the root canal in the various types of teeth.* As judged by the long-term results with this technique, this appears to be a worthwhile approach.

Another factor in canal instrumentation which appears to be of prognostic importance is enlargement of the apical foramen or over-instrumentation of the canal. This affects the prognosis negatively and stresses the fact that the *instrumentation should not include the foraminal area, but should terminate inside the root canal*. Teeth with root canals which cannot be instrumented to the desired apical level due to canal obliteration have a good prognosis, better than that of teeth that are instrumented through the foramen.

Microbiological status of the root canal.   Several studies have shown that the prognosis of endodontic treatment will be 15–20% poorer if the root canal is infected at the time of obturation. These studies were all carried out before the availability of molecular microbiological techniques for the identification of microorganisms from the root canal and it is doubtful at the present time how meaningful they are. There is, however, full agreement that root canal infection should be eliminated before the canal is filled. *Failures of endodontic treatment are almost invariably related to infection of the root canal system or the periapical lesion, or both.* In a study of endodontically treated teeth which were extracted because of endodontic failures, bacteria were found in the root canals and root dentin of all teeth. Similarly, all periapical granuloma refractory to endodontic treatment which have been studied so far by anaerobic culturing or molecular techniques were infected.

Clinical complications.   The occurrence of iatrogenic exacerbations during endodontic treatment seemingly has no influence on the prognosis of the treatment.

Root canal filling material.   In most follow-up studies, biologically acceptable root canal filling materials have been used. However, the results of one study suggest that the choice of sealer may influence the outcome of treatment. Also, from a large number of experimental studies as well as from clinical experience, the conclusion can be drawn that it is important for the prognosis of endodontic treatment to use tissue-compatible materials that do not irritate the periapical tissues. It is also equally important that a material is dimensionally stable for a long period of time and does not deteriorate under the influence of tissues and tissue fluids.

Technical standard of root canal filling.   In all studies, the technical standard of the root canal filling has been found to have a decisive influence on the result of the treatment. The apical level of the root filling is of importance in all teeth, but *especially in vital teeth*. However, even in nonvital teeth an excess of root filling material of more than 1 mm will cause a reduction in the success rate of more than 10%. An inadequate seal of the root canal results in more than 20% poorer prognosis of endodontic treatment. *This is the one single factor which has the greatest negative influence on the prognosis.* When the influence of an inadequate seal of the canal as judged radiographically is not even more devastating, it is probably because there is an effective seal somewhere between the apex of the tooth and the oral cavity that at least temporarily prevents the oral bacteria from reaching the periapical tissues.

Coronal restoration.   It has become increasingly clear that the coronal restoration of endodontically treated teeth is important for the long-term success of endodontic treatment. The coronal restoration will protect the rather sensitive materials in the root canal that provide the bacteria-tight seal, and in addition an adequate restoration may in itself prevent coronal leakage from occurring. Thus, in a recent retrospective study the best results of endodontic treatment were seen when both the root filling and the coronal restoration radiographically were judged to be adequate. And interestingly, an adequate coronal restoration improved upon the results of teeth with radiographically inadequate root fillings. The poorest results were seen in teeth with both inadequate seal of the root canal and bad coronal restorations.

Instrument fragment in root canal.   Root canal instruments, whether made of steel or nickel-titanium, are bound to break occasionally during use. With untrained operators (students) this occurs in about one in every 100 teeth treated. The fracture of an instrument in the canal may or may not have a serious negative influence on the outcome of the treatment. To a great extent the effect of the mishap is dependent on the preoperative diagnosis, i.e., on whether the instrument fractured in an uninfected vital tooth or in a nonvital tooth with an infected root canal. Moreover, it depends on where in the canal the instrument fragment is situated und during which stage of the canal instrumentation the fracture occurred. Thus, if a sterile instrument fractures in a bacteria-free root canal near the apical level of instrumentation, the mishap may not influence the outcome of the treatment. On the other hand, if the fracture occurs at a distance from the foramen in an infected canal, effectively preventing adequate treatment of the apical part of the canal, failure of the treatment is almost certain.

As appears from the above, *the prognosis of optimal endodontic treatment is excellent.* The techni-

cal quality of the treatment is of the utmost importance, and if less than adequate will negatively influence the prognosis of the treatment. In this regard it is important to understand that inadequacies in root canal instrumentation and obturation may allow bacteria to survive in or gain access to the root canal system and the periapical tissues. Thus, *the underlying reason for failure of endodontic treatment is practically always infection and the influence of bacteria and bacterial products on the periradicular tissues.*

Further Reading

Åkerblom A, Hasselgren G. The prognosis for endodontic treatment of obliterated root canals. J Endod 1988;14:565–67.

Caliskan MK, Sen BH. Endodontic treatment of teeth with apical periodontitis using calcium hydroxide: a long-term study. Endod Dent Traumatol 1996;12: 215–221.

Eckerbom M, Flygare L, Magnusson T. A 20-year follow-up study of endodontic variables and apical status in a Swedish population. Int Endod J 2007;40:940–948.

Eriksen HM, Ørstavik D, Kerekes K. Healing of apical periodontitis after endodontic treatment using three different root canal sealers. Endod Dent Traumatol 1988;4:114–117.

Friedman S. Prognosis of initial endodontic therapy. Endod Topics 2002;2:59–88.

Gatti JJ, Dobeck JH, Smith C, White RR, Socransky SS, Skobe Z. Bacteria of asymptomatic periradicular endodontic lesions identified by DNA-DNA hybridization. Endod Dent Traumatol 2000;16:197–204.

Kerekes K, Tronstad L. Long-term results of endodontic treatment performed with a standardized technique. J Endod 1979;5:83–90.

Kvist T, Rydin E, Reit C. The relative frequency of periapical lesions in teeth with root canal-retained posts. J Endod 1989;15:578–580.

Ng Y-L, Mann V, Rahbaran S, Lewsey J, Gulabivala K. Outcome of primary root canal treatment: systematic review of the literature–Part 1. Effects of study characteristics on probability of success. Int Endod J 2007;40:921–939.

Saunders WP, Saunders EM. Coronal leakage as a cause of failure in root canal therapy: a review. Endod Dent Traumatol 1994;10:105–1088.

Sjögren U, Hägglund B, Sundqvist G, Wing K. Factors affecting the long-term results of endodontic treatment. J Endod 1990;16:498–504.

Skudutyte-Rysstad R, Eriksen HM. Endodontic status amongst 35-year old Oslo citizens and changes over a 30-year period. Int Endod J 2006;39:637–642.

Smith CS, Setchell DJ, Harty FJ. Factors influencing the success of conventional root canal therapy—a five-year retrospective study. Int Endod J 1993;26:321–333.

Strindberg LZ. The dependence of the results of pulp therapy on certain factors. An analytic study based on radiographic and clinical follow-up examination. Acta Odont Scand 1956;14:Suppl 21.

Sunde PT, Tronstad L, Eribe ER, Lind PO, Olsen I. Assessment of periradicular microbiota by DNA-DNA hybridization. Endod Dent Traumatol 2000;16:191–196.

Tronstad L, Asbjørnsen K, Döving L, Pedersen I, Eriksen HM. Influence of coronal restorations on the periapical health of endodontically treated teeth. Endod Dent Traumatol 2000;16:218–221.

Tronstad L. Recent development in endodontic research. Scand J Dent Res 1992;100:52–9.

Vire DE. Failure of endodontically treated teeth: classification and evaluation. J Endod 1991;17:338–342.

Yared GM, Bon Dagher FE. Influence of apical enlargement on bacterial infection during treatment of apical periodontitis. J Endod 1994;20:535–537.

Index

Page numbers in *italics* refer to illustrations